T0362478

Spondyloarthritis: The Changing Landscape Today

Editors

XENOFON BARALIAKOS
MICHAEL H. WEISMAN

RHEUMATIC DISEASE CLINICS OF NORTH AMERICA

www.rheumatic.theclinics.com

Consulting Editor
MICHAEL H. WEISMAN

May 2020 • Volume 46 • Number 2

ELSEVIER

1600 John F. Kennedy Boulevard • Suite 1800 • Philadelphia, Pennsylvania, 19103-2899
http://www.theclinics.com

RHEUMATIC DISEASE CLINICS OF NORTH AMERICA Volume 46, Number 2
May 2020 ISSN 0889-857X, ISBN 13: 978-0-323-73377-9

Editor: Lauren Boyle
Developmental Editor: Casey Potter

Rheumatic Disease Clinics of North America (ISSN 0889-857X) is published quarterly by Elsevier Inc., 360 Park Avenue South, New York, NY 10010-1710. Months of issue are February, May, August, and November. Business and editorial offices: 1600 John F. Kennedy Boulevard, Suite 1800, Philadelphia, PA 19103-2899. Periodicals postage paid at New York, NY and additional mailing offices. Subscription prices are USD 362.00 per year for US individuals, USD 777.00 per year for US institutions, USD 100.00 per year for US students and residents, USD 427.00 per year for Canadian individuals, USD 971.00 per year for Canadian institutions, USD 100.00 per year for Canadian students/residents, USD 465.00 per year for international individuals, USD 971.00 per year for international institutions, and USD 230.00 per year for foreign students/residents. To receive student/resident rate, orders must be accompanied by name of affiliated institution, date of term, and the *signature* of program/ residency coordinator on institution letterhead. Orders will be billed at individual rate until proof of status received. Foreign air speed delivery is included in all *Clinics* subscription prices. All prices are subject to change without notice. **POSTMASTER:** Send address changes to *Rheumatic Disease Clinics of North America,* Elsevier Health Sciences Division, Subscription Customer Service, 3251 Riverport Lane, Maryland Heights, MO 63043. **Customer Service: 1-800-654-2452 (US and Canada). From outside of the US and Canada: 314-447-8871. Fax: 314-447-8029. For print support, e-mail: JournalsCustomerService-usa@elsevier.com. For online support, e-mail: JournalsOnlineSupport-usa@elsevier.com.**

Reprints. For copies of 100 or more of articles in this publication, please contact the Commercial Reprints Department, Elsevier Inc., 360 Park Avenue South, New York, New York, 10010-1710; Tel.: +1-212-633-3874, Fax: +1-212-633-3820, and E-mail: reprints@elsevier.com.

Rheumatic Disease Clinics of North America is covered in *MEDLINE/PubMed (Index Medicus), Current Contents/Clinical Medicine, Science Citation Index, ISI/BIOMED,* and *EMBASE/Excerpta Medica.*

Contributors

CONSULTING EDITOR

MICHAEL H. WEISMAN, MD
Professor of Medicine, Emeritus, Division of Rheumatology, Cedars-Sinai Medical Center, Distinguished Professor of Medicine, Emeritus, David Geffen School of Medicine at University of California, Los Angeles, California, USA

EDITORS

XENOFON BARALIAKOS, MD
Associate Professor, Rheumatology, Rheumazentrum Ruhrgebiet Herne, Ruhr-University Bochum, Germany

MICHAEL H. WEISMAN, MD
Professor of Medicine, Emeritus, Division of Rheumatology, Cedars-Sinai Medical Center, Distinguished Professor of Medicine, Emeritus, David Geffen School of Medicine at University of California, Los Angeles, California, USA

AUTHORS

KRYSTEL AOUAD, MD
Rheumatology Department, Saint-Joseph University, Hotel-Dieu de France Hospital, Beirut, Lebanon

ADAM BERLINBERG, MD
Rheumatology Fellow, Division of Rheumatology, University of Colorado School of Medicine, Aurora, Colorado, USA

PAUL BIRD, PhD, GradDipMRI, FRACP
Associate Professor, University of New South Wales, Randwick, New South Wales, Australia

ANNELIES BOONEN, MD, PhD
Division of Rheumatology, Department of Internal Medicine, Maastricht University Medical Centre (MUMC+), Maastricht and Care and Public Health Research Institute, Maastricht University, Maastricht, The Netherlands

PHILIPPE CARRON, MD, PhD
Rheumatology Department, Ghent University Hospital, VIB Center of Inflammation Research, Ghent, Belgium

MIN CHEN, MD
Department of Radiology, Ghent University Hospital, Ghent, Belgium

FRANCESCO CICCIA, MD, PhD
Division of Rheumatology, Department of Precision Medicine, University of Campania "Luigi Vanvitelli," Napoli, Italy

ANN-SOPHIE DE CRAEMER, MD
Rheumatology Department, Ghent University Hospital, VIB Center of Inflammation Research, Ghent, Belgium

MANOUK DE HOOGE, PhD
Post-Doc Scientist, Department of Rheumatology, Ghent University Hospital, VIB Center of Inflammation Research, Ghent University, Ghent, Belgium

MARÍA PAZ POBLETE DE LA FUENTE, MD
Medicine Faculty Clínica Alemana de Santiago, Universidad del Desarrollo, Santiago, Chile; Internal Medicine Department, Padre Hurtado Hospital, San Ramón, Santiago, Chile

MAUREEN DUBREUIL, MD, MSc
Assistant Professor, Section of Rheumatology, Boston University School of Medicine, Boston, Massachusetts, USA

EMILIE DUMAS, PhD
Faculty of Medicine and Health Sciences, Department of Internal Medicine and Pediatrics (Rheumatology Unit), Ghent University, Molecular Immunology and Inflammation Unit, VIB Center of Inflammatory Research, Ghent, Belgium

DIRK ELEWAUT, MD, PhD
Faculty of Medicine and Health Sciences, Department of Internal Medicine and Pediatrics (Rheumatology Unit), Ghent University, Molecular Immunology and Inflammation Unit, VIB Center of Inflammatory Research, Ghent, Belgium

JOERG ERMANN, MD
Division of Rheumatology, Inflammation and Immunity, Brigham and Women's Hospital, Boston, MA, USA

HANNA FAHED, MD
Department of Rheumatology, Saint-Joseph University, Hôtel-Dieu de France Hospital, Beirut, Lebanon

RHYS J. HAYWARD, BSc (Hons)
Department of Rheumatology, Northwick Park Hospital, London North West University Healthcare NHS Trust, London, United Kingdom; Rheumatology Department, Northwick Park Hospital, Harrow, Middlesex, United Kingdom

SEBASTIÁN EDUARDO IBÁÑEZ VODNIZZA, MD
Rheumatology Department, Clínica Alemana de Santiago, Chile; Rheumatology Department, Padre Hurtado Hospital, Medicine Faculty Clínica Alemana de Santiago, Universidad del Desarrollo, Santiago, Chile

LENNART JANS, MD, PhD
Professor, Department of Radiology, Ghent University Hospital, Ghent, Belgium

DAVID KIEFER, MD
Rheumazentrum Ruhrgebiet, Herne, Ruhr-University Bochum, Herne, Germany

UTA KILTZ, MD
Rheumazentrum Ruhrgebiet, Herne, Ruhr-University Bochum, Herne, Germany

KRISTINE A. KUHN, MD, PhD
Assistant Professor of Medicine, Division of Rheumatology, University of Colorado School of Medicine, Aurora, Colorado, USA

JEAN W. LIEW, MD
Acting Instructor/Senior Fellow, Division of Rheumatology, Department of Medicine, University of Washington, Seattle, Washington, USA

PEDRO M. MACHADO, MD, PhD
Department of Rheumatology, Northwick Park Hospital, London North West University Healthcare NHS Trust, Department of Rheumatology, University College London Hospitals NHS Foundation Trust, Department of Neuromuscular Diseases, Centre for Rheumatology, University College London, London, United Kingdom

SINEAD MAGUIRE, MB, BCh, BAO, LRCSI, MRCPI
Department of Rheumatology, St James' Hospital, Ushers Quay, Dublin, Ireland

HELENA MARZO-ORTEGA, MD, PhD
NIHR Leeds Biomedical Research Centre, Leeds Teaching Hospitals NHS Trust, Leeds Institute of Rheumatic and Musculoskeletal Medicine, University of Leeds, Chapel Allerton Hospital, Leeds, United Kingdom

DANIELE MAURO, MD, PhD
Division of Rheumatology, Department of Precision Medicine, University of Campania "Luigi Vanvitelli," Napoli, Italy

XABIER MICHELENA, MD
NIHR Leeds Biomedical Research Centre, Leeds Teaching Hospitals NHS Trust, Leeds Institute of Rheumatic and Musculoskeletal Medicine, University of Leeds, Chapel Allerton Hospital, Leeds, United Kingdom; Hospital Universitari de Bellvitge-IDIBELL, Hospitalet de Llobregat, Barcelona, Spain

FINBAR O'SHEA, MB, BCh, BAO
Department of Rheumatology, St James' Hospital, Ushers Quay, Dublin, Ireland

ELISA CATALINA PARRA CANCINO, MD
Medicine Faculty Clínica Alemana de Santiago, Universidad del Desarrollo, Santiago, Chile; Gastroenterology Department, Clínica Alemana de Santiago, Chile; Gastroenterology Department, Padre Hurtado Hospital, San Ramón, Santiago, Chile

DENIS PODDUBNYY, MD, MSc (Epi)
Department of Gastroenterology, Infectious Diseases and Rheumatology, Charité—Universitätsmedizin Berlin, German Rheumatism Research Centre, Berlin, Germany

JAMES T. ROSENBAUM, MD
Oregon Health & Science University, Legacy Devers Eye Institute, Portland, Oregon, USA

JOHANNES ROTH, MD, PhD, FRCPC, RhMSUS
Chief, Division of Pediatric Dermatology and Rheumatology, Children's Hospital of Eastern Ontario, Professor of Pediatrics, University of Ottawa, Ottawa, Ontario, Canada

LISA SEE, BA
The International Women's Forum of Southern California, Los Angeles, California; PEN America, PEN Center, New York, USA

RAJ SENGUPTA, MD
Royal National Hospital for Rheumatic Diseases, Royal United Hospitals, Bath, United Kingdom

RIANNE E. VAN BENTUM, MD
Department of Rheumatology, Amsterdam University Medical Centre - Location VU
University Medical Centre, Amsterdam, The Netherlands

IRENE E. VAN DER HORST-BRUINSMA, MD, PhD
Professor, Department of Rheumatology, Amsterdam University Medical Centre -
Location VU University Medical Centre, Amsterdam, The Netherlands

KOEN VENKEN, PhD
Faculty of Medicine and Health Sciences, Department of Internal Medicine and Pediatrics
(Rheumatology Unit), Ghent University, Molecular Immunology and Inflammation Unit,
VIB Center of Inflammatory Research, Ghent, Belgium

PAMELA F. WEISS, MD, MSCE
Associate Professor of Epidemiology and Pediatrics, Perelman School of Medicine
UPENN, Attending and Clinical Research Director, Division of Rheumatology, Children's
Hospital of Philadelphia, Philadelphia, Pennsylvania, USA

DIETER WIEK

NELLY R. ZIADE, MD, MPH, PhD, FRCP
Department of Rheumatology, Saint-Joseph University, Hôtel-Dieu de France Hospital,
Beirut, Lebanon

Contents

> Scientific breakthroughs have culminated in the development of the spondyloarthritis (SpA) concept as a family of rheumatic diseases, distinct from rheumatoid arthritis. The demonstration of inflammatory lesions in the sacroiliac joints and spine of SpA patients who lacked radiographic features of ankylosing spondylitis (AS) helped refine the SpA concept. Axial SpA includes patients with AS and patients with axial symptoms previously categorized as undifferentiated SpA. This review examines the sources of knowledge that inform axial SpA pathogenesis, highlighting current limitations, and presents a basic working model of axial SpA pathogenesis.

> New and emerging molecular techniques are expanding understanding of the pathophysiology of spondyloarthritis (SpA). Genome-wide association studies identified novel pathways in antigen processing and presentation as well as helper T cell type 17 (T_H17) immunity associated with SpA. Immune cell profiling techniques have supported T_H17 immune responses and increasingly are revealing intestinal mucosal immune cells as associated with disease. Emerging technologies in epigenetics, transcriptomics, microbiome, and proteomics/metabolomics are adding to these, refining disease pathways and potentially identifying biomarkers for diagnosis and treatment responses. This review describes many of the new molecular techniques that are being utilized to investigate SpA.

> Spondyloarthritis, although primarily a joint-centered disease, is associated with extra-articular features, such as gut inflammation, psoriasis, and/or uveitis. Evidence points to underlying genetic predisposing factors and/or environmental factors. This is most clear in the gut, with progress through 16S and metagenomics sequencing studies and the results of functional studies in preclinical arthritis models. Translation of these findings to the clinic is making progress based on encouraging results of fecal microbial transplant studies in several human diseases. This review elaborates on novel trends in host-microbial interplay in spondyloarthritis,

EAMs

To adequately and efficiently evaluate patients with gastrointestinal symptoms in the context of axial spondyloarthritis can be difficult, considering that many of these patients suffer from chronic pain, present high inflammatory parameters, and use drugs with possible gastrointestinal adverse effects. In addition, the immunosuppressive treatments that these patients can receive make it necessary to always consider infections within the differential diagnoses of inflammatory bowel disease. In this article, we propose a practical approach to patients diagnosed with axial spondyloarthritis and suspected inflammatory bowel disease.

Imaging

Imaging of the sacroiliac joint plays a critical role in the classification of patients with axial spondyloarthritis. New imaging techniques are emerging, changing the way clinicians look at the sacroiliac joint. This article introduces the novel techniques in imaging of spondyloarthritis, including dual-energy computed tomography and new MRI sequences, with a focus on the imaging of bone marrow edema and erosions of the sacroiliac joint.

This article discusses the current position of conventional radiography and MRI, the techniques recommended by the European League Against Rheumatism for use in imaging in axial spondyloarthritis (axSpA). Several challenges and areas of development regarding radiography and MRI in axSpA are considered. Also, a few interesting focus points for future research are noted. Besides the recommended techniques, this article discusses several nuclear imaging techniques and the usability of these techniques in daily practice.

Targeting clinical remission is currently the focus of the treat-to-target strategy. Defining clinical outcomes as the main achievable treatment goal questions whether imaging remission should also be considered in the treat-to-target concept. Imaging has gained a pivotal role in diagnosing and classifying axial spondyloarthritis at the earliest phase of the disease. Its importance has been expanded to monitoring and prognosticating spondyloarthritis. This article summarizes current evidence on the use of imaging for monitoring disease activity and predicting treatment response in axial spondyloarthritis, and discusses the concept of an imaging-driven treat-to-target strategy with a highlight on the newest imaging modalities in spondyloarthritis.

Treatment and Outcomes

Axial involvement in psoriatic arthritis is a well-recognized manifestation with a prevalence between 12.5% and 78%. This huge heterogeneity is due to the different criteria used by authors to define psoriatic arthritis with axial involvement combining clinical features with radiographic evidence of disease. Specific genetic and clinical attributes of axial psoriatic arthritis might differentiate it from axial spondyloarthritis with concurrent skin psoriasis. Few studies address the specific management. The purpose of this review is to acknowledge the current understanding of axial involvement in psoriatic arthritis and highlight the need for a definition to facilitate research and clinical recognition.

Treat to target describes a management paradigm that involves choosing a clinically relevant target, assessment with validated measures at a prespecified frequency, and a change in therapy if the target is not met. Although guidelines recommend treating to target in axial spondyloarthritis (axSpA), ideal methods to reach this target remain controversial. This review focuses on background for a treat-to-target strategy in axSpA. Potential targets of treatment, association of targets with outcomes, evidence of treatment impact on outcomes, and how treat to target has been incorporated into treatment guidelines are discussed. Treat-to-target trials and the research agenda for studies in axSpA are discussed.

Axial spondyloathritis (axSpA) treatment with biologic DMARDs was previously focused around anti-TNF agents. Significant advances in research have led to new therapeutic options, such as secukinumab, an IL-17 inhibitor, which has been approved for the treatment of axSpA. Two other biologic agents that are already licensed for rheumatoid and psoriatic arthritis, tofacitinib and ixekizumab, have demonstrated improved outcomes in axSpA. Several newer agents have been developed to inhibit IL-17, IL-23, and JAK. Early trials are promising; however, further research is needed. Rapid expansion of therapies available to treat axSpA could lead to improved disease control and decreased disease burden.

> In axial spondyloarthritis (axSpA), the first treatment is nonsteroidal anti-inflammatory drugs, and if insufficient, a biologic. Most evidence is available of tumour necrosis factor alpha inhibitors (TNFi), although recently, IL-17a inhibitors have also become available. In patients with sustained low disease activity, TNFi tapering can be considered. Importantly, the effect of axSpA treatment on extra-articular manifestations should be considered. Most TNFi are efficacious on spinal and extra-articular symptoms, but some differences exist for anterior uveitis and inflammatory bowel disease. Overall, it is recommended that axSpA treatment is individualised as much as possible, taking into account both spinal- and extra-articular symptoms.

> The most prevalent health concerns in patients with axial spondyloarthritis (axSpA) include spinal stiffness, spinal pain, mobility limitations, fatigue, and disturbed sleep. Many patients experience impairments related to extraspinal disease, extra-articular disease, or drug side effects. To capture overall life impact, self-reported measurement instruments assessing health-related quality of life (HRQoL) have been developed. This article summarizes the literature on relevant concepts and frameworks when measuring overall health or HRQoL, available measures assessing this outcome in axSpA, the hierarchical relations between overall health/HRQoL and specific axSpA impairments, and the role of context when interpreting interventions for overall health or HRQoL outcomes.

Patient's Perspective

> A patient who has had ankylosing spondylitis for 50 years describes her long journey to diagnosis, living with the disease, the different types of treatments she has tried (both traditional and nontraditional), and her participation in clinical studies. She describes her use of nonsteroidal anti-inflammatory drugs as well as biologics to help manage inflammation and the importance of diet and exercise—Pilates, yoga, and physical therapy—to maintain and improve movement and flexibility. She offers her own personal advice to those recently diagnosed.

> Being seriously affected by a rheumatic disease at the age of 16 seems a catastrophe that somehow must be learned to manage. And the challenges that come up when the illness worsens in the life course have to be coped with. So, this article tries to outline some of the points I have experienced and find relevant for patients with ankylosing spondylitis.

RHEUMATIC DISEASE CLINICS OF NORTH AMERICA

SERIES OF RELATED INTEREST

Medical Clinics of North America
https://www.medical.theclinics.com/
Neurologic Clinics
https://www.neurologic.theclinics.com/
Dermatologic Clinics
https://www.derm.theclinics.com/
Physical Medicine and Rehabilitation Clinics of North America
https://www.pmr.theclinics.com/

THE CLINICS ARE AVAILABLE ONLINE!
Access your subscription at:
www.theclinics.com

Preface

Spondyloarthritis: The Changing Landscape—Are We There Yet?

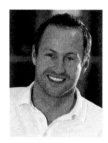 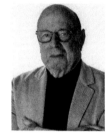

Xenofon Baraliakos, MD   Michael H. Weisman, MD
Editors

Dear friends, dear colleagues,

We are happy to provide you this issue of *Rheumatic Disease Clinics of North America*. This piece of work includes contributions of many of the leaders in the field of spondyloarthritis (SpA). Together with the authors, we have tried to address all aspects of the disease related to axial, peripheral, or combinations of both phenotypes. The authors achieved very nicely, in small pieces that at the end fit together like a puzzle, capturing the entire landscape of SpA, giving objective and their own views on the most recent changes but also describing the (possible) future directions. The contributions are dealing with the disease pathogenesis and biology, genetics and cellular interactions, differences between phenotypes and classification challenges, musculoskeletal and extraarticular manifestations, treatment options, treatment targets, imaging, clinical assessment, and precision medicine. Of great interest are also the perspectives of 2 patients, who describe the burden of the disease and the challenges of coping with it in everyday life. These contributions aim to capture all aspects that are relevant for physicians, researchers, and patients. Our aim was to update knowledge, inform about upcoming changes in the field, and stipulate discussions about what might be more or less relevant in the future of SpA, in order to achieve the best possible medical care for our patients.

Rheum Dis Clin N Am 46 (2020) xiii–xiv
https://doi.org/10.1016/j.rdc.2020.02.001
0889-857X/20/© 2020 Published by Elsevier Inc.

rheumatic.theclinics.com

We hope that you will enjoy reading this issue as much as we all enjoyed working on it together.

Sincerely,

Xenofon Baraliakos, MD
Rheumazentrum Ruhrgebiet Herne
Ruhr-University Bochum, Germany
Claudiusstr. 45
Herne 44649, Germany

Michael H. Weisman, MD
Division of Rheumatology
Cedars-Sinai Medical Center
David Geffen School of Medicine at University of California, Los Angeles
1545 Calmar Court
Los Angeles, CA 90024, USA

E-mail addresses:
Xenofon.Baraliakos@elisabethgruppe.de (X. Baraliakos)
michael.weisman@cshs.org (M.H. Weisman)

Genetics and Juvenile SpA

Pathogenesis of Axial Spondyloarthritis — Sources and Current State of Knowledge

Joerg Ermann, MD

KEYWORDS

- pathogenesis • disease model • axial spondyloarthritis • ankylosing spondylitis

KEY POINTS

- Models of disease pathogenesis are informed by multiple lines of investigation. Animal studies are just one of many sources of knowledge.
- The development of axial SpA involves the interplay of genetic and environmental factors likely including mechanical stress and intestinal dysbiosis.
- The lack of access to diseased human tissue has hampered progress in understanding the pathogenesis of axial SpA.
- Randomized controlled trials with biologics are explorations of disease pathogenesis. Combining therapeutic drug trials with mechanistic studies would be desirable.

INTRODUCTION

Scientific breakthroughs, such as the discovery of rheumatoid factor in the 1940s and the development of techniques for histocompatibility testing in the 1960s, culminated in the development of the spondyloarthritis (SpA) concept as a family of rheumatic diseases, distinct from rheumatoid arthritis (RA), with overlapping clinical features and genetic risk factors.[1,2] The demonstration, by magnetic resonance imaging (MRI), of inflammatory lesions in the sacroiliac (SI) joints and spine of patients with axial symptoms of SpA who lacked radiographic features of ankylosing spondylitis (AS),[3,4] helped further refine the SpA concept by introducing axial SpA as a new entity.[5] Axial SpA includes patients with AS (also referred to as radiographic axial SpA) and patients with axial symptoms previously categorized as undifferentiated SpA (now nonradiographic axial SpA). AS was described more than 100 years before

Division of Rheumatology, Inflammation and Immunity, Brigham and Women's Hospital, HBTM, Room 06002P, 60 Fenwood Road, Boston, MA 02115, USA
E-mail address: jermann@bwh.harvard.edu

Rheum Dis Clin N Am 46 (2020) 193–206
https://doi.org/10.1016/j.rdc.2020.01.016
0889-857X/20/© 2020 Elsevier Inc. All rights reserved.

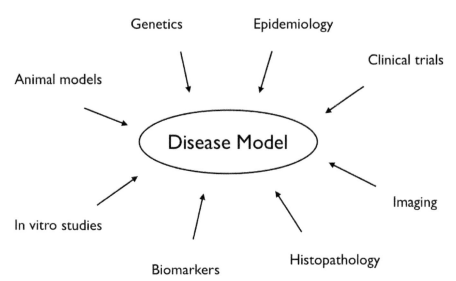

Fig. 1. Sources of knowledge informing the current (and future) understanding of axial SpA pathogenesis.

the development of the axial SpA concept and most clinical studies in axial SpA have been performed in AS. It is likely (although not proved) that the early events leading to axial inflammation are the same in all patients with axial SpA and that additional factors, environmental or genetic, drive progression to AS in a subset of patients. Ideas about pathogenesis, like disease concepts, evolve over time under the influence of new discoveries and changing scientific paradigms. This review examines the sources of knowledge that inform axial SpA pathogenesis (**Fig.1**), highlighting some of the current limitations and ending with a basic working model of axial SpA pathogenesis (**Fig. 2**).

EPIDEMIOLOGY

Axial SpA is a disease that typically begins in young adulthood and is equally common in men and women. In contrast, AS is more common in men, with a male:female ratio of 2 to 3:1 by current estimates.[6] This suggests that male sex controls the progression from inflammation to structural damage rather than susceptibility to axial inflammation. On the other hand, women with axial SpA tend to have higher disease activity and are less responsive to treatment with tumor necrosis factor (TNF) inhibitors.[7] The mechanistic understanding of these sexual dimorphisms is still in its infancy.[8] Relatively little is also known about environmental risk factors for the development of axial SpA, which may reflect the fact that genetic factors play a much greater role. A study from 2008 analyzed the occupational history of 397 patients with long-standing AS[9] and found an association between jobs requiring dynamic flexibility (repeated stretching, bending, twisting, or reaching) and functional impairment as measured by Bath Ankylosing Spondylitis Functional Index (BASFI). Moreover, certain types of workplace exposures, including whole-body vibration, were associated with worse radiographic disease. In light of the current interest in the role of mechanical stress in axial SpA, this study carries substantial weight, but confirmation in independent studies is required. Whether similar associations exist between workplace exposure and susceptibility to axial inflammation has not been studied. Smoking predominantly affects the progression from inflammation to structural damage.[10,11]

GENETICS

Twin studies in AS have demonstrated concordance rates in monozygotic twins greater than 50%, which is substantially higher than in other rheumatic diseases and suggests that genetic factors are the major determinant of disease risk in AS.[12] The association between HLA-B27 and AS was first described in 1973.[13,14] It is likely the strongest genetic association of any complex polygenic autoimmune/inflammatory disease with P values less than 10^{-100}.[15] Several hypothesis have been proposed but the precise mechanism underlying this association remains unknown.[16] Genome-wide association studies (GWAS) performed over the past 10–15 years in AS have identified multiple disease-associated loci outside of the major histocompatibility complex. In addition to genes involved in peptide processing and interleukin (IL)-23 receptor signaling, several disease-associated polymorphisms were found in genes relevant to lymphocyte biology, including RUNX3, TBX21, EOMES, ZMIZ1, IL7, IL7R, and BACH2. Currently, more than 100 risk loci for AS have been identified, which together explain 27.8% of the heritability of AS, with HLA-B27 contributing 20.4%.[17] Thus, much remains to be learned, including the identification of the actual risk variants in many of the identified risk loci.

The HLA-B27 association holds true for the broader category of axial SpA, although it is slightly lower than in AS.[18] GWAS studies have not been performed in (nonradiographic) axial SpA. One study applied a genetic risk score developed for AS to a cohort of patients with axial SpA and found a lower discriminatory capacity compared with AS.[19] The authors reasoned that this might indicate differences in the genetic make-up between the studied cohorts. Whether this truly reflects differences in genetic risk factors between nonradiographic axial SpA and AS remains to be shown. Heterogeneity of patient populations captured by the axial SpA criteria is a major problem for genetic studies.

IMAGING

MRI has revolutionized the axial SpA field by providing means to detect inflammation before skeletal changes become evident on radiographs.[3,4] Unfortunately, imaging studies have largely focused on diagnosis, and relatively few studies have utilized imaging to study disease pathogenesis.

Two types of lesions are frequently seen with MRI in patients with axial SpA—bone marrow edema (BME) and fat lesions. BME is considered to be the equivalent of inflammation whereas fat lesions are thought to represent a later lesion. Both types of lesions occur in the pelvic bone marrow adjacent to the SI joints as well as at the edges of vertebral bodies and in the posterior spinal elements. Observational studies have provided evidence that inflammatory vertebral corner lesions may either disappear or progress to become fat lesions, which are associated with an increased risk for subsequent syndesmophyte formation.[20,21] Fat lesions have also been observed as intermediary lesions in the SI joints filling in erosions (backfill) prior to progression to bony ankylosis.[22] Unfortunately (from the scientists' perspective), MRI entered the axial SpA world at about the same time as TNF inhibitors. Many patients in the aforementioned observational studies were thus treated with a TNF inhibitor and a comprehensive MRI account of the natural (untreated) history of sacroiliitis and vertebral corner inflammation in axial SpA is lacking.

The same caveat applies to recent studies that used serial computed tomography (CT) imaging to visualize and quantify syndesmophyte growth in AS.[23,24] These studies have shown that the distribution of syndesmophytes around the perimeter of the vertebral body is not random and that they occur most frequently at the postero-lateral aspect of the vertebral body.[25] A more recent study demonstrated that anterior syndesmophytes in the thoracolumbar spine were smaller and less frequent in close proximity to the aorta.[26] Together these data provide circumstantial evidence that me-chanical factors, intrinsic or extrinsic to the spine, may influence syndesmophyte formation.

Molecular imaging is an umbrella term for imaging modalities that permit insight into function.[27] Several studies have demonstrated the utility of PET-CT, PET-MRI or SPECT to identify inflammatory or bone forming lesions using ^{18}F-Fluorodeoxyglu-cose or ^{18}F-Sodium Fluoride tracers or [99m]Tc (Technetium)–labeled antibodies.[28–33] Radiation exposure associated with these approaches is likely a major reason that they have not used been more widely.

MRI studies in axial SpA typically rely on the standard sequences used in routine clinical practice. Newer MRI approaches, including 7T imaging or zero echo time MRI,[34] have not been applied in the axial SpA field yet and may offer higher spatial resolutions or insight into tissue properties that currently cannot be visualized.

CLINICAL TRIALS

While TNF inhibitors showed broad efficacy across many rheumatic diseases, including all diseases in the SpA family, subsequent studies of other inhibitors yielded more diverse results. IL-17A inhibitors (secukinumab and ixekizumab) showed clinical efficacy similar to TNF inhibitors in patient with active AS and non-radiographic axial SpA, including patients with AS who previously failed or were intolerant of TNF inhibitors.[35–38] In contrast, IL-6 antagonists (tocilizumab and sar-ilumab) failed to demonstrate efficacy in clinical trials in AS.[39,40] Perhaps even more surprising was finding that the IL-23p19 inhibitor rizankizumab and the IL-12/23p40 inhibitor ustekinumab did not meet their primary endpoints in clinical tri-als in AS and axial SpA, respectively.[41,42] Multiple lines of evidence point toward a role for the IL-23/IL-17A pathway in axial SpA, including the efficacy of IL-17A in-hibition in axial SpA, in vitro data documenting the reliance of IL-17A producing lymphocytes on IL-23 stimulation, association of AS with multiple genetic polymor-phisms in the IL-23 signaling pathway, and data from animal models.[43] Why then did IL-23 inhibition not work in axial SpA? Both rizankizumab and ustekinumab have demonstrated efficacy in other diseases of the SpA spectrum, including pso-riasis and Crohn disease (rizankizumab) and psoriasis, psoriatic arthritis, Crohn disease, and ulcerative colitis (ustekinumab), making pharmacokinetic problems less likely. The fact that both a p19 and a p40 inhibitor showed negative trial re-sults effectively rules out hypotheses invoking IL-23–related cytokines, such as IL-12 and IL-39 (a heterodimer of IL-23p19 and EBI3).[44] The most likely explana-tion might be that IL-23 plays a role during the initiation of axial inflammation but is dispensable at later time points, when factors other than IL-23 may drive the expression of IL-17A.[45]

As documented by these results, randomized controlled trials of biologics (typically monoclonal antibodies with high specificity) do not just test therapeutic efficacy, they also interrogate disease pathogenesis. Unfortunately, most clinical trials in axial SpA focus on clinical disease activity scores, serum C-reactive protein and standard

MRI of the SI joints as outcome measures and rarely collect additional mechanistic information. A lost opportunity.

TISSUE SPECIMENS

The importance and value of studying immune responses in the diseased tissue has been demonstrated in RA.[46,47] SpA research has been lagging behind because spine biopsies are considered unacceptable and too invasive for research purposes. Autopsies were an important source of biological specimens for research in the past, including in AS,[48] but are infrequently performed today. Moreover, except for rare circumstances,[49] autopsy specimens provide tissue only from late-stage disease, which is of limited value for understanding the critical early events in axial SpA pathogenesis. The same is true for specimens obtained during corrective spine surgery,[50,51] which occasionally is performed in patients with long-standing AS. Several studies have reported results from CT-guided needle biopsies of the SI joints.[52–55] These studies have demonstrated the presence of inflammation in the SI joints as well as evidence for cartilage erosion, pannus formation, and osteoproliferation. The value of this approach is limited, however, because the obtained specimens are small and the targeting of specific structures in the SI joints is challenging.[55]

An alternative more easily accessible biopsy target might be the pelvic BME lesions seen on MRI in patients with active axial SpA. BME is a radiological term that describes lesions in bone with low-intermediate signal on T1 and high signal on T2-weighted MRI sequences. On short tau inversion recovery (STIR) or similar sequences that suppress the high T2 signal of fat, BME lesions are hyperintense compared with regular BM. Since the original description in 1988,[56] BME has been observed in multiple conditions, including RA, SpA, trauma, degenerative disk disease, osteoarthritis, and primary BME syndrome.[57] Although the usage of the BME term across multiple conditions suggests shared pathology, histopathologic studies have demonstrated variable findings. A single study of surgical facet joint specimens from patients with long-standing AS described the "accumulation of eosinophilic fluid in the bone marrow interstitium" consistent with edema.[58] Studies performed in other diseases, however, do not support the idea that BME represents the accumulation of interstitial fluid as the name suggests. In osteoarthritis, BME seems to correlate with tissue fibrosis and necrosis[59,60] whereas studies in RA revealed the presence of inflammatory cell infiltrates in regions with BME on MRI.[61,62] The histopathologic equivalent of subchondral BME lesions in axial SpA or similar lesions in healthy individuals[63–65] is unclear. With regard to MRI fat lesions at vertebral corners, a recent histology study in advanced AS demonstrated that these lesions were indeed characterized by the accumulation of adipocytes[51].

BLOOD BIOMARKERS

Peripheral blood is easily accessible and can be sampled repeatedly with minor risk for morbidity.[66] Multiple cytokines and other soluble markers have been studied in AS. In order to understand these measurements in their relationship to the disease process in the axial skeleton, it would be important to assess disease status and activity at the time of blood sampling using appropriate imaging techniques (for instance whole body MRI) rather than rely on patient reported disease activity measures or serum C-reactive protein. To date such studies are lacking.[67] Many research groups have analyzed immune cells from patients with AS comparing them to healthy controls or patients with other rheumatic diseases. Numerical or functional abnormalities have been found in patients with AS in multiple lymphocyte subsets, including CD4$^+$ T cells, CD8$^+$ T cells, $\gamma\delta$ T cells, invariant natural killer (NK) T cells, NK cells, and mucosal-associated invariant T (MAIT) cells.[8,68–74] An expansion of IL-17A–producing cells has been a common finding in the more recent studies. This is consistent with the success of IL-17A inhibitors in AS clinical trials and supports a critical role for the IL-23/IL-17A axis in AS pathogenesis. However, the identity of the expanded IL-17A producing lymphocyte populations varied between studies. It is unclear whether this is due to differences in experimental design (each study only analyzed a limited spectrum of cell types) or patient selection. It is feasible that subsets of AS patients exist with abnormalities in distinct lymphocyte populations that reflect differences in disease pathogenesis. Alternatively, different cell types may play a role at different time points during the evolution of the disease.

IN VITRO STUDIES

In vitro studies represent a reductionist approach to study the "behavior" of certain cells types under defined conditions. Recent studies demonstrated that tissue-derived osteoblast precursors from AS patients more readily differentiated into osteoblasts in vitro than cells from controls; this was linked to increased JAK2/STAT3 and alkaline phosphatase activity in AS cells. [75–77] These are difficult studies to perform as one major drawback of experiments with primary cells is the difficulty obtaining these cells from patients and controls at the right time and from the right location. Experiments with cells isolated from patients cannot distinguish between primary abnormalities driving disease from secondary effects occurring as the result of disease. An alternative strategy is thus the introduction of genetic modifications in cell lines using clustered regularly interspaced short palindromic repeats (CRISPR)/Cas to study the impact of genetic variants under controlled conditions.

ANIMAL MODELS

The human HLA-B27 transgenic rat (of which several versions exist) has been a particularly influential animal model of SpA.[78] The fact that expressing a human risk gene in a different species resulted in disease was a major argument at that time that HLA-B27 itself and not a closely linked gene mediates the disease.[79] Findings in the human HLA-B27 transgenic rat model that influenced the thinking about SpA pathogenesis include (1) dependence of the disease on lymphocytes but not CD8+ T cells[80,81], (2) evidence for a critical role of intestinal microbiota[82], and (3) demonstration that an HLA-B27-induced unfolded protein response could trigger inflammation[83,84]. Arguably, the demonstration that CD8+ T cells were dispensable for disease development in HLA-B27 transgenic rats had a major impact on the field by focusing research activities on lymphocytes other than CD8+ T cells.

While mice transgenic for human HLA-B27 do not develop arthritis[85] several other models with SpA-like features exist including SKG mice, TNF transgenics, mice with proteoglycan-induced arthritis and IL-23 minicircle-induced arthritis.[78] Studies using these models have provided critical insight into disease mechanisms but have important limitations. For instance, mice are quadrupeds with a tail. The weight of an adult mouse is about 1/3000 of a human but its body structures are built with cells that are the same size as human cells. Even with the most sophisticated techniques to "humanize" mice, a murine vertebral body or Achilles enthesis models the biology of the equivalent human structures only to a certain extent. Recent studies demonstrating the impact of mechanical strain on the development of arthritis in mice thus need to be interpreted with caution with regard to their external validity for human disease.[86–88]

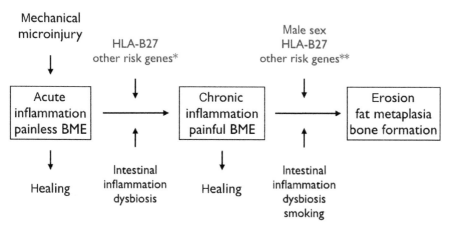

Fig. 2. A working model of axial SpA pathogenesis. Nonmodifiable risk factors (genes and sex) are in red; modifiable risk factors (intestinal inflammation, dysbiosis, and smoking) are in blue. Genetic risk factors controlling the development of chronic inflammation (*asterisk*) may be different from those controlling progression to structural damage (*double asterisk*).

A MODEL OF AXIAL SPONDYLOARTHRITIS PATHOGENESIS

The idea of enthesitis as the central lesion in AS was originally proposed by John Ball in 1971[89]. It was later resurrected and popularized through the work of Dennis McGonagle and colleagues.[90,91] Entheses are attachment sites of ligaments or tendons to bone which are constantly exposed to mechanical stress. This is thought to result in microinjury, which may in genetically predisposed individuals and influenced by environmental factors lead to chronic inflammation. Supporting evidence for this concept comes from recent studies that demonstrated the reciprocal impact of mechanical off-loading or running on arthritis development in mice[86–88]. However, an enthesis-centric disease model cannot explain axial SpA entirely, as early SI joint inflammation is primarily characterized by BME in the subchondral pelvic bone whereas enthesitis is rare.[92] A basic working model of axial SpA pathogenesis is presented in (**Fig. 2**) that focuses on the SI joints and surrounding pelvic bone. Clearly, this model contains multiple gaps and can only be considered as a preliminary framework for future experimental studies.

- The identification of pelvic BME lesions in healthy subjects, in particular athletes, military recruits and post-partum women suggests that mechanical stress may result in micro-injury giving rise to BME lesions on MRI. These lesions are typically not painful.[63–65] The sensitivity of currently available imaging modalities is limited and abnormalities may not be detectable in all cases.[54]
- Such micro-injuries may heal spontaneously, or in a genetically predisposed individual and under the influence of environmental factors progress to chronic inflammation. At some point the lesions become painful. Interestingly, the mechanism of inflammatory back pain in axial SpA is one of the least understood phenomena in this disease.
- The evolution from (sub)acute microinjury to chronic inflammation may be controlled by HLA-B27. The precise role of HLA-B27 in SpA pathogenesis is not understood[16]. One potential mechanism involves the presentation of tissue-specific antigens and activation of HLA-B27-restricted antigen-specific CD8+ T cells.[93] Subclinical inflammation in the gut may participate in this

process via travel of activated lymphocytes from the intestine to the early bone marrow lesion in the pelvis or via long-distance effects of microbial products leaking from the intestine into the blood stream.

- Inflammation may spread from the subchondral bone marrow into the SI joint space, either by direct invasion or through vascular channels[94], leading to synovitis, pannus formation and cartilage destruction.[95]
- Reparative processes continue to be activated. However, the ability to restore tissue homeostasis is lost at some point and resolution of inflammation (if it occurs) is accompanied by permanent structural damage visible on radiographs. Healing may involve the formation of an intermediary tissue dominated by fat cells ultimately leading to new bone formation and fusion of the SI joints (or syndesmophyte formation in the spine).

SUMMARY

Research efforts to understand the pathogenesis of axial SpA should focus primarily on the human disease. Mouse and rat models are extremely valuable by permitting detailed mechanistic studies that cannot be performed in humans. However, diseases in rodents at best resemble human disease. Limited access to biopsy specimens from the spine, in particular from patients with nonradiographic axial SpA, is a major obstacle. Novel molecular imaging techniques may circumvent the need for invasive procedures. Clinical trials with highly specific monoclonal antibodies have shown value as explorations of disease pathogenesis, which could be increased further by tagging on more mechanistic studies (beyond measuring standard parameters of inflammation). Ideally, pathogenetic studies should be coordinated across the whole spectrum of SpA diseases. A comparative analysis of patients with axial SpA, psoriatic arthritis, psoriasis, inflammatory bowel disease, uveitis, or combinations thereof can be expected to be extremely insightful.

DISCLOSURE

Supported by research grants from the Arthritis National Research Foundation and the National Psoriasis Foundation.

REFERENCES

1. Moll JM, Haslock I, Macrae IF, et al. Associations between ankylosing spondylitis, psoriatic arthritis, Reiter's disease, the intestinal arthropathies, and Behcet's syndrome. Medicine (Baltimore) 1974;53(5):343–64.
2. Zeidler H, Calin A, Amor B. A historical perspective of the spondyloarthritis. Curr Opin Rheumatol 2011;23(4):327–33.
3. Braun J, Bollow M, Eggens U, et al. Use of dynamic magnetic resonance imaging with fast imaging in the detection of early and advanced sacroiliitis in spondylarthropathy patients. Arthritis Rheum 1994;37(7):1039–45.
4. Jevtic V, Kos-Golja M, Rozman B, et al. Marginal erosive discovertebral "Romanus" lesions in ankylosing spondylitis demonstrated by contrast enhanced Gd-DTPA magnetic resonance imaging. Skeletal Radiol 2000;29(1):27–33.
5. Rudwaleit M, van der Heijde D, Landewe R, et al. The development of Assessment of SpondyloArthritis international Society classification criteria for axial spondyloarthritis (part II): validation and final selection. Ann Rheum Dis 2009; 68(6):777–83.

6. Sieper J, Poddubnyy D. Axial spondyloarthritis. Lancet 2017;390(10089):73–84.
7. Rusman T, van Vollenhoven RF, van der Horst-Bruinsma IE. Gender differences in axial spondyloarthritis: women are not so lucky. Curr Rheumatol Rep 2018; 20(6):35.
8. Gracey E, Yao Y, Green B, et al. Sexual dimorphism in the Th17 signature of anky-losing spondylitis. Arthritis Rheumatol 2016;68(3):679–89.
9. Ward MM, Reveille JD, Learch TJ, et al. Occupational physical activities and long-term functional and radiographic outcomes in patients with ankylosing spondylitis. Arthritis Rheum 2008;59(6):822–32.
10. Poddubnyy D, Haibel H, Listing J, et al. Cigarette smoking has a dose-dependent impact on progression of structural damage in the spine in patients with axial spondyloarthritis: results from the German SPondyloarthritis Inception Cohort (GESPIC). Ann Rheum Dis 2013;72(8):1430–2.
11. Akar S, Kaplan YC, Ecemis S, et al. The role of smoking in the development and progression of structural damage in axial SpA patients: a systematic review and meta-analysis. Eur J Rheumatol 2018;6(4):184–92.
12. Brown MA, Kennedy LG, MacGregor AJ, et al. Susceptibility to ankylosing spon-dylitis in twins: the role of genes, HLA, and the environment. Arthritis Rheum 1997;40(10):1823–8.
13. Brewerton DA, Hart FD, Nicholls A, et al. Ankylosing spondylitis and HL-A 27. Lancet 1973;1(7809):904–7.
14. Schlosstein L, Terasaki PI, Bluestone R, et al. High association of an HL-A anti-gen, W27, with ankylosing spondylitis. N Engl J Med 1973;288(14):704–6.
15. Cortes A, Pulit SL, Leo PJ, et al. Major histocompatibility complex associations of ankylosing spondylitis are complex and involve further epistasis with ERAP1. Nat Commun 2015;6:7146.
16. Bowness P. Hla-B27. Annu Rev Immunol 2015;33:29–48.
17. Costantino F, Breban M, Garchon HJ. Genetics and functional genomics of spon-dyloarthritis. Front Immunol 2018;9:2933.
18. Sieper J, van der Heijde D. Review: nonradiographic axial spondyloarthritis: new definition of an old disease? Arthritis Rheum 2013;65(3):543–51.
19. Thomas GP, Willner D, Robinson PC, et al. Genetic diagnostic profiling in axial spondyloarthritis: a real world study. Clin Exp Rheumatol 2017;35(2):229–33.
20. Song IH, Hermann KG, Haibel H, et al. Relationship between active inflammatory lesions in the spine and sacroiliac joints and new development of chronic lesions on whole-body MRI in early axial spondyloarthritis: results of the ESTHER trial at week 48. Ann Rheum Dis 2011;70(7):1257–63.
21. Chiowchanwisawakit P, Lambert RG, Conner-Spady B, et al. Focal fat lesions at vertebral corners on magnetic resonance imaging predict the development of new syndesmophytes in ankylosing spondylitis. Arthritis Rheum 2011;63(8): 2215–25.
22. Maksymowych WP, Wichuk S, Chiowchanwisawakit P, et al. Fat metaplasia and backfill are key intermediaries in the development of sacroiliac joint ankylosis in patients with ankylosing spondylitis. Arthritis Rheumatol 2014;66(11):2958–67.
23. Tan S, Yao J, Flynn JA, et al. Quantitative measurement of syndesmophyte vol-ume and height in ankylosing spondylitis using CT. Ann Rheum Dis 2014;73(3): 544–50.
24. Tan S, Yao J, Flynn JA, et al. Quantitative syndesmophyte measurement in anky-losing spondylitis using CT: longitudinal validity and sensitivity to change over 2 years. Ann Rheum Dis 2015;74(2):437–43.

25. Tan S, Dasgupta A, Yao J, et al. Spatial distribution of syndesmophytes along the vertebral rim in ankylosing spondylitis: preferential involvement of the posterolateral rim. Ann Rheum Dis 2016;75(11):1951–7.

26. Tan S, Dasgupta A, Flynn JA, et al. Aortic-vertebral interaction in ankylosing spondylitis: syndesmophyte development at the juxta-aortic vertebral rim. Ann Rheum Dis 2019;78(7):922–8.

27. Kircher MF, Willmann JK. Molecular body imaging: MR imaging, CT, and US. Part II. Applications. Radiology 2012;264(2):349–68.

28. Bruijnen STG, Verweij NJF, van Duivenvoorde LM, et al. Bone formation in ankylosing spondylitis during anti-tumour necrosis factor therapy imaged by 18F-fluoride positron emission tomography. Rheumatology (Oxford) 2018;57(4):631–8.

29. Buchbender C, Ostendorf B, Ruhlmann V, et al. Hybrid 18F-labeled fluoride positron emission tomography/magnetic resonance (MR) imaging of the sacroiliac joints and the spine in patients with axial spondyloarthritis: a pilot study exploring the link of MR bone pathologies and increased osteoblastic activity. J Rheumatol 2015;42(9):1631–7.

30. Fischer DR, Pfirrmann CW, Zubler V, et al. High bone turnover assessed by 18F-fluoride PET/CT in the spine and sacroiliac joints of patients with ankylosing spondylitis: comparison with inflammatory lesions detected by whole body MRI. EJNMMI Res 2012;2(1):38.

31. Taniguchi Y, Arii K, Kumon Y, et al. Positron emission tomography/computed tomography: a clinical tool for evaluation of enthesitis in patients with spondyloarthritides. Rheumatology (Oxford) 2010;49(2):348 51.

32. Carron P, Lambert B, Van Praet L, et al. Scintigraphic detection of TNF-driven inflammation by radiolabelled certolizumab pegol in patients with rheumatoid arthritis and spondyloarthritis. RMD Open 2016;2(1):e000265.

33. Carron P, Renson T, de Hooge M, et al. Immunoscintigraphy in axial spondyloarthritis: a new imaging modality for sacroiliac inflammation. Ann Rheum Dis 2020.

34. Argentieri EC, Koff MF, Breighner RE, et al. Diagnostic accuracy of zero-echo time MRI for the evaluation of cervical neural foraminal stenosis. Spine (Phila Pa 1976) 2018;43(13):928–33.

35. Baeten D, Sieper J, Braun J, et al. Secukinumab, an interleukin-17A inhibitor, in ankylosing spondylitis. N Engl J Med 2015;373(26):2534–48.

36. van der Heijde D, Cheng-Chung Wei J, Dougados M, et al. Ixekizumab, an interleukin-17A antagonist in the treatment of ankylosing spondylitis or radiographic axial spondyloarthritis in patients previously untreated with biological disease-modifying anti-rheumatic drugs (COAST-V): 16 week results of a phase 3 randomised, double-blind, active-controlled and placebo-controlled trial. Lancet 2018; 392(10163):2441–51.

37. Deodhar A, Poddubnyy D, Pacheco-Tena C, et al. Efficacy and safety of ixekizumab in the treatment of radiographic axial spondyloarthritis: sixteen-week results from a phase III randomized, double-blind, placebo-controlled trial in patients with prior inadequate response to or intolerance of tumor necrosis factor inhibitors. Arthritis Rheumatol 2019;71(4):599–611.

38. Deodhar A, van der Heijde D, Gensler LS, et al. Ixekizumab for patients with non-radiographic axial spondyloarthritis (COAST-X): a randomised, placebo-controlled trial. Lancet 2020;395(10217):53–64.

39. Sieper J, Porter-Brown B, Thompson L, et al. Assessment of short-term symptomatic efficacy of tocilizumab in ankylosing spondylitis: results of randomised, placebo-controlled trials. Ann Rheum Dis 2014;73(1):95–100.

40. Sieper J, Braun J, Kay J, et al. Sarilumab for the treatment of ankylosing spondylitis: results of a Phase II, randomised, double-blind, placebo-controlled study (ALIGN). Ann Rheum Dis 2015;74(6):1051–7.

41. Baeten D, Ostergaard M, Wei JC, et al. Risankizumab, an IL-23 inhibitor, for ankylosing spondylitis: results of a randomised, double-blind, placebo-controlled, proof-of-concept, dose-finding phase 2 study. Ann Rheum Dis 2018;77(9): 1295–302.

42. Deodhar A, Gensler LS, Sieper J, et al. Three multicenter, randomized, double-blind, placebo-controlled studies evaluating the efficacy and safety of ustekinumab in axial spondyloarthritis. Arthritis Rheumatol 2019;71(2):258–70.

43. Smith JA, Colbert RA. Review: the interleukin-23/interleukin-17 axis in spondyloarthritis pathogenesis: Th17 and beyond. Arthritis Rheumatol 2014;66(2):231–41.

44. Wang X, Wei Y, Xiao H, et al. A novel IL-23p19/Ebi3 (IL-39) cytokine mediates inflammation in Lupus-like mice. Eur J Immunol 2016;46(6):1343–50.

45. van Tok MN, Na S, Lao CR, et al. The Initiation, but not the persistence, of experimental spondyloarthritis is dependent on interleukin-23 signaling. Front Immunol 2018;9:1550.

46. Rao DA, Gurish MF, Marshall JL, et al. Pathologically expanded peripheral T helper cell subset drives B cells in rheumatoid arthritis. Nature 2017;542(7639):110–4.

47. Zhang F, Wei K, Slowikowski K, et al. Defining inflammatory cell states in rheumatoid arthritis joint synovial tissues by integrating single-cell transcriptomics and mass cytometry. Nat Immunol 2019;20(7):928–42.

48. Geiler G. [Spondylarthritis ankylopoietica from the viewpoint of pathologic anatomy]. Dtsch Med Wochenschr 1969;94(22):1185–8.

49. Aufdermaur M. Pathogenesis of square bodies in ankylosing spondylitis. Ann Rheum Dis 1989;48(8):628–31.

50. Appel H, Kuhne M, Spiekermann S, et al. Immunohistologic analysis of zygapophyseal joints in patients with ankylosing spondylitis. Arthritis Rheum 2006;54(9): 2845–51.

51. Baraliakos X, Boehm H, Bahrami R, et al. What constitutes the fat signal detected by MRI in the spine of patients with ankylosing spondylitis? A prospective study based on biopsies obtained during planned spinal osteotomy to correct hyperkyphosis or spinal stenosis. Ann Rheum Dis 2019;78(9):1220–5.

52. Bollow M, Fischer T, Reisshauer H, et al. Quantitative analyses of sacroiliac biopsies in spondyloarthropathies: T cells and macrophages predominate in early and active sacroiliitis- cellularity correlates with the degree of enhancement detected by magnetic resonance imaging. Ann Rheum Dis 2000;59(2):135–40.

53. Marzo-Ortega H, O'Connor P, Emery P, et al. Sacroiliac joint biopsies in early sacroiliitis. Rheumatology (Oxford) 2007;46(7):1210–1.

54. Gong Y, Zheng N, Chen SB, et al. Ten years' experience with needle biopsy in the early diagnosis of sacroiliitis. Arthritis Rheum 2012;64(5):1399–406.

55. Wang DM, Lin L, Peng JH, et al. Pannus inflammation in sacroiliitis following immune pathological injury and radiological structural damage: a study of 193 patients with spondyloarthritis. Arthritis Res Ther 2018;20(1):120.

56. Wilson AJ, Murphy WA, Hardy DC, et al. Transient osteoporosis: transient bone marrow edema? Radiology 1988;167(3):757–60.

57. Patel S. Primary bone marrow oedema syndromes. Rheumatology (Oxford) 2014; 53(5):785–92.

58. Appel H, Loddenkemper C, Grozdanovic Z, et al. Correlation of histopathological findings and magnetic resonance imaging in the spine of patients with ankylosing spondylitis. Arthritis Res Ther 2006;8(5):R143.

59. Zanetti M, Bruder E, Romero J, et al. Bone marrow edema pattern in osteoarthritic knees: correlation between MR imaging and histologic findings. Radiology 2000; 215(3):835–40.

60. Martig S, Boisclair J, Konar M, et al. MRI characteristics and histology of bone marrow lesions in dogs with experimentally induced osteoarthritis. Vet Radiol Ultrasound 2007;48(2):105–12.

61. Jimenez-Boj E, Nobauer-Huhmann I, Hanslik-Schnabel B, et al. Bone erosions and bone marrow edema as defined by magnetic resonance imaging reflect true bone marrow inflammation in rheumatoid arthritis. Arthritis Rheum 2007; 56(4):1118–24.

62. Dalbeth N, Smith T, Gray S, et al. Cellular characterisation of magnetic resonance imaging bone oedema in rheumatoid arthritis; implications for pathogenesis of erosive disease. Ann Rheum Dis 2009;68(2):279–82.

63. Varkas G, de Hooge M, Renson T, et al. Effect of mechanical stress on magnetic resonance imaging of the sacroiliac joints: assessment of military recruits by magnetic resonance imaging study. Rheumatology (Oxford) 2018;57(3):508–13.

64. Weber U, Jurik AG, Zejden A, et al. Frequency and anatomic distribution of magnetic resonance imaging features in the sacroiliac joints of young athletes: exploring "background noise" toward a data-driven definition of sacroiliitis in early spondyloarthritis. Arthritis Rheumatol 2018;70(5):736–45.

65. Seven S, Ostergaard M, Morsel-Carlsen L, et al. Magnetic resonance imaging of lesions in the sacroiliac joints for differentiation of patients with axial spondyloarthritis from control subjects with or without pelvic or buttock pain: a prospective, cross-sectional study of 204 participants. Arthritis Rheumatol 2019;71(12): 2034–46.

66. Ermann J, Rao DA, Teslovich NC, et al. Immune cell profiling to guide therapeutic decisions in rheumatic diseases. Nat Rev Rheumatol 2015;11(9):541–51.

67. Maksymowych WP. Biomarkers for diagnosis of axial spondyloarthritis, disease activity, prognosis, and prediction of response to therapy. Front Immunol 2019; 10:305.

68. Duftner C, Dejaco C, Kullich W, et al. Preferential type 1 chemokine receptors and cytokine production of CD28- T cells in ankylosing spondylitis. Ann Rheum Dis 2006;65(5):647–53.

69. Kenna TJ, Davidson SI, Duan R, et al. Enrichment of circulating interleukin-17-secreting interleukin-23 receptor-positive gamma/delta T cells in patients with active ankylosing spondylitis. Arthritis Rheum 2012;64(5):1420–9.

70. Venken K, Jacques P, Mortier C, et al. RORgammat inhibition selectively targets IL-17 producing iNKT and gammadelta-T cells enriched in Spondyloarthritis patients. Nat Commun 2019;10(1):9.

71. Chan AT, Kollnberger SD, Wedderburn LR, et al. Expansion and enhanced survival of natural killer cells expressing the killer immunoglobulin-like receptor KIR3DL2 in spondylarthritis. Arthritis Rheum 2005;52(11):3586–95.

72. Gracey E, Qaiyum Z, Almaghlouth I, et al. IL-7 primes IL-17 in mucosal-associated invariant T (MAIT) cells, which contribute to the Th17-axis in ankylosing spondylitis. Ann Rheum Dis 2016;75(12):2124–32.

73. Hayashi E, Chiba A, Tada K, et al. Involvement of mucosal-associated invariant T cells in ankylosing spondylitis. J Rheumatol 2016;43(9):1695–703.

74. Al-Mossawi MH, Chen L, Fang H, et al. Unique transcriptome signatures and GM-CSF expression in lymphocytes from patients with spondyloarthritis. Nat Commun 2017;8(1):1510.

75. Jo S, Kang S, Han J, et al. Accelerated osteogenic differentiation of human bone-derived cells in ankylosing spondylitis. J Bone Miner Metab 2018;36(3):307–13.

76. Jo S, Wang SE, Lee YL, et al. IL-17A induces osteoblast differentiation by activating JAK2/STAT3 in ankylosing spondylitis. Arthritis Res Ther 2018;20(1):115.

77. Jo S, Han J, Lee YL, et al. Regulation of osteoblasts by alkaline phosphatase in ankylosing spondylitis. Int J Rheum Dis 2019;22(2):252–61.

78. Vieira-Sousa E, van Duivenvoorde LM, Fonseca JE, et al. Review: animal models as a tool to dissect pivotal pathways driving spondyloarthritis. Arthritis Rheumatol 2015;67(11):2813–27.

79. Hammer RE, Maika SD, Richardson JA, et al. Spontaneous inflammatory disease in transgenic rats expressing HLA-B27 and human beta 2m: an animal model of HLA-B27-associated human disorders. Cell 1990;63(5):1099–112.

80. May E, Dorris ML, Satumtira N, et al. CD8 alpha beta T cells are not essential to the pathogenesis of arthritis or colitis in HLA-B27 transgenic rats. J Immunol 2003;170(2):1099–105.

81. Maksymowych WP, Wichuk S, Dougados M, et al. Modification of structural lesions on MRI of the sacroiliac joints by etanercept in the EMBARK trial: a 12-week randomised placebo-controlled trial in patients with non-radiographic axial spondyloarthritis. Ann Rheum Dis 2018;77(1):78–84.

82. Taurog JD, Richardson JA, Croft JT, et al. The germfree state prevents development of gut and joint inflammatory disease in HLA-B27 transgenic rats. J Exp Med 1994;180(6):2359–64.

83. Turner MJ, Delay ML, Bai S, et al. HLA-B27 up-regulation causes accumulation of misfolded heavy chains and correlates with the magnitude of the unfolded protein response in transgenic rats: implications for the pathogenesis of spondylarthritis-like disease. Arthritis Rheum 2007;56(1):215–23.

84. DeLay ML, Turner MJ, Klenk EI, et al. HLA-B27 misfolding and the unfolded protein response augment interleukin-23 production and are associated with Th17 activation in transgenic rats. Arthritis Rheum 2009;60(9):2633–43.

85. Nickerson CL, Hanson J, David CS. Expression of HLA-B27 in transgenic mice is dependent on the mouse H-2D genes. J Exp Med 1990;172(4):1255–61.

86. Jacques P, Lambrecht S, Verheugen E, et al. Proof of concept: enthesitis and new bone formation in spondyloarthritis are driven by mechanical strain and stromal cells. Ann Rheum Dis 2014;73(2):437–45.

87. Cambre I, Gaublomme D, Burssens A, et al. Mechanical strain determines the site-specific localization of inflammation and tissue damage in arthritis. Nat Commun 2018;9(1):4613.

88. Cambre I, Gaublomme D, Schryvers N, et al. Running promotes chronicity of arthritis by local modulation of complement activators and impairing T regulatory feedback loops. Ann Rheum Dis 2019;78(6):787–95.

89. Ball J. Enthesopathy of rheumatoid and ankylosing spondylitis. Ann Rheum Dis 1971;30(3):213–23.

90. McGonagle D, Gibbon W, Emery P. Classification of inflammatory arthritis by enthesitis. Lancet 1998;352(9134):1137–40.

91. McGonagle D, Lories RJ, Tan AL, et al. The concept of a "synovio-entheseal complex" and its implications for understanding joint inflammation and damage in psoriatic arthritis and beyond. Arthritis Rheum 2007;56(8):2482–91.

92. de Hooge M, van den Berg R, Navarro-Compan V, et al. Magnetic resonance imaging of the sacroiliac joints in the early detection of spondyloarthritis: no added value of gadolinium compared with short tau inversion recovery sequence. Rheumatology (Oxford) 2013;52(7):1220–4.

93. Winchester R, FitzGerald O. The many faces of psoriatic arthritis: their genetic determinism. Rheumatology (Oxford) 2020;59(Supplement_1):i4–9.
94. Binks DA, Gravallese EM, Bergin D, et al. Role of vascular channels as a novel mechanism for subchondral bone damage at cruciate ligament entheses in osteoarthritis and inflammatory arthritis. Ann Rheum Dis 2015;74(1):196–203.
95. Francois RJ, Gardner DL, Degrave EJ, et al. Histopathologic evidence that sacroiliitis in ankylosing spondylitis is not merely enthesitis. Arthritis Rheum 2000; 43(9):2011–24.

Molecular Biology Approaches to Understanding Spondyloarthritis

Adam Berlinberg, MD, Kristine A. Kuhn, MD, PhD*

KEYWORDS

- Spondyloarthritis • Genetics • Epigenetics • microRNA • Microbiome
- Metabolomics • Immunophenotyping • Transcriptomics

KEY POINTS

- Recent advances in genetics, omics technologies, and immune profiling methods have contributed to significant advances in the clinical and scientific understanding of spondyloarthritis.
- Genetic studies have shifted from genome-wide association studies to newer technologies, such as whole-genome sequencing and identification of epigenetic modifications.
- Single-cell sequencing and time-of-flight cytometry allow identification of novel cell populations in tissues.
- Multiomic analyses will further integrate large data sets and inform pathophysiologic mechanisms.

INTRODUCTION

Numerous factors involved with the pathogenesis of spondyloarthritis (SpA) from genetic predisposition, transcriptional expression of genes, immune function, and environmental factors like the microbiome increasingly are identified as potential contributors to the pathophysiology. Recent advances in molecular techniques, including omics technologies and improved immune profiling methods, have allowed for further elucidation of important pathways and cell types, expanding understanding of diseases like ankylosing spondylitis (AS) and psoriatic arthritis (PsA). This article describes some of the molecular approaches utilized as well as some of the recent advances that are helping to progress the field and provide more targets for intervention.

Division of Rheumatology, University of Colorado School of Medicine, 1775 Aurora Court Mail Stop B115, Aurora, CO 80045, USA
* Corresponding author.
E-mail address: kristine.kuhn@cuanschutz.edu

Rheum Dis Clin N Am 46 (2020) 207–215
https://doi.org/10.1016/j.rdc.2020.01.001
0889-857X/20/© 2020 Elsevier Inc. All rights reserved.

GENETICS

The genetic landscape has evolved over the past 5 years away from traditional mendelian approaches toward genome-wide association studies (GWASs), next-generation sequencing (NGS), and epigenetics. These new molecular approaches have led to significant advances in science and have provided a powerful platform for studies in SpA, extending genetic understanding of SpA well beyond HLA-B27, which contributes only 20.1% of the heritability of AS.[1]

Genome-Wide Association Studies and Next-Generation Sequencing

GWASs are a complex genetic analysis tool that allows for the detailed profiling of genetic variants. GWASs allow for the analysis of hundreds of thousands of single-nucleotide polymorphisms (SNPs) to be assessed for association with a given disease.[2] A GWAS is performed most commonly as a case-control study design with a group of patients diagnosed with a disease of interest compared with healthy controls. For this type of study, DNA usually is isolated from peripheral blood and subsequently genotyped using commercial chip platforms. After data quality control, which can be assessed by several computational programs, data are analyzed for associations between SNPs and disease. Generally, an analysis is followed by replicating associations in an independent population sample.[3]

GWASs have been used extensively in SpA to identify genes linked to signaling pathways not previously identified.[4–6] This is further exemplified nicely in the study by Ellinghaus and colleagues,[7] in which 86,000 individuals of European ancestry with AS, inflammatory bowel diseases, primary sclerosing cholangitis, or psoriasis were compared with healthy controls. The analysis allowed identification of 27 new genetic susceptibility loci, 17 in AS alone, and demonstrated shared risk among these related diseases. Studies like this have identified novel pathways of disease based on susceptibility loci, such as interleukin (IL)-23 receptor (R), IL-12B, and chemokine receptor 6, which affect CD4+ effector function.[8] Numerous other genes related to the IL-23/IL-17 pathway also have been identified through GWASs, including CARD9, PTGER4, TYK2, and STAT3[8] as well as ERAP1 and ERAP2, which relate to peptide trimming in the endoplasmic reticulum for peptide loading onto HLA class 1 molecules, such as HLA-B27.[9] Although these data have vastly expanded understanding of genetic susceptibility for SpA, GWASs are limited by their sample size and heterogeneity. They best identify common genetic variants but can miss rare polymorphisms and are unable to identify genetic interactions with other loci.

Better identification of rare genetic variants of clinical importance can be achieved through NGS methodologies like whole-exome and genome sequencing. In these methods, DNA is extracted from white blood cells, broken into short fragments and the DNA sequence determined through various sequencing technologies.[10] These fragments then are read as millions of short sequencing DNA reads, followed by alignment to the human genome reference sequence via a variety of available computational tools. In this manner, DNA composition can be determined in a specific order with individual nucleotides. Overall, NGS is a valuable tool for detecting single-nucleotide substitutions and/or insertions as well as differences in gene composition.[10] One study of exosome sequencing in AS confirmed previously identified susceptibility polymorphisms, such as ERAP1 and IL-23R; however, the study was underpowered to identify novel rare variants.[11]

Epigenetics: Methylation and Histone Acetylation/Deacetylation

DNA methylation is an epigenetic modification in which methyl groups are added to cysteine or adenine residues, thereby controlling transcription.[12]

Age, sex, smoking, medications, alcohol, and diet are known to affect DNA methylation.[13] Methylation patterns have been implicated in numerous biologic processes, such as aging, and several diseases, including SpA.[12] DNA methyltransferase 1 (DNMT1) is an enzyme that regulates patterns of methylated cytosine residues. Expression of DNMT1 is decreased in the setting of increased methylation of the DNMT1 promoter in AS patients compared with healthy controls, which is of unclear etiology in AS pathogenesis, because this did not correlate with clinical manifestations.[14] Furthermore, numerous genes in AS have been found to be differentially methylated, with hypermethylation of HLA-DQB1 having the most significant signal.[15] Another gene, B-cell chronic lymphocytic leukemia/lymphoma 11B (BCL11B), also was found to have increased methylation and decreased transcription in AS compared with healthy controls.[16] More recently, the first study to assess the role of HLA-B27 in methylation status of AS was performed. This study found hypomethylation of HCP5, tubulin folding cofactor A, and phospholipase D family member 6 in AS patients.[17] Thus, methylation studies have identified additional genes that may be important in disease development.

Histone modification allows activation (euchromatin) and deactivation (heterochromatin) of chromatin by histone acetyltransferases (HATs) and histone deacetylases (HDACs).[18] These different acetylation patterns allow for chromatin stability, gene regulation, and transcription silencing. The concept of histone modification has been minimally studied in SpA. In peripheral blood mononuclear cells from patients with AS, HAT and HDAC activity were significantly reduced compared with healthy controls.[19] HDAC inhibitors, such as sirtinol, were able to decrease HDAC expression in healthy controls but not in AS. Sirtinol decreased production of tumor necrosis factor (TNF) in AS patients, suggesting an intriguing treatment strategy in AS requiring further study.[19] Targeting modifiable states, such as histone acetylation, versus unmodifiable states, such as genetic composition, is an attractive strategy that likely will be studied further in the future. For example, HDAC inhibitors have shown anti-inflammatory effects in vitro in rheumatoid arthritis (RA) models[20,21] but have not been studied thus far in SpA.

MicroRNA

MicroRNA (miRNA) is a type of small, noncoding RNA of approximately 22 nucleotides that can form complex networks that regulate cell differentiation, development, and homeostasis.[22] MiRNAs have been proposed to be involved in the pathogenesis of numerous rheumatic diseases, such as RA, systemic lupus erythematosus (SLE), and osteoarthritis.[23–25] The role of miRNA in the pathogenesis of AS has indicated a variety of expression variability of miRNAs. Common miRNA profiles in AS have identified individuals with increased miR-146a and miR-155.[26] Mechanistically, increased miR-146a expression has been studied in terms of gene regulation, in that miR-146a has been shown to inhibit dickkopf 1 (DKK1), which also has been implicated in AS pathogenesis, and miR-146a knockdown models can hinder AS progression.[27] Other miRNAs that have been implicated in AS include miR-125a-5p, miR-151a-3p, and miR-22-3p based on higher expression compared with healthy controls.[28]

Given that there is increased specific miRNA expression in patients with AS compared with healthy controls, miRNAs represent a potential biomarker for diagnosis, disease activity, or potential therapeutic targets. The previously discussed miRNAs, miR-146a and miR-155, have been found to correlate with disease activity using the Bath Ankylosing Spondylitis Disease Activity Index (BASDAI).[26] Additional correlations with BASDAI and miR-625-3p and miR-29a also have been identified.[29,30] Other miRNAs have been identified in AS patients with down-regulated miR-199a-5p correlating with increased TNF, IL-17, and IL-23.[31] This finding implies that miRNAs could distinguish SpA phenotypes responsive to inhibitors of TNF, IL-17, or IL-23.[32] This concept also has been assessed in PsA with specific miRNA signatures noted in patients with PsA compared with healthy controls, which have been proposed as biomarkers or potential therapeutic targets.[33]

PROTEOMICS AND METABOLOMICS

Proteomics and metabolomics are omics tools that focus on unbiased identification and measurement of the proteins or small molecule metabolites in a biologic system. These approaches rely on high-pressure liquid chromatography and mass spectrometry of a sample followed by alignment of results with a database of known proteins and metabolites for identification. Addition of known concentrations of specific proteins and metabolites allows further quantification within samples. These approaches have potential to identify biomarkers for disease diagnosis and activity as well as pathogenic mechanisms. For example, proteomics identified several candidate biomarkers for either the diagnosis of or conversion from psoriasis to PsA[34–36]; however, none of these candidates has been confirmed in independent cohorts. Similarly, in AS, 2 proteomic studies suggested biologic processes of cytotoxicity and vitamin D binding in the pathogenesis of AS,[37,38] although these have yet to be validated. With regard to metabolomics, analysis of multiple tissue, including plasma, urine, and hip ligament, found alterations in fat, glucose, and choline metabolism.[39,40] Given the known dysbiosis in the fecal microbiota that have been identified in SpA compared with controls,[41–43] metabolites also have been studied in fecal samples in a pediatric population with enthesitis-related arthritis. The investigaton of fecal metabolites in pediatric enthesis-related arthritis found decreased metabolic diversity and alterations in the tryptophan metabolism pathway relative to healthy controls.[44]

MICROBIOME

Alterations in intestinal bacterial communities (dysbiosis) have been identified in SpA, although the etiology and consequence of dysbiosis is not elucidated.[41–43] The microbiome represents an emerging area in SpA given the presumed gut-joint relationship in disease pathogenesis. There are numerous approaches toward studying the microbiome in patients with SpA: 16S sequencing identifies bacteria through limited sequencing of regions within the bacterial 16S ribosomal RNA gene and alignment with sequence databases; this approach limits identification of bacteria to the level of genera. Similar methods exist for sequencing fungi using the internal transcribed spacer. Shotgun metagenomics allows species-level identification through untargeted sequencing using random primer sets. This technique also provides the functional potential of a community after analysis of genetic pathways identified by sequencing. Metatranscriptomics and single-cell RNA sequencing (scRNA-seq) are still being optimized to microbiome analysis and will provide another level of analysis.

A limitation of microbiome studies to date in AS has been the variability of findings from one study cohort to another.[41,43,45] For example, Breban and colleagues[43] identified a significant expansion of *Ruminococcus gnavus* by 16S sequencing of stool in patients with AS compared with controls. Tito and colleagues,[46] however, identified a significant expansion of *Dialister* by 16S sequencing of intestinal biopsies from individuals with AS that correlated with disease activity scores. The variation of findings may be related to tissue sampling (eg, stool vs mucosa-associated bacteria), geographic differences, or other confounding factors that need to be considered when designing and interpreting microbiome studies in AS. Furthermore, the specific microbiota may not be as important as the community function, which may be better assessed with newer technologies, such as metagenomics and metatranscriptomics.

IMMUNE PHENOTYPING

Numerous new techniques have been utilized in discovering novel immune phenotypes in SpA. Traditional immune cell profiling through flow cytometry has led to the identification of cells hypothesized to contribute to disease pathogenesis. These immune phenotypes include expanded helper T cell type 22, helper T cell type 17, γδ T cells, and mucosal-associated invariant T cells in the peripheral blood[47–50] as well as IL-17–producing natural killer cells in the intestine of AS patients.[51] As general knowledge of immune cells and function has expanded, traditional techniques have revealed additional cell types, such as innate lymphoid cells. Increased levels of type 3 innate lymphoid cells that produce IL-17 and IL-22 have been identified in the intestine, peripheral blood, synovial fluid, and bone marrow of AS patients[48] and in the peripheral blood of patients with PsA that correlate with clinical disease activity.[52] Newer molecular approaches, namely mass cytometry and scRNA-seq, have additive potential to reveal unique cell types and pathways.

Cytometry by Time-of-Flight and Imaging Mass Cytometry

Traditional flow cytometry is limited by use of fluorescent dyes that have overlapping spectra, thus limiting the resolution between dyes and number of antibody markers that can be combined (usually <20). Cytometry by time-of-flight (CyTOF) is a technology for single-cell analysis that relies on using heavy metal ions as antibody labels without the limitations of fluorescence,[53] allowing combinations of greater numbers of antibodies, upwards of approximately 40. Recently CyTOF was used to identify an expansion of unique $CD8^+$ T cells in the synovial fluid of patients with AS. These $CD8^+$ T cells expressed integrins β7, CD103, CD29, and CD49a.[54] Thus, CyTOF has the power to characterize immune cell populations more thoroughly. Coupling CyTOF technology with histology, imaging mass cytometry has the ability to add spatial information, which will be a powerful tool in understanding the function of immune cells in tissues relevant to SpA.

Single-Cell RNA Sequencing and Cellular Indexing of Transcriptomes and Epitopes by Sequencing

scRNA-seq allows more refined profiling of immune cells compared to flow cytometry and CyTOF. There are numerous different methods, each with specific strengths and weaknesses, for single-cell isolation followed by amplification and NGS of transcribed RNA, as reviewed by Papalexi and Satija.[55] Analysis of the data allows for characterization of distinct cell subsets, uncovering the heterogeneity within a population, and dissecting cell fate branch points.[55] The power of scRNA-seq is best highlighted by the efforts of the Accelerating Medicines Partnership in profiling peripheral blood and tissue cells in patients with RA and SLE,[56] which has revealed novel cellular functions for further study in the pathogenesis of these diseases. A significant limitation of scRNA-seq is that immune cells are characterized by cell surface proteins that are not highly expressed mRNAs and thus not easily detected through transcriptional sequencing. Cellular indexing of transcriptomes and epitopes by sequencing (CITE-Seq) adds on scRNA-seq through the use of nucleotide barcode-labeled antibodies targeting cell surface markers. These barcodes are sequenced along with the transcriptome of each cell, allowing the coupling of protein marker information in the analysis of cellular populations. Although studies utilizing scRNA-seq in SpA have yet to be published, this represents an approach that could lead to significant advances in the field of SpA in terms of pathophysiology, diagnosis, and pharmacology.

INTEGRATED OMICS

With the rise of multiple omics technologies, integration of data from these approaches represents a powerful analysis for understanding aspects of SpA. This method can be used to study pathophysiology as well as identify candidate biomarkers for diagnostic purposes. For example, a recent study in inflammatory bowel disease utilized the techniques of multiomics to study microbial dysbiosis with regard to host factors toward dysregulation of microbial transcription, metabolite pools, and levels of antibodies in the serum.[57] A similar approach was used in the rat HLA-B27 transgenic model of AS in which microbiome analysis and host bulk RNA sequencing revealed correlations between specific bacteria and cytokine dysregulation, and bacterial metagenomics predicted pathways associated with inflammation.[58] Such approaches have great potential to expand understanding of SpA.

SUMMARY

With an ever-evolving scientific landscape, emerging molecular techniques continue to elucidate important pathways in complex diseases, such as SpA. Within SpA, many of the techniques, described in this article, are offering new approaches toward diagnosis, such as metabolites, miRNA, or immune cell profiling, as well as identifying new therapeutic approaches, such as epigenetic modifications. In addition to the development of new techniques is the expansion of analysis tools in handling data generated from the methodologies. Altogether, these approaches provide exciting pathways forward in the study of SpA.

ACKNOWLEDGMENTS

The authors are supported by grants through the National Institutes of Health (T32AR007534, K08DK107905, R01AR075033), the Rheumatology Research Foundation, and the Boettcher Foundation Webb-Waring Biomedical Research Award.

DISCLOSURE

The authors have nothing to disclose.

REFERENCES

1. Busch R, Kollnberger S, Mellins ED. HLA associations in inflammatory arthritis: emerging mechanisms and clinical implications. Nat Rev Rheumatol 2019; 15(6):364–81.
2. Manolio TA. Genomewide association studies and assessment of the risk of disease. N Engl J Med 2010;363(2):166–76.
3. Pearson TA, Manolio TA. How to interpret a genome-wide association study. JAMA 2008;299(11):1335–44.
4. Parkes M, Cortes A, van Heel DA, et al. Genetic insights into common pathways and complex relationships among immune-mediated diseases. Nat Rev Genet 2013;14(9):661–73.
5. Tsoi LC, Spain SL, Knight J, et al. Identification of 15 new psoriasis susceptibility loci highlights the role of innate immunity. Nat Genet 2012;44(12):1341–8.

6. Cortes A, Hadler J, Pointon JP, et al. Identification of multiple risk variants for ankylosing spondylitis through high-density genotyping of immune-related loci. Nat Genet 2013;45(7):730–8.

7. Ellinghaus D, Jostins L, Spain SL, et al. Analysis of five chronic inflammatory diseases identifies 27 new associations and highlights disease-specific patterns at shared loci. Nat Genet 2016;48(5):510–8.

8. Coffre M, Roumier M, Rybczynska M, et al. Combinatorial control of Th17 and Th1 cell functions by genetic variations in genes associated with the interleukin-23 signaling pathway in spondyloarthritis. Arthritis Rheum 2013;65(6):1510–21.

9. Kanaseki T, Blanchard N, Hammer GE, et al. ERAAP synergizes with MHC class I molecules to make the final cut in the antigenic peptide precursors in the endoplasmic reticulum. Immunity 2006;25(5):795–806.

10. Biesecker LG, Green RC. Diagnostic clinical genome and exome sequencing. N Engl J Med 2014;371(12):1170.

11. Robinson PC, Leo PJ, Pointon JJ, et al. Exome-wide study of ankylosing spondylitis demonstrates additional shared genetic background with inflammatory bowel disease. NPJ Genome Med 2016;1:16008.

12. Dor Y, Cedar H. Principles of DNA methylation and their implications for biology and medicine. Lancet 2018;392(10149):777–86.

13. Whyte JM, Ellis JJ, Brown MA, et al. Best practices in DNA methylation: lessons from inflammatory bowel disease, psoriasis and ankylosing spondylitis. Arthritis Res Ther 2019;21(1):133.

14. Aslani S, Mahmoudi M, Garshasbi M, et al. Evaluation of DNMT1 gene expression profile and methylation of its promoter region in patients with ankylosing spondylitis. Clin Rheumatol 2016;35(11):2723–31.

15. Hao J, Liu Y, Xu J, et al. Genome-wide DNA methylation profile analysis identifies differentially methylated loci associated with ankylosis spondylitis. Arthritis Res Ther 2017;19(1):177.

16. Karami J, Mahmoudi M, Amirzargar A, et al. Promoter hypermethylation of BCL11B gene correlates with downregulation of gene transcription in ankylosing spondylitis patients. Genes Immun 2017;18(3):170–5.

17. Coit P, Kaushik P, Caplan L, et al. Genome-wide DNA methylation analysis in ankylosing spondylitis identifies HLA-B*27 dependent and independent DNA methylation changes in whole blood. J Autoimmun 2019.

18. Allis CD, Jenuwein T. The molecular hallmarks of epigenetic control. Nat Rev Genet 2016;17(8):487–500.

19. Toussirot E, Abbas W, Khan KA, et al. Imbalance between HAT and HDAC activities in the PBMCs of patients with ankylosing spondylitis or rheumatoid arthritis and influence of HDAC inhibitors on TNF alpha production. PLoS One 2013; 8(8):e70939.

20. Joosten LA, Leoni F, Meghji S, et al. Inhibition of HDAC activity by ITF2357 ameliorates joint inflammation and prevents cartilage and bone destruction in experimental arthritis. Mol Med 2011;17(5–6):391–6.

21. Angiolilli C, Kabala PA, Grabiec AM, et al. Histone deacetylase 3 regulates the inflammatory gene expression programme of rheumatoid arthritis fibroblast-like synoviocytes. Ann Rheum Dis 2017;76(1):277–85.

22. Gebert LFR, MacRae IJ. Regulation of microRNA function in animals. Nat Rev Mol Cell Biol 2019;20(1):21–37.

23. Duroux-Richard I, Jorgensen C, Apparailly F. What do microRNAs mean for rheumatoid arthritis? Arthritis Rheum 2012;64(1):11–20.

24. Dai Y, Huang YS, Tang M, et al. Microarray analysis of microRNA expression in peripheral blood cells of systemic lupus erythematosus patients. Lupus 2007; 16(12):939–46.

25. Murata K, Yoshitomi H, Tanida S, et al. Plasma and synovial fluid microRNAs as potential biomarkers of rheumatoid arthritis and osteoarthritis. Arthritis Res Ther 2010;12(3):R86.

26. Qian BP, Ji ML, Qiu Y, et al. Identification of serum miR-146a and miR-155 as novel noninvasive complementary biomarkers for ankylosing spondylitis. Spine (Phila Pa 1976) 2016;41(9):735–42.

27. Di G, Kong L, Zhao Q, et al. MicroRNA-146a knockdown suppresses the progression of ankylosing spondylitis by targeting dickkopf 1. Biomed Pharmacother 2018;97:1243–9.

28. Perez-Sanchez C, Font-Ugalde P, Ruiz-Limon P, et al. Circulating microRNAs as potential biomarkers of disease activity and structural damage in ankylosing spondylitis patients. Hum Mol Genet 2018;27(5):875–90.

29. Prajzlerová K, Grobelná K, Hušáková M, et al. Association between circulating miRNAs and spinal involvement in patients with axial spondyloarthritis. PLoS One 2017;12(9):e0185323.

30. Li X, Lv Q, Tu L, et al. Aberrant expression of microRNAs in peripheral blood mononuclear cells as candidate biomarkers in patients with axial spondyloarthritis. Int J Rheum Dis 2019;22(7):1188–95.

31. Wang Y, Luo J, Wang X, et al. MicroRNA-199a-5p induced autophagy and inhibits the pathogenesis of ankylosing spondylitis by modulating the mTOR signaling via directly targeting Ras homolog enriched in brain (Rheb). Cell Physiol Biochem 2017;42(6):2481–91.

32. Jethwa H, Bowness P. The interleukin (IL)-23/IL-17 axis in ankylosing spondylitis: new advances and potentials for treatment. Clin Exp Immunol 2016;183(1):30–6.

33. Pelosi A, Lunardi C, Fiore PF, et al. MicroRNA expression profiling in psoriatic arthritis. Biomed Res Int 2018;2018:7305380.

34. Reindl J, Pesek J, Krüger T, et al. Proteomic biomarkers for psoriasis and psoriasis arthritis. J Proteomics 2016;140:55–61.

35. Gęgotek A, Domingues P, Wroński A, et al. Proteomic plasma profile of psoriatic patients. J Pharm Biomed Anal 2018;155:185–93.

36. Butt AQ, McArdle A, Gibson DS, et al. Psoriatic arthritis under a proteomic spotlight: application of novel technologies to advance diagnosis and management. Curr Rheumatol Rep 2015;17(5):35.

37. Cai A, Qi S, Su Z, et al. Quantitative proteomic analysis of peripheral blood mononuclear cells in ankylosing spondylitis by iTRAQ. Clin Transl Sci 2015;8(5): 579–83.

38. Fischer R, Trudgian DC, Wright C, et al. Discovery of candidate serum proteomic and metabolomic biomarkers in ankylosing spondylitis. Mol Cell Proteomics 2012;11(2). M111.013904.

39. Gao P, Lu C, Zhang F, et al. Integrated GC-MS and LC-MS plasma metabonomics analysis of ankylosing spondylitis. Analyst 2008;133(9):1214–20.

40. Wang W, Yang GJ, Zhang J, et al. Plasma, urine and ligament tissue metabolite profiling reveals potential biomarkers of ankylosing spondylitis using NMR-based metabolic profiles. Arthritis Res Ther 2016;18(1):244.

41. Stoll ML, Kumar R, Morrow CD, et al. Altered microbiota associated with abnormal humoral immune responses to commensal organisms in enthesitis-related arthritis. Arthritis Res Ther 2014;16(6):486.

42. Costello ME, Ciccia F, Willner D, et al. Brief report: intestinal dysbiosis in ankylosing spondylitis. Arthritis Rheumatol 2015;67(3):686–91.
43. Breban M, Tap J, Leboime A, et al. Faecal microbiota study reveals specific dysbiosis in spondyloarthritis. Ann Rheum Dis 2017;76(9):1614–22.
44. Stoll ML, Kumar R, Lefkowitz EJ, et al. Fecal metabolomics in pediatric spondyloarthritis implicate decreased metabolic diversity and altered tryptophan metabolism as pathogenic factors. Genes Immun 2016;17(7):400–5.
45. Wen C, Zheng Z, Shao T, et al. Quantitative metagenomics reveals unique gut microbiome biomarkers in ankylosing spondylitis. Genome Biol 2017;18(1):142.
46. Tito RY, Cypers H, Joossens M, et al. Brief report: dialister as a microbial marker of disease activity in spondyloarthritis. Arthritis Rheumatol 2017;69(1):114–21.
47. Zhang L, Li YG, Li YH, et al. Increased frequencies of Th22 cells as well as Th17 cells in the peripheral blood of patients with ankylosing spondylitis and rheumatoid arthritis. PLoS One 2012;7(4):e31000.
48. Ciccia F, Guggino G, Rizzo A, et al. Type 3 innate lymphoid cells producing IL-17 and IL-22 are expanded in the gut, in the peripheral blood, synovial fluid and bone marrow of patients with ankylosing spondylitis. Ann Rheum Dis 2015; 74(9):1739–47.
49. Gracey E, Yao Y, Green B, et al. Sexual dimorphism in the Th17 signature of ankylosing spondylitis. Arthritis Rheumatol 2016;68(3):679–89.
50. Kenna TJ, Davidson SI, Duan R, et al. Enrichment of circulating interleukin-17-secreting interleukin-23 receptor-positive γ/δ T cells in patients with active ankylosing spondylitis. Arthritis Rheum 2012;64(5):1420–9.
51. Venken K, Jacques P, Mortier C, et al. RORγt inhibition selectively targets IL-17 producing iNKT and $\gamma\delta$-T cells enriched in Spondyloarthritis patients. Nat Commun 2019;10(1):9.
52. Soare A, Weber S, Maul L, et al. Cutting edge: homeostasis of innate lymphoid cells is imbalanced in psoriatic arthritis. J Immunol 2018;200(4):1249–54.
53. Yao Y, Liu R, Shin MS, et al. CyTOF supports efficient detection of immune cell subsets from small samples. J Immunol Methods 2014;415:1–5.
54. Qaiyum Z, Gracey E, Yao Y, et al. Integrin and transcriptomic profiles identify a distinctive synovial CD8+ T cell subpopulation in spondyloarthritis. Ann Rheum Dis 2019;78(11):1566–75.
55. Papalexi E, Satija R. Single-cell RNA sequencing to explore immune cell heterogeneity. Nat Rev Immunol 2018;18(1):35–45.
56. Arazi A, Rao DA, Berthier CC, et al. The immune cell landscape in kidneys of patients with lupus nephritis. Nat Immunol 2019;20(7):902–14.
57. Lloyd-Price J, Arze C, Ananthakrishnan AN, et al. Multi-omics of the gut microbial ecosystem in inflammatory bowel diseases. Nature 2019;569(7758):655–62.
58. Gill T, Brooks SR, Rosenbaum JT, et al. Novel inter-omic analysis reveals relationships between diverse gut microbiota and host immune dysregulation in HLA-B27-induced experimental spondyloarthritis. Arthritis Rheumatol 2019;71(11): 1849–57.

Intestinal Microbiota, HLA-B27, and Spondyloarthritis
Dangerous Liaisons

Emilie Dumas, PhD[a,b,1], Koen Venken, PhD[a,b,1],
James T. Rosenbaum, MD[c,d], Dirk Elewaut, MD, PhD[a,b,*]

KEYWORDS

- Spondyloarthritis • HLA-B27 • Microbiota • Innate mucosal immunity

KEY POINTS

- Spondyloarthritis (SpA) is a rheumatic disease commonly associated with extra-articular features, such as gut inflammation.
- Gut microbial changes have been detected in patients with SpA.
- Alterations in mucosal immunity potentially driven by HLA-B27 and microbiome interactions could potentially underly SpA disease development.

INTESTINAL MICROBIOTA IN SPONDYLOARTHRITIS: GOOD, BAD, AND UGLY

The human gut harbors a tremendously diverse microbial community that correlates with and even modulates many health-related processes. Disruption of this ecological equilibrium leads to dysbiosis, which is involved in a growing list of diseases, particularly inflammatory and autoimmune disease. Intriguingly, spondyloarthritis (SpA) patients frequently develop extra-articular manifestations, such as acute anterior uveitis, psoriasis, and inflammatory bowel disease (IBD). Moreover, microscopic signs of intestinal inflammation were observed in 50% of patients with SpA without gastrointestinal symptoms,[1] from which a fraction develops Crohn disease (CD) over time.[1,2] The presence of microscopic gut inflammation has been linked to early onset disease, high disease activity, and degree of bone marrow edema in sacroiliac joints.[3,4] Conversely, patients with

[a] Faculty of Medicine and Health Sciences, Department of Internal Medicine and Pediatrics (Rheumatology Unit), Ghent University, Corneel Heymanslaan 10, Gent 9000, Belgium; [b] Molecular Immunology and Inflammation Unit, VIB Center for Inflammatory Research, Ghent, Belgium; [c] Oregon Health & Science University, Portland, OR, USA; [d] Legacy Devers Eye Institute, Portland, OR, USA
[1] Joint first author.
* Corresponding author. Faculty of Medicine and Health Sciences, Department of Internal Medicine and Pediatrics (Rheumatology Unit), Ghent University, Corneel Heymanslaan 10, Gent 9000, Belgium.
E-mail address: dirk.elewaut@ugent.be

Rheum Dis Clin N Am 46 (2020) 217–228
https://doi.org/10.1016/j.rdc.2020.01.007
0889-857X/20/© 2020 Elsevier Inc. All rights reserved.

IBD commonly develop joint inflammation with features of SpA.[5] Thus, there is an unclear relationship between joint and gut inflammation in SpA disease.

Experiments done on animal models of SpA provide compelling evidence for the involvement of indigenous microbiota in the disease. Rats transgenic for HLA-B27, a well-known risk factor for SpA (discussed later), develop SpA-like disease when exposed to specific pathogen-free enteric bacteria but not when raised under germ-free conditions.[6] A gut microbiota dysbiosis has been reported in HLA-B27 rats with notably an increase of *Akkermansia muciniphila* and *Bacteroides vulgatus*.[7,8] Both of these bacteria have mucolytic activity, which facilitates the access and the invasion of the gut epithelium by other microorganisms that may contribute to distant joint inflammation. Similarly, in the ankylosing enthesopathy model, mice do not develop joint disease in germ-free conditions.[9] Under conventional microbial conditions, SKG mice spontaneously develop chronic autoimmune arthritis. In contrast, under specific pathogen-free conditions, only the injection of curdlan (a major component of bacterial and yeast cell walls) can provoke severe arthritis, ileitis resembling CD, and unilateral uveitis.[10,11]

Gut dysbiosis has been demonstrated in several SpA subtypes (**Table 1**). It is challenging to compare and identify a simple, common dysbiosis detected in SpA studies. Several factors can explain these differences: the technology used to access the microbiome diversity, the level of taxonomic identification, the functional complementation and redundancy (proteins from different bacteria can achieve the same functions), patient characteristics (eg, diet, geography, medications, disease duration, or genotype), and the nature of the samples analyzed (feces or biopsies). In studies analyzing fecal samples, the microbial diversity observed was reduced in patients with SpA compared with healthy control subjects (see **Table 1**). Two studies analyzed (ileal/colonic) biopsies as starting material. Intriguingly, in both studies, a higher microbial diversity was observed in patients with SpA. Of note (functional) dysbiosis in the gut microbiome of patients with IBD has also been extensively reported (see **Table 1**; for extended details we refer to recent reviews[12,13]).

Two bacterial genus/species have been proposed as a marker of disease activity in axial SpA. Breban and colleagues[14] evidenced an increase of the species *Ruminococcus gnavus* abundance in patient feces compared with healthy control subjects. This species is also positively correlated with disease activity in patients having a history of IBD. *R gnavus* display a mucolytic activity, and this ability may contribute to trigger or maintain inflammation. Tito and colleagues[15] evidenced a strong association between the intestinal inflammation status and the mucosal microbiota profile of patients with SpA. Furthermore, the authors highlighted a positive correlation between the abundance of the bacterial genus *Dialister* with the Ankylosing Spondylitis Disease Activity Score. Manasson and colleagues[16] reported that *Dialister* bacteria was independently enriched in reactive arthritis patients with sacroiliitis and those with uveitis. Wen and colleagues,[17] also demonstrated dysbiosis between axial SpA and healthy control subjects analyzing shotgun sequencing data from feces. The authors reported an increase of abundance of the bacterial class Actinobacteria in ankylosing spondylitis compared with healthy control subjects. Actinobacteria are able to modify proteins by ubiquitination, targeting the proteins for degradation by proteasomes.[18] The authors proposed that Actinobacteria may activate the nuclear factor-κB pathway via the ubiquitination of the inhibitor molecule IκB inducing the accumulation of inflammatory factors in patients with ankylosing spondylitis.

Despite the identification of promising candidates and linking gut to joint inflammation, no single organism has been identified as inducing SpA or IBD. In both diseases, it is still not known if the gut microbiota is involved in the initiation of the disease or is a

Table 1
Overview of microbiome studies in patients with SpA

Reference	Disease	Technology	Sample	Number of Participants	Alpha-Diversity Compared with Healthy Control Subjects	Increased Compared with Healthy Control Subjects	Decreased Compared with Healthy Control Subjects	Interaction with Disease Parameter
Scher et al,[55] 2015	Psoriatic arthritis	16S rRNA amplicon seq	Feces	16 (+17 control subjects)	Decreased diversity		p_Verrucomicrobia, c_Verrucomicrobiae, c_Clostridia, o_Verrucomicrobiales, g_Pseudobutyrivibrio, g_Akkermansia, g_Ruminococcus	
Manasson et al,[16] 2018	Reactive arthritis	16S rRNA amplicon seq	Feces	30 (+32 control subjects)	No significant difference	g_Ewinia, g_Pseudomonas		Bacteria candidate (unranked) TM7, p_Firmicutes, c_Clostridia, c_Fusobacteria, o_Fusobacteriales, g_Dialister, g_Erwinia, g_Campylobacter
Breban et al,[14] 2017	SpA	16S rRNA amplicon seq	Feces	49 (+18 control subjects) + validation: 38 (+51 control subjects)	Decreased diversity	f_Coriobacteriaceaea, g_Coprococcus, g_Ruminococcus, s_Bifidobacterium longum, s_Blautia pruducta, s_Ruminococcus gnavus		s_Ruminococcus gnavus

(continued on next page)

Table 1
(continued)

Reference	Disease	Technology	Sample	Number of Participants	Alpha-Diversity Compared with Healthy Control Subjects	Increased Compared with Healthy Control Subjects	Decreased Compared with Healthy Control Subjects	Interaction with Disease Parameter
Tito et al,[15] 2017	Axial SpA	16S rRNA amplicon seq	Ileal and colonic biopsies	27 (+15 control subjects)	Trend to increased diversity (specially for patients with acute gut inflammation)			g_Dialister
Costello et al,[56] 2015	AS	16S rRNA amplicon seq	Ileal biopsies	9 (+9 control subjects)	Increased diversity	f_Bocteroidaceae[a], f_Rikenelloceae[a], f_Lachnospiraceae[a], f_Ruminococcaceae[a], f_Porphyromonadaceae[a]	f_Actinomycetaceae[a], f_Gemellaceae[a], f_Streptoccoceae[a], f_Veillonellaceae[a], f_Prevotellaceae[a]	
Stoll et al,[57] 2018	SpA (mainly AS)	16S rRNA amplicon seq	Feces	11 (+10 control subjects)	ND		s_Faecalibacterium prausnitzii A2-165	
Wen et al,[17] 2017	AS	Shotgun seq	Feces	73 (+83 control subjects) + validation: 24 (+31 control subjects)	Decreased diversity	g_Collinsella, g_Neisseria, g_Bifidobacterium, g_Rothia, g_Actinomyces	g_Entrobacter, g_Citrobacter, g_Fusobacterium, s_Prevotella meloninogenica, s_Prevotella copri, s_Prevotella sp C561	

Halfvarson et al,[58] 2017	IBD	16S rRNA amplicon seq	Feces	109 (+9 control subjects)	o_Alteromonadales, s_Alistipes massiliensis	f_Ruminococcaceae, f_Lactospiraceae, g_Coprococcus, g_Ruminococcus, g_Methano-brevibacter, s_Faecalibacterium prausnitzii, s_Prevotella copri
Lloyd-Price et al,[59] 2019	IBD	16S rRNA amplicon seq + Shotgun seq	Feces + ileal and rectal biopsies	105 (+27 control subjects)	s_Prevotella copri, s_Bacteroides fragilis, s_Escherichia coli, s_Klebsiella pneumonia[b]	s_Faecalibacterium prausnitzii, s_Bacteroides uniformis, s_Eubacterium rectale, s_Alistipes putredinis[b]

Taxonomic abbreviations: phylum (p), class (c), order (o), family (f), genus (g), species (s).
Abbreviations: AS, ankylosing spondylitis; ND, not determined.
[a] No multiple test correction (q-value).
[b] Here are only represented the 4 most dysbiotic species out of 87 in total.
Data from Refs.[14–17,55–59]

consequence of the disease development. Moreover, other microorganisms within the microbial communities may play a role in SpA disease, such as fungi, virus, or protist. Additionally, a specific combination of genetic, microbiota, and other environmental factors can be involved and contribute to the disease. Evidence indicates that gut dysbiosis-induced intestinal inflammation leads to a compromised intestinal barrier in patients with SpA.[19] This could lead to translocation of bacterial components, some of which may traffic to the joints causing local inflammation.[20] Alternatively, intestinal T cells and macrophages, primed by the dysbiotic microbiota, might travel to the joints where they induce inflammation in the synovium.[21]

These observations suggest that restoring immune homeostasis in the gut by modulating the microbiota is a promising therapeutic strategy for targeting remote sites of inflammation, such as articular joints in rheumatic disorders. One of the treatment options is the use of probiotics. A noncontrolled pilot study found a positive effect of supplementing a probiotic consisting of a mixture of *Lactobacillus acidophilus* and *Lactobacillus salivarius* to patients with SpA with quiescent ulcerative colitis.[22] In this study, significant reductions were noted in two disease activity indices: Bath Ankylosing Spondylitis Functional Index and Visual Analogue Scale scores. However, other studies failed to document significant beneficial effects of probiotics. As an alternative to probiotic treatment, the use of fecal microbiota transplants may be explored to restore the microbiota equilibrium. More research and clinical testing are needed to fully explore the use and efficacy of microbiome-tailored approaches in the treatment of SpA pathology.

INNATE(-LIKE) LYMPHOCYTE RESPONSES IN THE GUT: SENSORS OF INTESTINAL DYSBIOSIS IN SPONDYLOARTHRITIS?

The human gut mucosal immune system has largely evolved to maintain an essentially symbiotic relationship with a complex microbial community. Commensal microbiota plays a key role in the development and maturation of the host immune system, in this way indirectly leading to protection against the deleterious effect of pathogenic microorganisms.[23] The size of the intestinal immune system is substantial (about 70%–80% of all the immune cells are found in the gut wall) and a diverse and mostly unique composition of cell subsets are present even early in life as recently underscored by advanced high-dimensional cytometric analyses of human gut biopsies.[24,25]

The understanding of the innate immune responses involved in the protection of tissue homeostasis and the immune response to infection at mucosal surfaces has evolved over the last years, but many questions remain on the tight regulation of multiple cellular interactions. Although resident mononuclear phagocytes (mainly macrophages and dendritic cells) are key inducers of primary immune responses, a clear separation of adaptive and innate immunity in the intestinal milieu is more challenging to define because also highly differentiated lymphocytes seem to possess innate-like immune cell functions. An essential first layer of host defense against pathogens is the epithelial layer, in which absorptive enterocytes, mucus-producing goblet cells, enteroendocrine cells and Paneth cells (predominantly found in the small intestine), and particular T-cell subsets are present. The latter, the so-called intraepithelial lymphocytes, include cells from the T-cell receptor (TCR) $\alpha\beta+$ and TCR$\gamma\delta+$ lineages, comprise a considerable fraction of the total body's T cells, and play a key role in host (innate) immune responses (extensively reviewed in[26]). Scattered throughout the lamina propria or organized in tissue-specific lymphoid structures, such as Peyer patches, isolated lymphoid follicles, and cryptopatches, other innate(-like) intestinal lymphocytes are found.[27] These include TCR$\gamma\delta+$ T cells, more recently identified populations of innate lymphoid cells (ILC), invariant natural killer T cells (iNKT), and mucosal associated invariant T (MAIT) cells (reviewed in[28,29]).

ILCs form a rare population of (lineage negative) lymphoid cells lacking rearranged antigen-specific receptors, which are found in blood circulation but predominantly present in mucosal areas. ILCs include natural killer cells with cytotoxic properties and noncytotoxic "helper-like" ILCs, which express the interleukin-7 receptor (CD127).[30] The activity of ILCs is shaped by multiple tissue-specific signals, including nutrients, microbial factors, and cytokines and therefore they are important players in (gut) tissue homeostasis and inflammation.[30] iNKT and MAIT cells are classified as unconventional T cells (to which also subsets of $\gamma\delta$ and CD1a and CD1b restricted T cells belong) and both express a semi-invariant TCR and show antigen restriction toward nonpolymorphic MHC-like molecules (CD1d and MR1 respectively) by which they can respond to microbial-derived products. iNKT cells recognize bacterial-derived glycolipid molecules, whereas MAIT cells are activated by vitamin B_2 (riboflavin) metabolites, such as ribityllumazines and pyrimidines. Many vitamin biosynthetic pathways are unique to bacteria and yeast organisms, suggesting that MAIT cells recognize these ligands to detect microbial infections. iNKT and MAIT cells can also be activated independently of their TCR stimulation, mainly by cytokine-mediated signaling events.[31] Similar to the classic delineation of T-helper subsets, ILC, iNKT, and MAIT cells have been categorized into distinct subsets based on shared transcription factors and cytokine signatures including: ILC1/iNKT1/MAIT1 cells expressing the transcription factor T-bet and producing interferon-γ, ILC2/iNKT2 regulated by GATA3 and secreting interleukin (IL)-5 and IL-13, and finally ILC3/iNKT17/MAIT17 cells characterized by the key Th17-related transcription factor RORγt and IL-17 and IL-22 expression.[32–34] Of note, it is at the moment unclear whether a subpopulation of MAIT2 cells exists, but MAIT cells expressing high levels of IL-13 have been described recently.[35] This classification holds true to some extent (being also less clear for human-derived cells) because they show a general plasticity *in vivo* and the existence of discrete functional compartments within the known subsets have been reported.[35,36]

Strong evidence suggests that host-microbial interactions play a key role in the development and function of these lymphoid cells. From experiments with germ-free and antibiotic-treated mice, it is clear that ILC, iNKT, and MAIT cells experience maturation in the gut mucosal surfaces.[10,37,38] ILC diversity seems maintained on encounter with microbiota, by epigenetic mechanisms of ILC specification.[36,39] Furthermore, it was recently shown rather unexpectedly that commensal microbiota-derived metabolites can even control the development of thymic MAIT cells in mice, in a process where a MAIT ligand (5-OP-RU: 5-[2-oxopropylideneamino]-6-d-ribitylaminouracil) is able to travel from mucosal surfaces to the thymus, there being presented by MR1 expressing cells.[40] In this regard, one might speculate that gut dysbiosis as observed in patients with SpA could have significant immunologic effects potentially contributing to SpA pathology. This might be especially relevant in the context of an aberrant IL-23/IL-17 (type 3) immunity strongly associated with SpA disease.[31,41] Indeed, several studies have highlighted that MAIT, ILC, $\gamma\delta$, and iNKT cells, of which some express Rorγt, can act as major contributors to IL-17-mediated pathology in SpA joints.[42–45] Whether local gut interactions between these immune cells and microbiota might potentially contribute to SpA pathology warrants further investigation.[31]

HLA-B27 AND THE MICROBIOTA: THE NEW KID ON THE BLOCK?

It has been known for a long time that the MHC class I gene HLA-B27 is an important genetic risk factor for the development of SpA, still its exact contribution to the disease development remains enigmatic. Given the potential role for microbiota in the pathogenesis of SpA as described, it is plausible to hypothesize that HLA-B27 might affect the composition of the microbial community in susceptible patients. From a teleologic perspective, the major histocompatibility complex is easily the most polymorphic set of genes in the human species. Some have proposed that this diversity helps to reduce the chance that any single infectious agent would eliminate the human race. If so, it is logical to believe that HLA molecules would present bacterial antigens such that one's HLA type would impact the ecosystem that constitutes the gut microbiota. Experimental evidence supports this hypothesis. Using samples obtained during colonoscopy on healthy individuals, Asquith and colleagues[46] reported that the gut microbiome of HLA-B27-positive individuals differed from those with other HLA types. This study also supports the contention that the change in the microbiota is primary rather than secondary to a change in intestinal mucosa. The same study also demonstrated that HLA-DRB1, which predisposes to rheumatoid arthritis, likewise has an effect to shape the microbiota.[46] Other publications on sprue,[47] diabetes,[48] and CD[48] have also reported that HLA molecules affect the composition of the microbiota.

The simplest hypothesis to explain the mechanism of this effect of HLA is to cite its known function in antigen presentation. The diversity of HLA results in differential immunity to specific bacteria, which in turn skews the composition of the microbiota. A seminal study by Paun and colleagues[48] indicates that the antibody immune responses to specific commensal bacteria are impacted by one's HLA alleles. With regard to HLA-B27 specifically one might assume this is linked to particular changes in adaptive CD8 T-cell responses. Although this idea was abandoned for some time with the notion that CD8+ T cells are not essential for joint and gut disease manifestations in a B27 transgenic rat model,[49] several recent reports have resurrected the potential importance of CD8+ T cells in human SpA disease.[50–52] Studies directly linking B27-CD8+ T cells responses to alterations in intestinal microbiota are therefore of interest. It is possible that this is not the only mechanism by which HLA-B27 impacts the microbiota. For example, in HLA-B27 transgenic rats, antimicrobial peptides are increased in the gut before the onset of bowel or joint inflammation.[7] Because HLA-B27 tends to misfold,[53] some evidence indicates that it activates the unfolded protein response, which in turn could affect the synthesis of antimicrobial peptides and thus alter the microbiota. In addition, this could underlie alterations in type 3 responses observed in SpA,[54] affecting intestinal antimicrobial responses. In this regard, a further understanding of the mechanisms by which HLA-B27 alters gut microbiota could lead to strategies to suppress or even prevent SpA pathology.

CONCLUDING REMARKS

The precise relationship between intestinal changes and joint inflammation as observed in patients with SpA is still ill defined but it is clear from clinical and experimental data that underlying genetic predisposing factors (eg, HLA-B27) and/or environmental factors (microbiota) might play a key role herein. Future research approaches including in-depth (paired) microbial and immune cell profiling of gut tissue samples from patients with SpA and control individuals will shed further light on this matter. Moreover, this will lead to better knowledge regarding the presence of specialized immune subsets in the SpA gut mucosae and potentially their role in antimicrobial responses. Unraveling the underlying cellular and molecular pathways in SpA disease models will help to clarify the precise nature of the relationship among microbiota, mucosal, and HLA-B27-mediated immunity and their complex contribution to gut and joint pathology.

ACKNOWLEDGMENTS

E. Dumas is the holder of an individual Marie Skłodowska Curie Actions grant. K. Venken is supported by Fonds voor Wetenschappelijk Onderzoek Vlaanderen (FWO-VI) and Flanders Innovation & Entrepreneurship (VLAIO). D. Elewaut is supported by FWO-VI, Research Council of Ghent University, and interuniversity Attraction Pole grant Devrepair from Belspo Agency (project P7/07) and an FWO Excellence of Science Grant. J.T. Rosenbaum received support from NIH (grant RO EY029266) and the William and Mary Bauman Foundation, the Stan and Madelle Rosenfeld Family Trust, and the Grandmaison Fund for Autoimmunity Research.

DISCLOSURE

The authors have nothing to declare.

REFERENCES

1. Mielants H, Veys E, Cuvelier C, et al. The evolution of spondyloarthropathies in relation to gut histology. II. Histological aspects. J Rheumatol 1995;22(12): 2273–81.
2. De Vos M, Mielants H, Cuvelier C, et al. Long-term evolution of gut inflammation in patients with spondyloarthropathy. Gastroenterology 1996;110(6):1696–703.
3. Van Praet L, Van Den Bosch FE, Jacques P, et al. Microscopic gut inflammation in axial spondyloarthritis: a multiparametric predictive model. Ann Rheum Dis 2013; 72(3):414–7.
4. Van Praet L, Jans L, Carron P, et al. Degree of bone marrow oedema in sacroiliac joints of patients with axial spondyloarthritis is linked to gut inflammation and male sex: results from the GIANT cohort. Ann Rheum Dis 2014;73(6):1186–9.
5. Van Praet L, Jacques P, Van Den Bosch F, et al. The transition of acute to chronic bowel inflammation in spondyloarthritis. Nat Rev Rheumatol 2012;8(5):288–95.
6. Taurog JD, Richardson JA, Croft JT, et al. The germfree state prevents development of gut and joint inflammatory disease in HLA-B27 transgenic rats. J Exp Med 1994;180(6):2359–64.
7. Asquith MJ, Stauffer P, Davin S, et al. Perturbed mucosal immunity and dysbiosis accompany clinical disease in a rat model of spondyloarthritis. Arthritis Rheumatol 2016;68(9):2151–62.
8. Lin P, Bach M, Asquith M, et al. HLA-B27 and human β2-microglobulin affect the gut microbiota of transgenic rats. PLoS One 2014;9(8):e105684.
9. Řeháková Z, Čapková J, Štěpánková R, et al. Germ-free mice do not develop ankylosing enthesopathy, a spontaneous joint disease. Hum Immunol 2000; 61(6):555–8.
10. Sakaguchi N, Takahashi T, Hata H, et al. Altered thymic T-cell selection due to a mutation of the ZAP-70 gene causes autoimmune arthritis in mice. Nature 2003; 426(6965):454–60.
11. Yoshitomi H, Sakaguchi N, Kobayashi K, et al. A role for fungal β-glucans and their receptor Dectin-1 in the induction of autoimmune arthritis in genetically susceptible mice. J Exp Med 2005;201(6):949–60.
12. Zuo T, Ng SC. The gut microbiota in the pathogenesis and therapeutics of inflammatory bowel disease. Front Microbiol 2018;9:2247.
13. Basso PJ, Câmara NOS, Sales-Campos H. Microbial-based therapies in the treatment of inflammatory bowel disease: an overview of human studies. Front Pharmacol 2019;9:1571.

14. Breban M, Tap J, Leboime A, et al. Faecal microbiota study reveals specific dysbiosis in spondyloarthritis. Ann Rheum Dis 2017;76(9):1614–22.

15. Tito RY, Cypers H, Joossens M, et al. Brief report: *Dialister* as a microbial marker of disease activity in spondyloarthritis. Arthritis Rheumatol 2017;69(1):114–21.

16. Manasson J, Shen N, Garcia Ferrer HR, et al. Gut microbiota perturbations in reactive arthritis and postinfectious spondyloarthritis. Arthritis Rheumatol 2018; 70(2):242–54.

17. Wen C, Zheng Z, Shao T, et al. Quantitative metagenomics reveals unique gut microbiome biomarkers in ankylosing spondylitis. Genome Biol 2017;18(1):1–13.

18. Thaiss CA, Zmora N, Levy M, et al. The microbiome and innate immunity. Nature 2016;535(7610):65–74.

19. Ciccia F, Guggino G, Rizzo A, et al. Dysbiosis and zonulin upregulation alter gut epithelial and vascular barriers in patients with ankylosing spondylitis. Ann Rheum Dis 2017;76(6):1123–32.

20. Asquith M, Schleisman M, Davin S, et al. FRI0148 A study of microbial translocation in an animal model of spondyloarthritis. Ann Rheum Dis 2018;77:618, 1-618.

21. Wong MT, Ong DEH, Lim FSH, et al. A high-dimensional atlas of human T cell diversity reveals tissue-specific trafficking and cytokine signatures. Immunity 2016; 45(2):442–56.

22. Sanges M, Valente G, Rea M, et al. Probiotics in spondyloarthropathy associated with ulcerative colitis: a pilot study. Eur Rev Med Pharmacol Sci 2009;13(3): 233–4.

23. Lazar V, Ditu LM, Pircalabioru GG, et al. Aspects of gut microbiota and immune system interactions in infectious diseases, immunopathology, and cancer. Front Immunol 2018;9:1–18.

24. van Unen V, Li N, Molendijk I, et al. Mass cytometry of the human mucosal immune system identifies tissue- and disease-associated immune subsets. Immunity 2016;44(5):1227–39.

25. Li N, van Unen V, Guo N, et al. Early-life compartmentalization of immune cells in human fetal tissues revealed by high-dimensional mass cytometry. Front Immunol 2019;10:1932.

26. Cheroutre H, Lambolez F, Mucida D. The light and dark sides of intestinal intraepithelial lymphocytes. Nat Rev Immunol 2012;11(7):445–56.

27. Eberl G, Lochner M. The development of intestinal lymphoid tissues at the interface of self and microbiota. Mucosal Immunol 2009;2(6):478–85.

28. Sonnenberg GF, Hepworth MR. Functional interactions between innate lymphoid cells and adaptive immunity. Nat Rev Immunol 2019;19(10):599–613.

29. Toubal A, Nel I, Lotersztajn S, et al. Mucosal-associated invariant T cells and disease. Nat Rev Immunol 2019;19(10):643–57.

30. Sonnenberg GF, Artis D. Innate lymphoid cells in the initiation, regulation and resolution of inflammation. Nat Med 2015;21:698.

31. Mortier C, Govindarajan S, Venken K, et al. It takes "guts" to cause joint inflammation: role of innate-like T cells. Front Immunol 2018;9:1489.

32. Diefenbach A, Colonna M, Koyasu S. Development, differentiation, and diversity of innate lymphoid cells. Immunity 2014;41(3):354–65.

33. Lee YJ, Holzapfel KL, Zhu J, et al. Steady-state production of IL-4 modulates immunity in mouse strains and is determined by lineage diversity of iNKT cells. Nat Immunol 2013;14:1146.

34. Lantz O, Legoux F. MAIT cells: programmed in the thymus to mediate immunity within tissues. Curr Opin Immunol 2019;58:75–82.

35. Koay HF, Gherardin NA, Xu C, et al. Diverse MR1-restricted T cells in mice and humans. Nat Commun 2019;10(1):1–15.
36. Gury-BenAri M, Thaiss CA, Serafini N, et al. The spectrum and regulatory landscape of intestinal innate lymphoid cells are shaped by the microbiome. Cell 2016;166(5):1231–46.e13.
37. Olszak T, An D, Zeissig S, et al. Microbial exposure during early life has persistent effects on natural killer T cell function. Science 2012;336(6080):489–93.
38. Wingender G, Stepniak D, Krebs P, et al. Intestinal microbes affect phenotypes and functions of invariant natural killer T cells in mice. Gastroenterology 2012; 143(2):418–28.
39. Minton K. ILC diversity maintained by microbiota. Nat Rev Immunol 2016;16:593.
40. Legoux F, Bellet D, Daviaud C, et al. Microbial metabolites control the thymic development of mucosal-associated invariant T cells. Science 2019;366(6464): 494–9.
41. Venken K, Elewaut D. New immune cells in spondyloarthritis: key players or innocent bystanders? Best Pract Res Clin Rheumatol 2015;29(6):706–14.
42. Gracey E, Qaiyum Z, Almaghlouth I, et al. IL-7 primes IL-17 in mucosal-associated invariant T (MAIT) cells, which contribute to the Th17-axis in ankylosing spondylitis. Ann Rheum Dis 2016;75(12):2124–32.
43. Ciccia F, Guggino G, Zeng M, et al. Proinflammatory CX3CR1+CD59+tumor necrosis factor–like molecule 1A+interleukin-23+ monocytes are expanded in patients with ankylosing spondylitis and modulate innate lymphoid cell 3 immune functions. Arthritis Rheumatol 2018;70(12):2003–13.
44. Venken K, Jacques P, Mortier C, et al. RORγt inhibition selectively targets IL-17 producing iNKT and γδ-T cells enriched in spondyloarthritis patients. Nat Commun 2019;10(1):9.
45. Al-Mossawi MH, Chen L, Fang H, et al. Unique transcriptome signatures and GM-CSF expression in lymphocytes from patients with spondyloarthritis. Nat Commun 2017;8(1):1510.
46. Asquith M, Sternes PR, Costello M, et al. HLA alleles associated with risk of ankylosing spondylitis and rheumatoid arthritis influence the gut microbiome. Arthritis Rheumatol 2019;71(10):1642–50.
47. Olivares M, Neef A, Castillejo G, et al. The HLA-DQ2 genotype selects for early intestinal microbiota composition in infants at high risk of developing coeliac disease. Gut 2015;64(3):406–17.
48. Paun A, Yau C, Meshkibaf S, et al. Association of HLA-dependent islet autoimmunity with systemic antibody responses to intestinal commensal bacteria in children. Sci Immunol 2019;4(32):eaau8125.
49. May E, Dorris ML, Satumtira N, et al. CD8αβ T cells are not essential to the pathogenesis of arthritis or colitis in HLA-B27 transgenic rats. J Immunol 2003;170(2): 1099–105.
50. Qaiyum Z, Gracey E, Yao Y, et al. Integrin and transcriptomic profiles identify a distinctive synovial CD8+ T cell subpopulation in spondyloarthritis. Ann Rheum Dis 2019;78(11):1566–75.
51. Zheng M, Zhang X, Zhou Y, et al. TCR repertoire and CDR3 motif analyses depict the role of αβ T cells in ankylosing spondylitis. EBioMedicine 2019;47:414–26.
52. Faham M, Carlton V, Moorhead M, et al. Discovery of T cell receptor β motifs specific to HLA–B27–positive ankylosing spondylitis by deep repertoire sequence analysis. Arthritis Rheumatol 2017;69(4):774–84.
53. Colbert RA, Tran TM, Layh-Schmitt G. HLA-B27 misfolding and ankylosing spondylitis. Mol Immunol 2014;57(1):44–51.

54. Venken K, Elewaut D. IL-23 responsive innate-like T cells in spondyloarthritis: the less frequent they are, the more vital they appear. Curr Rheumatol Rep 2015; 17(5):30.
55. Scher JU, Ubeda C, Artacho A, et al. Decreased bacterial diversity characterizes the altered gut microbiota in patients with psoriatic arthritis, resembling dysbiosis in inflammatory bowel disease. Arthritis Rheumatol 2015;67(1):128–39.
56. Costello ME, Ciccia F, Willner D, et al. Brief report: intestinal dysbiosis in ankylosing spondylitis. Arthritis Rheumatol 2015;67(3):686–91.
57. Stoll ML, Weiss PF, Weiss JE, et al. Age and fecal microbial strain-specific differences in patients with spondyloarthritis. Arthritis Res Ther 2018;20(1):14.
58. Halfvarson J, Brislawn CJ, Lamendella R, et al. Dynamics of the human gut microbiome in inflammatory bowel disease. Nat Microbiol 2017;2:17004.
59. Lloyd-Price J1, Arze C, Ananthakrishnan AN, et al. Multi-omics of the gut microbial ecosystem in inflammatory bowel diseases. Nature 2019;569(7758):655–62.

What Does Human Leukocyte Antigen B27 Have to Do with Spondyloarthritis?

Hanna Fahed, MD[a], Daniele Mauro, MD, PhD[b],
Francesco Ciccia, MD, PhD[b], Nelly R. Ziade, MD, MPH, PhD, FRCP[a],*

KEYWORDS

- HLA-B27 • Spondyloarthritis • Diagnosis • Prognosis • Genetics
- Disease phenotype

KEY POINTS

- Human leukocyte antigen (HLA) B27 plays a central role in axial spondyloarthritis (axSpA) diagnosis and constitutes a significant part of previous and current classification criteria.
- HLA-B27 plays a role in the physiopathology of axSpA, although the exact mechanism is not yet fully elucidated.
- HLA-B27 is correlated with spondyloarthritis phenotype, with a consistent positive association with family history, early disease onset, shorter diagnostic delay, and acute anterior uveitis, and a controversial association with disease activity.
- HLA-B27 does not seem to be a poor prognostic factor for radiographic progression and response to treatment.

INTRODUCTION

Spondyloarthritis (SpA) is a common disease, potentially disabling, with a serious socioeconomic burden.[1,2] However, despite this significant impact, particularly in young adults, a substantial diagnostic delay is observed, mostly caused by the ubiquitous and nonspecific primary manifestation of the disease (ie, low back pain), and by the scarcity of diagnostic laboratory markers.[3–5]

Since its first report in 1973,[6,7] human leukocyte antigen (HLA) B27 has been considered the key laboratory parameter for axial SpA (axSpA) and has been used as a supplemental diagnostic test in patients with suspicion of axSpA. Among the typical manifestations of axSpA, HLA-B27 has a sensitivity of 83% to 96% and a

[a] Department of Rheumatology, Saint-Joseph University, Hôtel-Dieu de France Hospital, BP 166830, Achrafieh, Beirut, Lebanon; [b] Division of Rheumatology, Department of Precision Medicine, University of Campania "Luigi Vanvitelli", Via Sergio Pansini 5, Napoli 80131, Italy
* Corresponding author. Tour des Consultations Externes, Hôtel-Dieu de France Hospital, 6th floor, Alfred Naccache Avenue, Achrafieh, Beirut, Lebanon.
E-mail addresses: nelly.zoghbi@usj.edu.lb; nellziade@yahoo.fr

Rheum Dis Clin N Am 46 (2020) 229–243
https://doi.org/10.1016/j.rdc.2020.01.002
0889-857X/20/© 2020 Elsevier Inc. All rights reserved.

specificity of 90% to 95% in European white populations with chronic low back pain and an age of onset of less than 45 years.[8]

Its diagnostic importance is reflected by its inclusion in several classification criteria. It is a double-weighted criterion in the 1990 Amor criteria for spondyloarthropathy,[9] and one of 2 major entry criteria in the 2009 Assessment of Spondyloarthritis International Society (ASAS) classification criteria for axSpA, allowing the classification through a clinical arm, even in the absence of radiological manifestations.[8]

In the latter classification criteria, sensitivity and specificity for axSpA were 56.6% and 83.3% respectively, slightly lower than the imaging arm (66.2% and 97.3% respectively). HLA-B27 positivity had a high likelihood ratio of 9, similar to sacroiliitis on MRI.

However, these properties may not be applicable in other populations who have a different HLA-B27 background prevalence than the European white population, in which the ASAS classification criteria were validated.

This article discusses the epidemiologic distribution of HLA-B27, the methods of testing, the relationship with SpA epidemiology, physiopathology, disease phenotype, and prognosis, as well as its role in referral strategies.

WHAT IS THE EPIDEMIOLOGIC DISTRIBUTION OF HUMAN LEUKOCYTE ANTIGEN B27 AROUND THE GLOBE?

Large differences in HLA-B27 prevalence have been described across different geographic areas and ethnicities.[10] In general, the incidence and prevalence of axSpA mirror the frequency of HLA-B27 in the population[11] (**Table 1**).

Axial Spondyloarthritis Prevalence in the Population

Low rates of axSpA have been described in southern Africa, Japan, and Arab countries, compared with higher rates in Europe and very high rates among the native people of circumpolar arctic and subarctic regions of Eurasia and North America. Among Europeans, higher rates of ankylosing spondylitis (AS) were reported in Norway compared with other European countries.[11,12]

Table 1
Human leukocyte antigen B27 and axial spondyloarthritis mirroring prevalence across different populations

	axSpA Prevalence in the General Population (%)	HLA-B27 Prevalence in the General Population (%)	HLA-B27 Prevalence in the axSpA Patients (%)
Africa	0.07	2–9	—
Arab countries	0.30	0.3–6.8	41–84
Asia	0.17–0.18	—	—
Eskimos	0.40–2	25–50	—
Haida Indians	6.10	50	—
Latin America	0.10–0.12	—	—
North America	0.32–0.5	6–8	80–95
Western Europe (Norway)	0.20–0.90 1.10–1.40	8–9 14	75–95

Data from Refs.[2,10,12–20]

Human Leukocyte Antigen B27 Prevalence in the Population

In parallel, in the general population, lower rates of HLA-B27 were reported in Japanese and most Arab populations (0.3%–6.8%) compared with Western European and North American populations (6% to 25%), possibly caused by different genetic backgrounds.[12,13,21,22] The highest rates of HLA-B27 were reported in the population of Papua New Guinea (13%–53%)[23] and Eskimos (25%–50%).[24] In the United States, the prevalence of HLA-B27 in the population was higher in non-Hispanic white Americans (7.5%) compared with other US races/ethnicities combined (3.5%), according to the 2009 US National Health and Nutrition Examination Survey (NHANES) cross-sectional survey.[21]

Human Leukocyte Antigen B27 Prevalence in Patients with Axial Spondyloarthritis

In patients with axSpA, higher rates of HLA-B27 were found in North America and Western Europe (80%–95%)[10] compared with lower rates in Japan and Arab countries (41%–84%).[12,25]

However, despite the lower background prevalence in these populations, HLA-B27 is characterized by high specificity and a high positive Likelihood Ratio, with a significant strength of association, similar to European and North American studies. These properties make this test highly valuable for axSpA diagnosis, particularly when found positive, but may affect its value in primary screening and referral strategies (see **Table 1**).

HOW IS HUMAN LEUKOCYTE ANTIGEN B27 TESTED?

The strong genetic association between HLA-B27 positivity and SpA after its discovery in 1973 and the role of HLA-B27 testing in the diagnostic work-up of SpA generated a growing increase in the demand for testing worldwide.[6,7] It has been suggested that some of the change of the HLA-B27 prevalence with time may be related to changes in testing methods.

In 1964, Terasaki and McClelland[26] established a complement-dependent cytotoxicity (CDC) test for HLA. Patient lymphocytes are exposed to a panel of sera containing characterized HLA-specific antibodies obtained from multiparous women immunized against HLA-B present on the cells of the fetus. The addition of rabbit serum was used as a source of complement, and the binding of alloantibodies to the HLA triggers complement-dependent cell death detected, at the time, by ethidium bromide positivity and microscopic evaluation.[26] One of the most critical limitations was the lack of specificity toward each HLA-B27 variant, among which only a limited set is associated with SpA.

At present, more than 160 subtypes of HLA-B27 have been identified. These subtypes are distributed according to race and ethnicity and may be associated differently with axSpA.

The most common disease-associated subtypes are B*2702 (Mediterranean population), B*2705 (white people and American Indians), and B*2704 (Asians). Most of the subtypes are disease associated, which makes identifying them in individuals of little utility. However, some subtypes are not associated with disease, such as HLA-B27*09 in Sardinia and HLA-B27*06 in Southeast Asia.[20,27,28]

The CDC test for HLA requires viable cells and poses the risk of false-negative results when the antigen is downregulated or masked. In addition, the assay is extremely sensitive to sample storage conditions and timing.

The development of specific monoclonal antibodies toward HLA-B27 and the increased accessibility of molecular biology techniques allowed the diffusion of flow cytometry and polymerase chain reaction (PCR) in place of the CDC-based assay.

Monoclonal antibodies targeting HLA-B27 (ie, clones ABC-m3, GS145.2, and FD705) conjugated with fluorochromes (fluorescein isothiocyanate) are used to detect the expression of HLA-B27 on T lymphocytes identified by cluster of differentiation 3 (CD3) positivity (phycoerythrin), commonly comparing the mean fluorescent intensity with positive and negative reference microspheres.[29] This approach is widely used worldwide because it is fast and inexpensive and grants acceptable performance in the hands of experienced professionals.[29–31] However, similarly to other immunoassays, flow cytometry is not suitable for the distinction between the HLA-B27 variants and the downregulation of HLA-B27 or the masking by autoantibodies can lead to false-negative results. Note that HLA-B27 belongs to the large cross-reacting group (CREG); thus, the currently used clones can cross react with other CREG members, mainly B7 and B37, leading to false-positivity.[32]

PCR-based genetic testing is a valuable alternative to immunoassays. The HLA-B gene is amplified, and the PCR product is hybridized with multiple sequence-specific oligonucleotides, allowing the detection of the HLA-B27 and providing information on the HLA-B27 variants discriminating the associated SpA.[33] Alternatively, the PCR product can undergo Sanger sequencing, providing the HLA-B sequence at a single-base-pair resolution. More recently, a faster single-step method has been developed involving a specific set of directly conjugated probes for real-time PCR (TaqMan assay).[34]

Overall, the specificity and the resolution of DNA-based assay could replace or at least integrate the flow cytometry data for research purposes or in case of ambiguous results.

DOES HUMAN LEUKOCYTE ANTIGEN B27 HAVE A PHYSIOPATHOLOGIC ROLE AS WELL?

The strong association between axSpA and the positivity for HLA-B27 led to speculation about a causative effect of HLA-B27 risk variants in the pathogenesis of the disease. A definitive explanation of the mechanisms behind this association is still lacking, and a detailed systematic review of the molecular mechanisms by which HLA-B27 could increase the susceptibility to AS goes beyond the scope of this article. However, the mechanisms postulated can be summarized in 3 theories, perhaps not mutually exclusive:

- The main highly polymorphic sites associated with SpA are responsible for determining the amino acidic residue in positions 67 and 97 of the HLA-B that takes part in the formation of the peptide-binding domain, involved in both antigen presentation and protein folding.[35,36] The arthritogenic peptide theory postulates a response toward peptides expressed in axSpA joints and other sites of the disease. The HLA-B27 could mediate the presentation of peptides, possibly of microbial origin to cytotoxic CD8+ T cells mounting, because of molecular mimicry, an autoimmune response triggering AS manifestation including spondylitis and arthritis.[37] This theory was partially supported by the detection of CD8+ T cells reactive toward *Chlamydia* in the joints of patients with reactive arthritis.[38] However, many groups failed to identify an arthritogenic peptide in AS and animal models showed that CD8+ T cells are dispensable for the manifestation of the disease.
  [39]The natural function of HLA-B27 in presenting foreign antigens is consistent

with the suggested role for the microbiota in the development or perpetuation of the disease. Different lines of research showed subclinical gut inflammation in patients affected by AS and quantitative and qualitative perturbations of the gut microbiota.[40] Interestingly, the variation in the gut microbial content has been associated with the AS disease activity and is influenced by anti–tumor necrosis factor (TNF) therapy.[41,42] In keeping with the arthritogenic peptide theory, the altered gut microbiome could be a source of multiple autoantigens.[43]

- Typically, the HLA-B27 complex consists of heavy chains forming heterodimers with the with b2-microglobulin (b2m) and, as stated earlier, the complex binds and presents peptides to cytotoxic T cells. The homodimerization theory developed after the observation that the HLA-B27 chains can form homodimers via disulfide bonds through its unpaired cysteine at position 67 without the b2m ($B27_2$).[44] Once at the cell surface, $B27_2$ can be recognized by killer immunoglobulin–like receptors expressed on natural killer cells and CD4+ T cells, possibly triggering the activation and polarization toward a T-helper 17 phenotype.[45] How this process could affect only the target organs such as the joints is still not explained.

- The unfolded protein response (UPR) theory hypothesized that because the HLA-B27 is more prone to misfolding during its assembly in the endoplasmic reticulum (ER), it can form aberrant protein complexes that activate the UPR in the ER.[46] The UPR is known to be associated with a proinflammatory phenotype, leading to the production of inflammatory cytokines, including TNF and interleukin-23. However, the evidence of the increased activation of UPR in AS is so far conflicting.[47]

More recently, nonimmunologic functions of HLA-B27 have been suggested. MRI has shown a link between HLA-B27 positivity and pathologic response to biomechanical stress.[48] However, the cellular mechanisms linking the HLA-B27 to stress-induced inflammation and ossification remain elusive.[49]

DOES HUMAN LEUKOCYTE ANTIGEN B27 INFLUENCE SPONDYLOARTHRITIS PHENOTYPE?

Although the physiopathologic theories are still debated, several studies have established that HLA-B27 positivity can influence the patient clinical phenotype (**Fig. 1**).

Family History

It has long been established that a family history of SpA is common in patients with axSpA. Also, HLA-B27–positive first-degree relatives of HLA-B27–positive patients with axSpA are 16 times more likely to develop axSpA than HLA-B27–positive individuals in the general population.[14,50] In 2 European cohorts of patients with chronic back pain suspected of axSpA, a positive family history (PFH) for axSpA and acute anterior uveitis (AAU) was associated with positive HLA-B27, unlike the PFH for reactive arthritis, inflammatory bowel disease (IBD), or psoriasis.[51] In line with those findings, an analysis of the ASAS cohort, which includes more variable ethnicities, showed that a PFH of axSpA was strongly associated with positive HLA-B27 in both white and Asian patients and in both first-degree and second-degree relatives, but this association was stronger with white ethnicity and with a PFH in first-degree relatives.[52]

A study of Finnish patients with axSpA found higher relative risk of developing axSpA in HLA-B27 homozygotes, with those showing, surprisingly, a less severe disease course.[53] However, 1 Dutch and 1 Korean study found no significant difference between homozygous and heterozygous patients.[14,54]

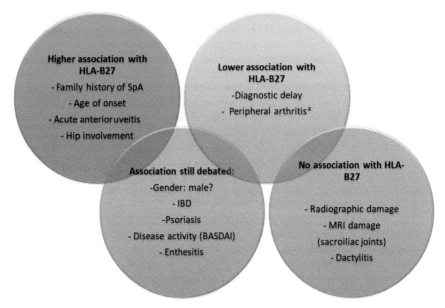

Fig. 1. Classification of axSpA parameters based on their association with HLA-B27. [a] Association between HLA-B27 and peripheral SpA is significant, but it is lower than the association with axSpA. BASDAI, Bath Ankylosing Spondylitis Disease Activity Index; IBD, inflammatory bowel disease.

Moreover, in HLA-B27–positive first-degree relatives of patients with axSpA, the risk of developing axSpA is 12%, whereas the risk in HLA-B27–negative relatives is very low ($\leq$1%).[55]

Age of Onset

Several studies have reported that HLA-B27 was associated with earlier onset of disease,[3,56,57] a finding that was confirmed in the more recent DEvenir des Spondylarthropathies Indifférenciées Récentes cohort.[58] This association is an interesting feature of axSpA, because it may play a predictive role in evaluating the disease evolution and prognosis.

Diagnostic Delay

In early axSpA cohort studies, HLA-B27 positivity was associated with shorter delay to diagnosis.[3,58] Therefore, its presence, as an objective marker, may prompt earlier diagnosis.

Gender

Several studies showed a higher male prevalence in HLA-B27–positive patients with axSpA, but the data are conflicting on this point.[59–62]

Disease Activity

HLA-B27–positive patients with axSpA showed no higher clinical burden of the disease. On the contrary, 1 study found significantly higher Bath Ankylosing Spondylitis Disease Activity Index (BASDAI) and Bath Ankylosing Spondylitis Functional Index

(BASFI) scores in HLA-B27–negative patients, even without differences in biological parameters (erythrocyte sedimentation rate and C-reactive protein [CRP]).[53]

Other cohort studies reported similar BASDAI and BASFI scores in HLA-B27–positive and HLA-B27–negative patients,[53,54,63] except for the DESIR cohort, which found slightly worse BASDAI, BASFI, and Bath Ankylosing Spondylitis Metrology Index scores in the HLA-B27–negative population.[58] Findings of a positive correlation with high CRP level were not confirmed.[64,65]

Joint Topography Pattern

Hip arthritis was more frequently reported in HLA-B27–positive patients with AS in most of the studies.[54,60,63]

Association with peripheral disease pattern is less than for axial SpA.[56,58,61] In cohorts with psoriatic arthritis, HLA-B27 was positive in only 29.3% of patients.[65]

From 30% to 80% of patients with reactive arthritis and 20% to 35% of patients with psoriatic arthritis were HLA-B27 positive.[66,67]

Regarding enthesitis, few studies showed their significantly higher prevalence among patients with AS with positive HLA-B27,[58,68] but this pattern was not observed in other studies.[54,60,63]

For dactylitis, no significant differences were noted between HLA-B27–positive and HLA-B27–negative patients with AS in the few studies mentioning it.

Extra-Articular Manifestations

Acute anterior uveitis

AAU prevalence in HLA-B27–positive individuals is estimated at around 1%. This risk is 2.6 to 4.2 times higher in HLA-B27–positive patients with SpA.[69,70] In contrast, the prevalence of HLA-B27 in patients presenting with AAU is around 50%. Moreover, in HLA-B27–positive patients with axSpA, the prevalence of AAU increases to 40%, whereas it is between 26% and 30% in general axSpA studies.[71] Also, Juanola and colleagues[72] recently found that SpA existed in 41% of patients presenting with more than 1 episode of AAU separated by at least 3 months.

Taken from the AAU angle, in patients with AAU who are HLA-B27 positive, the risk of developing SpA is between 35% and 66%, in contrast with HLA-B27-negative patients with AAU, in whom it is between 3.8% and 6%.[73]

Even HLA-B27–positive AAU seems to have a unique clinical presentation: unilateral; sudden in onset; and symptomatic, with blurred vision, photophobia, ocular redness, and pain. On examination it presents a significant anterior segment inflammation, often including hypopyon, posterior synechiae, and fibrin; it is typically nongranulomatous, episodic, and can alternate between eyes.[74]

Moreover, it has different characteristics than the negative one, independent of its association with axSpA: earlier onset (32–35 years), male preponderance (1.5:1–2.5:1), familial aggregation.[74,75]

Also, the incidence of ocular complications seems to be frequent in HLA-B27–associated uveitis: posterior synechiae and posterior subcapsular cataracts at presentation, ocular hypertension and posterior subcapsular cataract during follow-up, epiretinal membrane, cystoid macular edema, and band keratopathy more rarely.[76]

Whether the incidence of those complications and the visual outcomes differ between patients with HLA-B27–positive and HLA-B27–negative uveitis remains controversial, with some studies finding a higher rate of visual loss with HLA-B27–positive uveitis,[77] and others, including a large meta-analysis, showing no differences.[78]

Therefore, counseling about the risk of development of SpA should be undertaken in patients found to have HLA-B27–associated uveitis, because the ability to identify and treat HLA-B27–associated uveitis and concomitant SpA can limit the ocular and systemic morbidity.

Inflammatory bowel diseases
The gastrointestinal inflammation associated with axSpA ranges from microscopic (subclinical but found on ileocolonoscopic and histologic studies) to clinically overt IBD, with a prevalence, respectively, of 25% to 69% and 3% to 10%.[20] In contrast, stratifying patients by the level of gastrointestinal involvement, HLA-B27 positivity was observed in 35% to 95% of individuals with subclinical inflammation and in 27% to 78% of patients with a diagnosis of IBD.

However, no clear evidence has been found to prove that, in HLA-B27–positive patients with axSpA, the risk of developing IBD or subclinical IBD is higher.

In contrast, in patients with IBD, many data show that there is an increasing trend of HLA-B27 prevalence, ranging from 9.6% in inflammatory back pain (IBP), to 40% in radiographic sacroiliitis, to 73% in axSpA.[79] These data suggest that being HLA-B27 positive can be taken as a predisposing factor for sacroiliitis or axSpA in patients with IBD.[80]

However, some studies suggest a negative association with IBD, which deserves further investigation regarding the gene-environment interaction hypothesis.[67,81]

In addition, in patients with IBD, the presence of HLA-B27 is associated with a higher risk of developing extraintestinal disease manifestations, including sacroiliitis, spondylitis, peripheral arthritis, and enthesitis.[82]

Psoriasis
In a multivariate analysis of an early SpA cohort, psoriasis data showed a negative association with HLA-B27 (odds ratio, 0.59; 95% confidence interval, 0.39, 0.90; $P = .01$),[58] which suggests a 22% to 58% reduction in the odds of having psoriasis when HLA-B27 is positive in patients with axSpA.

However, a contradictory trend is found in some other studies, with an increasing prevalence of HLA-B27 in psoriasis, psoriatic arthritis (PsA), and axial PsA/psoriatic SpA at 5%, 20%,[66] and 23.4% to 34.5%,[83,84] respectively.

The recent review by Queiro and colleagues[66] also suggested that HLA-B27 is a genetic biomarker of joint disease in patients with psoriasis, and a marker for disease expression in PsA. It is also associated with a shorter interval between the development of skin eruptions and musculoskeletal symptoms; a higher risk of enthesitis, dactylitis, and uveitis; and a tendency toward peripheral and axial joint damage over time.[66,84–86]

A recent study also showed that, in patients with PsA, positive HLA-B27 was associated with more severe sonographic enthesitis, particularly in patients with longer disease duration.[87] However, there is an ongoing debate over the definition of psoriatic axial disease and axSpA with associated psoriasis.

Radiologic Signs
Despite a common perception that HLA-B27 is associated with disease severity in AS, its role in structural progression and disease severity has not been sufficiently proved.

The first study to compare clinical features of HLA-B27–positive versus HLA-B27–negative patients with AS was that of Khan and colleagues[88] in 1977, finding no significant differences.

In the setting of early IBP cohorts, an association with the persistence of MRI-identified inflammation at the sacroiliac joints (SIJs) and lumbar spine in early IBP was reported.[58,89] In this kind of setting, HLA-B27 represented a predictive value for axSpA in patients with IBP.

Association with Behçet Disease

Although major histocompatibility complex class I, especially HLA-B5/B51, is the most associated gene with Behçet disease (BD), HLA-B27 has also been studied.

A recent meta-analysis found that the risk of HLA-B27 positivity for BD progression is increased by a factor of 1.55, which is weak compared with the odds ratio of 5.78 in carriers of HLA-B5/B51.[90]

Paradoxically, uveitis occurring in BD is milder in patients with both the HLA-B5/B51 and HLA-B27 genes, probably because of less posterior segment involvement and complications, and a less chronic course of the disease.[91]

IS HUMAN LEUKOCYTE ANTIGEN B27 ASSOCIATED WITH SPONDYLOARTHRITIS PROGNOSIS?

Some recent data suggested that HLA-B27 is a marker associated with more severe axial bone-forming phenotypes of the SpA disease spectrum (AS and axial PsA/peripheral spondyloarthritis (psSpa)).[20]

These data are contradicted by other studies suggesting that HLA-B27 does not seem to be associated with radiographic progression.[92] Data from the DESIR cohort did not find an association between HLA-B27 and MRI structural lesions of the SIJ.[58]

Moreover, the prevalence of HLA-B27 does not seem to be different between AS and nonradiographic axSpA.[93]

Furthermore, in early axSpA, data from the DESIR cohort showed that HLA-B27 is associated with less delay in diagnosis, which may indirectly affect disease prognosis positively.[58] In contrast, the presence of the HLA-B27 antigen does not seem to be associated with response to biologic treatment.[94]

HOW DOES HUMAN LEUKOCYTE ANTIGEN B27 AFFECT REFERRAL STRATEGIES FROM THE PRIMARY CARE SETTING?

In the past couple of decades, referral strategies were developed for primary care settings, with the aim of reducing the diagnostic delay, thus ensuring adequate management in the early stage of the disease and improving disease prognosis. These strategies have a common clinical starting point: chronic and/or inflammatory chronic low back pain. In addition, HLA-B27 is considered a major criterion in most of these strategies, whether in the primary screening step or in the second line, after documenting clinical criteria.[95]

Globally, in a target population consisting of patients with chronic low back pain and onset before 45 years of age, referring a patient based on HLA-B27 positivity yields in axSpA diagnosis in one-third of the cases in European white populations. Adding HLA-B27 positivity to IBP increases the diagnosis of axSpA from 34% to 62%.[95]

HLA-B27 is an interesting screening parameter because it is easy to prescribe, clear to interpret (positive or negative), and has a moderate 1-time cost. However, its value depends largely on its prevalence in the general population and the strength of its association with SpA across geographic regions and ethnicities. However, most of the published strategy studies were conducted in European populations and their results cannot be extrapolated to other populations, particularly where HLA-B27 prevalence is lower.

SUMMARY

HLA-B27 plays a central role in axSpA diagnosis and constitutes a significant part of previous and current classification criteria.

It has a certain role in the physiopathology of axSpA, although the exact mechanism is not yet fully elucidated. HLA-B27 is correlated with SpA phenotype, with a consistent positive association with family history, early disease onset, shorter diagnostic delay, and AAU. However, it does not seem to be associated with either higher disease activity or with a poor prognostic factor for radiographic progression and response to treatment.

Because of its strong association with axSpA, HLA-B27 can be a pivotal parameter in referral strategies. However, in countries with lower background HLA-B27 prevalence, these strategies should be studied further, and data for other sensitive and specific markers in populations with low prevalence are needed.

DISCLOSURE

The authors have nothing to disclose.

REFERENCES

1. Boonen A, van der Linden SM. The burden of ankylosing spondylitis LIFE. J Rheumatol 2006;33:4–11.
2. Dean LE, Jones GI, Macdonald AG, et al. Global prevalence of ankylosing spondylitis. Rheumatol (United Kingdom) 2014;53(4):650–7.
3. Feldtkeller E, Khan MA, van der Heijde D, et al. Age at disease onset and diagnosis delay in HLA-B27 negative vs. positive patients with ankylosing spondylitis. Rheumatol Int 2003;23(2):61–6.
4. Hoy D, March L, Brooks P. The global burden of low back pain: estimates from the Global Burden of Disease 2010 study. Ann Rheum Dis 2014 Jun;73(6):968–74.
5. Jordan KP, Kadam UT, Hayward R, et al. Annual consultation prevalence of regional musculoskeletal problems in primary care: An observational study. BMC Musculoskelet Disord 2010;11. https://doi.org/10.1186/1471-2474-11-144.
6. Schlosstein L, Terasaki PI, Bluestone R, et al. High Association of an HL-A Antigen, W27, with Ankylosing Spondylitis. N Engl J Med 1973;288:704–6.
7. Brewerton DA, Hart FD, Nicholls A, et al. Ankylosing Spondylitis and Hl-a 27. Lancet 1973;301(7809):904–7.
8. Rudwaleit M, van der Heijde D, Landewé R, et al. The development of Assessment of SpondyloArthritis international Society classification criteria for axial spondyloarthritis (part II): validation and final selection. Ann Rheum Dis 2009; 68(part II):777–83.
9. Amor B, Dougados M, Mijiyawa M. Criteria of the classification of spondylarthropathies. Rev Rhum Mal Osteoartic 1990;57(2):85–9 [in French] Available at: http://www.ncbi.nlm.nih.gov/pubmed/2181618. Accessed January 23, 2015.
10. Reveille JD. HLA-B27 and the Seronegative Spondyloarthropathies. Am J Med Sci 1998;316(4):239–49.
11. Gabriel SE, Michaud K. Epidemiological studies in incidence, prevalence, mortality, and comorbidity of the rheumatic diseases. Arthritis Res Ther 2009;11(3). https://doi.org/10.1186/ar2669.
12. Ziade NR. HLA B27 antigen in Middle Eastern and Arab countries: Systematic review of the strength of association with axial spondyloarthritis and methodological

gaps. BMC Musculoskelet Disord 2017;18(1). https://doi.org/10.1186/s12891-017-1639-5.

13. Khan MA. HLA-B27 and its subtypes in world populations. Curr Opin Rheumatol 1995;7(4):263–9. Available at: http://www.ncbi.nlm.nih.gov/pubmed/7547102.

14. van der Linden SM, Valkenburg HA, de Jongh BM, et al. The risk of developing ankylosing spondylitis in HLA-B27 positive individuals. A comparison of relatives of spondylitis patients with the general population. Arthritis Rheum 1984;27(3): 241–9. Available at: http://www.ncbi.nlm.nih.gov/pubmed/6608352.

15. Braun J, Bollow M, Remlinger G, et al. Prevalence of spondylarthropathies in HLA-B27 positive and negative blood donors. Arthritis Rheum 1998;41(1):58–67.

16. Gofton JP, Robinson HS, Trueman GE. Ankylosing spondylitis in a Canadian Indian population. Ann Rheum Dis 1966;25(6):525–7.

17. Khan MA. HLA-B27 and its pathogenic role. J Clin Rheumatol 2008;14(1):50–2.

18. Helmick CG, Felson DT, Lawrence RC, et al. Estimates of the prevalence of arthritis and other rheumatic conditions in the United States. Part I. Arthritis Rheum 2008;58(1):15–25.

19. Gran JT, Husby G, Hordvik M. Prevalence of ankylosing spondylitis in males and females in a young middle-aged population of Tromsø, northern Norway. Ann Rheum Dis 1985;44(6):359–67.

20. Edwin Lim CS, Sengupta R, Gaffney K. The clinical utility of human leucocyte antigen B27 in axial spondyloarthritis. Rheumatol (United Kingdom) 2018;57(6): 959–68.

21. Reveille JD, Hirsch R, Dillon CF, et al. The prevalence of HLA–B27 in the US: Data From the US National Health and Nutrition Examination Survey, 2009. Arthritis Rheum 2012;64(5):1407–11.

22. Rachid B, El Zorkany B, Youseif E, et al. Early diagnosis and treatment of ankylosing spondylitis in Africa and the Middle East. Clin Rheumatol 2012;31(11): 1633–9.

23. Bhatia K, Richens J, Prasad ML, et al. High prevalence of the haplotype HLA-A11, B27 in arthritis patients from the highlands of Papua New Guinea. Tissue Antigens 1988;31(2):103–6.

24. Erdesz S, Shubin SV, Shoch BP, et al. Spondyloarthropathies in circumpolar populations of chukotka (Eskimos and Chukchi): Epidemiology and clinical characteristics. J Rheumatol 1994;21(6):1101–4.

25. Ziade N, Abi Karam G, Merheb G, et al. HLA-B27 prevalence in axial spondyloarthritis patients and in blood donors in a Lebanese population: Results from a nationwide study. Int J Rheum Dis 2019;22(4):708–14.

26. Terasaki PI, McClelland JD. Microdroplet assay of human serum cytotoxins [38]. Nature 1964;204(4962):998–1000.

27. Khan MA. An Update on the Genetic Polymorphism of HLA-B*27 With 213 Alleles Encompassing 160 Subtypes (and Still Counting). Curr Rheumatol Rep 2017; 19(2):1–7.

28. Reveille JD. Major histocompatibility genes and ankylosing spondylitis. Best Pract Res Clin Rheumatol 2006;20(3):601–9.

29. Neumüller J, Schwartz DWM, Dauber E, et al. Evaluation of four monoclonal antibodies against HLA-B27 for their reliability in HLA-B27 typing with flow cytometry (FC): Comparison with the classic microlymphocytotoxic test (MLCT). Commun Clin Cytom 1996;26(3):209–15.

30. Zeng Y, Hiti A, Moranville S, et al. Human HLA-B27 Typing Using the BDTM HLA-B27 Kit on the BD FACSViaTM System: A Multicenter Study. Cytometry Part B 2018;94B:651–7.

31. Skalska U, Kozakiewicz A, Mäliński W, et al. HLA-B27 detection - comparison of genetic sequence-based method and flow cytometry assay. Reumatologia 2015; 53(2):74–8.
32. Hoffmann JJML, Janssen WCM. HLA-B27 phenotyping with flow cytometry: Further improvement by multiple monoclonal antibodies. Clin Chem 1997; 43(10):1975–81.
33. Chheda P, Warghade S, Mathias J, et al. HLA-B27 testing: a journey from flow cytometry to molecular subtyping. J Clin Lab Anal 2018;32(5):1–9.
34. Sylvain K, Aurélie H, Marc M, et al. Rapid screening for HLA-B27 by a TaqMan-PCR assay using sequence-specific primers and a minor groove binder probe, a novel type of TaqMan™ probe. J Immunol Methods 2004;287(1–2):179–86.
35. Cortes A, Pulit SL, Leo PJ, et al. Major histocompatibility complex associations of ankylosing spondylitis are complex and involve further epistasis with ERAP1. Nat Commun 2015. https://doi.org/10.1038/ncomms8146.
36. Blanco-Gelaz MA, Suárez-Alvarez B, González S, et al. The amino acid at position 97 is involved in folding and surface expression of HLA-B27. Int Immunol 2006;18(1):211–20.
37. Schwimmbeck PL, Oldstone MBA. Molecular mimicry between human leukocyte antigen B27 and klebsiella. Consequences for spondyloarthropathies. Am J Med 1988. https://doi.org/10.1016/0002-9343(88)90385-3.
38. Appel H, Kuon W, Kuhne M, et al. Use of HLA-B27 tetramers to identify low-frequency antigen-specific T cells in Chlamydia-triggered reactive arthritis. Arthritis Res Ther 2004;6(6). https://doi.org/10.1186/ar1221.
39. Taurog JD, Dorris ML, Satumtira N, et al. Spondylarthritis in HLA-B27/human β2-microglobulin- transgenic rats is not prevented by lack of CD8. Arthritis Rheum 2009;60(7):1977–84.
40. Mauro D, Macaluso F, Fasano S, et al. ILC3 in Axial Spondyloarthritis: the Gut Angle. Curr Rheumatol Rep 2019;21(7). https://doi.org/10.1007/s11926-019-0834-9.
41. Tito RY, Cypers H, Joossens M, et al. Brief Report: Dialister as a Microbial Marker of Disease Activity in Spondyloarthritis. Arthritis Rheumatol 2017;69(1):114–21.
42. Yin J, Sternes PR, Wang M, et al. Shotgun metagenomics reveals an enrichment of potentially cross-reactive bacterial epitopes in ankylosing spondylitis patients, as well as the effects of TNFi therapy and the host's genotype upon microbiome composition. bioRxiv 2019;571430. https://doi.org/10.1101/571430.
43. Rizzo A, Guggino G, Ferrante A, et al. Role of subclinical gut inflammation in the pathogenesis of spondyloarthritis. Front Med 2018;5. https://doi.org/10.3389/fmed.2018.00063.
44. Lin P, Bach M, Asquith M, et al. HLA-B27 and human β2-microglobulin affect the gut microbiota of transgenic rats. PLoS One 2014;9(8). https://doi.org/10.1371/journal.pone.0105684.
45. Huizinga T, Nigrovic P, Ruderman E, et al. Th17 cells expressing KIR3DL2+ and responsive to HLA-B27 homodimers are increased in ankylosing spondylitis: Commentary. Int J Adv Rheumatol 2011;186(4):2672–80.
46. Turner MJ, Sowders DP, DeLay ML, et al. HLA-B27 misfolding in transgenic rats is associated with activation of the unfolded protein response. J Immunol 2005. https://doi.org/10.4049/jimmunol.175.4.2438.
47. Ciccia F, Accardo-Palumbo A, Rizzo A, et al. Evidence that autophagy, but not the unfolded protein response, regulates the expression of IL-23 in the gut of patients with ankylosing spondylitis and subclinical gut inflammation. Ann Rheum Dis 2014;73(8):1566–74.

48. McGonagle D, Marzo-Ortega H, O'Connor P, et al. The role of biomechanical factors and HLA-B27 in magnetic resonance imaging-determined bone changes in plantar fascia enthesopathy. Arthritis Rheum 2002;46(2):489–93.

49. Neerinckx B, Kollnberger S, Shaw J, et al. No evidence for a direct role of HLA-B27 in pathological bone formation in axial SpA. RMD Open 2017;3(1):1–10.

50. Bedendo A, Glorioso S, Pasini CV, et al. A family study of ankylosing spondylitis. Rheumatol Int 1984;5(1):29–32.

51. Ez-Zaitouni Z, Hilkens A, Gossec L, et al. Is the current ASAS expert definition of a positive family history useful in identifying axial spondyloarthritis? Results from the SPACE and DESIR cohorts. Arthritis Res Ther 2017;19(1):4–9.

52. van Lunteren M, Sepriano A, Landewé R, et al. Do ethnicity, degree of family relationship, and the spondyloarthritis subtype in affected relatives influence the association between a positive family history for spondyloarthritis and HLA-B27 carriership? Results from the worldwide ASAS cohort. Arthritis Res Ther 2018; 20(1):4–9.

53. Jaakkola E, Herzberg I, Laiho K, et al. Finnish HLA studies confirm the increased risk conferred by HLA-B27 homozygosity in ankylosing spondylitis. Ann Rheum Dis 2006;65(6):775–80.

54. Kim TJ, Na KS, Lee HJ, et al. HLA-B27 homozygosity has no influence on clinical manifestations and functional disability in ankylosing spondylitis. Clin Exp Rheumatol 2009;27(4):574–9.

55. Brown MA, Laval SH, Brophy S, et al. Recurrence risk modelling of the genetic susceptibility to ankylosing spondylitis. Ann Rheum Dis 2000;59(11):883–6.

56. Rudwaleit M, Haibel H, Baraliakos X, et al. The early disease stage in axial spondylarthritis: results from the german spondyloarthritis inception cohort. Arthritis Rheum 2009;60(3):717–27.

57. Mou Y, Zhang P, Li Q, et al. Clinical features in juvenile-onset ankylosing spondylitis patients carrying different B27 subtypes. Biomed Res Int 2015;2015. https://doi.org/10.1155/2015/594878.

58. Chung HY, Machado P, Van Der Heijde D, et al. HLA-B27 positive patients differ from HLA-B27 negative patients in clinical presentation and imaging: Results from the DESIR cohort of patients with recent onset axial spondyloarthritis. Ann Rheum Dis 2011;70(11):1930–6.

59. Akkoç N, Yarkan H, Kenar G, et al. Ankylosing Spondylitis: HLA-B*27-Positive Versus HLA-B*27-Negative Disease. Curr Rheumatol Rep 2017;19(5). https://doi.org/10.1007/s11926-017-0654-8.

60. Yang M, Xu M, Pan X, et al. Epidemiological comparison of clinical manifestations according to HLA-B*27 carrier status of Chinese Ankylosing Spondylitis patients. Tissue Antigens 2013;82(5):338–43.

61. Arévalo M, Gratacós Masmitjà J, Moreno M, et al. Influence of HLA-B27 on the Ankylosing Spondylitis phenotype: Results from the REGISPONSER database. Arthritis Res Ther 2018;20(1):1–6.

62. Akassou A, Bakri Y. Does HLA-B27 status influence ankylosing spondylitis phenotype? Clin Med Insights Arthritis Musculoskelet Disord 2018;11. https://doi.org/10.1177/1179544117751627.

63. Kim TJ, Kim TH. Clinical spectrum of ankylosing spondylitis in Korea. Jt Bone Spine 2010;77(3):235–40.

64. Sheehan NJ. HLA-B27: what's new? Rheumatology 2010;49(4):621–31.

65. Ruiz DG, de Azevedo MNL, Lupi O. HLA-B27 frequency in a group of patients with psoriatic arthritis. An Bras Dermatol 2012;87(6):847–50.

66. Queiro R, Morante I, Cabezas I, et al. HLA-B27 and psoriatic disease: A modern view of an old relationship. Rheumatol (United Kingdom) 2015;55(2):221–9.

67. Ajene AN, Fischer Walker CL, Black RE. Enteric pathogens and reactive arthritis: A systematic review of Campylobacter, Salmonella and Shigella-associated reactive arthritis. J Heal Popul Nutr 2013;31(3):299–307.

68. Sampaio-Barros PD, Bertolo MB, Kraemer MHS, et al. Primary ankylosing spondylitis: Patterns of disease in a Brazilian population of 147 patients. J Rheumatol 2001;28(3):560–5.

69. Wendling D, Prati C, Demattei C, et al. Impact of uveitis on the phenotype of patients with recent inflammatory back pain: Data from a prospective multicenter French cohort. Arthritis Care Res 2012;64(7):1089–93.

70. Canouï-Poitrine F, Lekpa Kemta F, Farrenq V, et al. Prevalence and factors associated with uveitis in spondylarthritis patients in France: Results from an observational survey. Arthritis Care Res 2012;64(6):919–24.

71. Zeboulon N, Dougados M, Gossec L. Prevalence and characteristics of uveitis in the spondyloarthropathies: A systematic literature review. Ann Rheum Dis 2008; 67(7):955–9.

72. Juanola X, Loza Santamaría E, Cordero-Coma M. Description and Prevalence of Spondyloarthritis in Patients with Anterior Uveitis: The SENTINEL Interdisciplinary Collaborative Project. Ophthalmology 2016;123(8):1632–6.

73. Accorinti M, Iannetti L, Liverani M, et al. Clinical features and prognosis of HLA B27-associated acute anterior uveitis in an Italian patient population. Ocul Immunol Inflamm 2010;18(2):91–6.

74. Jhaj G, Kopplin LJ. Ocular features of the HLA-B27-positive seronegative spondyloarthropathies. Curr Opin Ophthalmol 2018;29(6):552–7.

75. McCluskey PJ, Wakefield D. Acute anterior uveitis and HLA-B27. Surv Ophthalmol 2005;50(4):364–88.

76. Loh AR, Acharya NR. Incidence Rates and Risk Factors for Ocular Complications and Vision Loss in HLA-B27-Associated Uveitis. Am J Ophthalmol 2010;150(4): 534–42.

77. Power WJ, Rodriguez A, Pedroza-Seres M, et al. Outcomes in anterior uveitis associated with the HLA-B27 haplotype. Ophthalmology 1998;105(9):1646–51.

78. D'Ambrosio EM, La Cava M, Tortorella P, et al. Clinical Features and Complications of the HLA-B27-associated Acute Anterior Uveitis: A Metanalysis. Semin Ophthalmol 2017;32(6):689–701.

79. Palm Ø, Moum B, Ongre A, et al. Prevalence of ankylosing spondylitis and other spondyloarthropathies among patients with inflammatory bowel disease: A population study (the IBSEN study). J Rheumatol 2002;29(3):511–5.

80. Rudwaleit M, Baeten D. Ankylosing spondylitis and bowel disease. Best Pract Res Clin Rheumatol 2006;20(3):451–71.

81. Brakenhoff LKPM, van der Heijde DM, Hommes DW, et al. The joint-gut axis in inflammatory bowel diseases. J Crohn's Colitis 2010;4(3):257–68.

82. Turkcapar N, Toruner M, Soykan I, et al. The prevalence of extraintestinal manifestations and HLA association in patients with inflammatory bowel disease. Rheumatol Int 2006;26(7):663–8.

83. Chandran V, Barrett J, Schentag CT, et al. Axial psoriatic arthritis: Update on a longterm prospective study. J Rheumatol 2009;36(12):2744–50.

84. Queiro R, Sarasqueta C, Belzunegui J, et al. Psoriatic spondyloarthropathy: A comparative study between HLA-B27 positive and HLA-B27 negative disease. Semin Arthritis Rheum 2002;31(6):413–8.

85. Chandran V, Tolusso DC, Cook RJ, et al. Risk factors for axial inflammatory arthritis in patients with psoriatic arthritis. J Rheumatol 2010;37(4):809–15.
86. Baraliakos X, Coates LC, Braun J. The involvement of the spine in psoriatic arthritis. Clin Exp Rheumatol 2015;33(7):31–5.
87. Polachek A, Cook R, Chandran V, et al. The Association Between HLA Genetic Susceptibility Markers and Sonographic Enthesitis in Psoriatic Arthritis. Arthritis Rheumatol 2018;70(5):756–62.
88. Khan M, Kushner I, Braun WE. Comparison of clinical features in HLA-B27 positive and negative patients with ankylosing spondylitis. Arthritis Rheum 1977;20(4):909–12. Available at: http://www.ncbi.nlm.nih.gov/pubmed/558764.
89. Marzo-Ortega H, McGonagle D, O'Connor P, et al. Baseline and 1-year magnetic resonance imaging of the sacroiliac joint and lumbar spine in very early inflammatory back pain. Relationship between symptoms, HLA-B27 and disease extent and persistence. Ann Rheum Dis 2009;68(11):1721–7.
90. Khabbazi A, Vahedi L, Ghojazadeh M, et al. Association of HLA-B27 and Behcet's disease: a systematic review and meta-analysis. Autoimmun Highlights 2019;10(1). https://doi.org/10.1186/s13317-019-0112-x.
91. Jae KA, Yeoung GP. Human leukocyte antigen B27 and B51 double-positive Behçet uveitis. Arch Ophthalmol 2007;125(10):1375–80.
92. Poddubnyy D, Rudwaleit M, Haibel H, et al. Effect of non-steroidal anti-inflammatory drugs on radiographic spinal progression in patients with axial spondyloarthritis: Results from the German Spondyloarthritis Inception Cohort. Ann Rheum Dis 2012;71(10):1616–22.
93. Kiltz U, Baraliakos X, Karakostas P, et al. The degree of spinal inflammation is similar in patients with axial spondyloarthritis who report high or low levels of disease activity: a cohort study. Ann Rheum Dis 2012;1207–12. https://doi.org/10.1136/annrheumdis-2011-200508.
94. Haroon N, Inman RD, Learch TJ, et al. The impact of tumor necrosis factor α inhibitors on radiographic progression in ankylosing spondylitis. Arthritis Rheum 2013;65(10):2645–54.
95. Rudwaleit M, Sieper J. Referral strategies for early diagnosis of axial spondyloarthritis. Nat Rev Rheumatol 2012;8(5):262–8.

Juvenile-Versus Adult-Onset Spondyloarthritis
Similar, but Different

Pamela F. Weiss, MD, MSCE[a,b,*],
Johannes Roth, MD, PhD, FRCPC, RhMSUS[c]

KEYWORDS

- Juvenile spondyloarthritis • Enthesitis-related arthritis • Psoriatic arthritis • Imaging
- MRI • Ultrasonography

KEY POINTS

- Key differences in nomenclature and classification criteria between children and adults with spondyloarthritis are important to understand, as they can make transition from pediatric to adult care challenging.
- In comparison to adult-onset disease, juvenile-onset disease has a lower prevalence of human leukocyte antigen B27 positivity and acute anterior uveitis, more peripheral arthritis and enthesitis, and less axial involvement.
- As with adult-onset disease, MRI is the preferred modality for assessment of early axial disease; however age-related maturation changes must be considered when assessing for pathology.
- Ultrasonography is the preferred modality for assessment of peripheral joints and entheses. Knowledge of age-related changes in the cartilage are imperative for accurate interpretation.

CLASSIFICATION AND NOMENCLATURE

The term "spondyloarthritis" (SpA) encompasses a heterogeneous group of diseases characterized by varying degrees of peripheral and axial arthritis, enthesitis, bowel inflammation, psoriasis, acute and painful uveitis, human leukocyte antigen (HLA) B27 positivity, and psoriasis. However, the term "spondyloarthritis" is not used in clinical practice by pediatric rheumatologists. In pediatric clinical practice the

[a] Perelman School of Medicine UPENN, Philadelphia, PA, USA; [b] Division of Rheumatology, Children's Hospital of Philadelphia, Philadelphia, PA, USA; [c] Division of Pediatric Dermatology and Rheumatology, Children's Hospital of Eastern Ontario, University of Ottawa, 401 Smyth Road, Ottawa, Ontario K1H8L1, Canada
* Corresponding author. Roberts Center for Pediatric Clinical Research, Room 11121, 2716 South Street, Philadelphia, PA 19146.
E-mail address: weisspa@email.chop.edu

Rheum Dis Clin N Am 46 (2020) 245–261
https://doi.org/10.1016/j.rdc.2020.01.003
0889-857X/20/© 2020 Elsevier Inc. All rights reserved.

Table 1
International League of Associations for Rheumatology classification criteria for enthesitis-related arthritis and psoriatic arthritis

Enthesitis-Related Arthritis	Psoriatic Arthritis
Arthritis and enthesitis OR Arthritis or enthesitis plus at least 2 of the following: • Sacroiliac joint tenderness or inflammatory back pain • HLA-B27 positivity • Family history (first-degree relative) with HLA-B27–associated disease • Acute and symptomatic anterior uveitis • Arthritis in a boy older than 6 y	Arthritis and psoriasis OR Arthritis and at least 2 of the following: • Dactylitis • Nail pitting or onycholysis • Family history of psoriasis (first-degree relative)
Exclusions: psoriasis in self or first-degree relative, rheumatoid factor positivity, systemic JIA	*Exclusions*: Onset of arthritis in an HLA-B27 positive man after age 6 y, family history (first-degree relative) with HLA-B27–associated disease, rheumatoid factor positivity, systemic JIA

inflammatory arthritides are classified into 6 mutually exclusive and phenotypically distinct categories based on the International League of Associations for Rheumatology (ILAR) criteria for juvenile idiopathic arthritis (JIA).[1] There is also a seventh category, "undifferentiated," for those children fulfilling criteria for more than one category. Of the JIA categories, the 2 that are encompassed by the umbrella term "spondyloarthritis" are enthesitis-related arthritis and psoriatic arthritis (PsA) (**Table 1**). To be classified as JIA the arthritis must be present for at least 6 weeks and onset of symptoms must begin before age 16 years. The JIA criteria do not specifically account for inflammatory bowel disease–associated arthritis, juvenile ankylosing spondylitis, or reactive arthritis.

Enthesitis-related arthritis classification criteria are listed in **Table 1**. There are 2 sets of Assessment of Spondyloarthritis International Society (ASAS) classification criteria for use in adults, one for those with a predominance of peripheral symptoms and the other for those with axial involvement.[2] The primary differences between the pediatric and adult criteria are highlighted in **Table 2**. In comparison to the adult ASAS criteria the pediatric criteria do not address axial disease, and there is no inclusion of imaging, markers of inflammation, or therapeutic response criteria. The pediatric criteria are also inclusive of any tender enthesis as part of the JIA criteria, whereas the adult

Table 2
Comparison of pediatric and adult spondyloarthritis classification criteria

Criteria	ILAR: Enthesitis-Related Arthritis	ASAS: Nonradiographic Axial SpA
Clinical	+	+
Imaging	-	+
Genetic	+	+
Markers of inflammation	-	+
Therapeutic response	-	+

criteria limit inclusion of enthesitis to enthesitis of the heel (Achilles tendon or plantar fascia). Further, the adult ASAS criteria are inclusive of inflammatory bowel disease, dactylitis, and psoriasis, whereas these are specific exclusion criteria for enthesitis-related arthritis.

The ILAR pediatric PsA criteria are listed in **Table 1**. In comparison to the adult classification criteria for psoriatic arthritis,[3] the pediatric criteria limit relevant family history of psoriasis to a first-degree relative (vs including second-degree relatives) and do not include imaging evidence of juxta-articular new bone formation. The differences between adult and pediatric classification criteria make the transition between pediatric and adult care tricky for both patients and providers.

Classification of Juvenile Spondyloarthritis and the Role of Imaging

In adults, axial SpA and PsA are grouped under the same disease category, but even in this group of patients imaging indicates potential differences in the pathogenesis and manifestations of structures that can be affected in both conditions as the enthesis.[4] In juvenile SpA the current ILAR classification of JIA is trying to accommodate an even more complex clinical picture, with JIA-PsA being a separate category from enthesitis-related JIA and many patients who have overlapping features ending up in the JIA subgroup of "unclassified." Imaging of peripheral disease in juvenile SpA is therefore important in recognizing the range of structures that may be affected by the disease and the complexity within a given structure. For the inflammatory process synovial joints, the tendon sheath, the paratenon, bursae, and the enthesis may be affected. For the associated damage cartilage and bone are the primary target structures but the tendon and enthesis can also be affected.

CLINICAL FEATURES

Juvenile- and adult-onset diseases have many similarities in clinical presentation but there are also important differences. The peak age of onset of SpA in children is age 12 years and there is male predominance. In one study of ankylosing spondylitis, male sex and HLA-B27 positivity were associated with earlier disease onset[5]; this finding has not been replicated in other larger studies.[6] Multiple studies have shown that disease onset before age 16 years is associated with more peripheral arthritis, more root arthritis, and less frequent axial symptoms.[5-8] In a multicenter inception cohort of children fulfilling criteria for enthesitis-related arthritis, 91% and 75% had peripheral arthritis and at least 1 tender enthesis, respectively.[9] The most commonly affected joints were the knees, ankles, wrists, and hip.[9] Three-quarters had oligoarticular onset of disease and 60% were HLA-B27positive.[9] In that study 15% had a family history of HLA-B27–associated disease (range 6%–43%) and acute anterior uveitis was present in only 6% of children. Approximately two-thirds of children have gastrointestinal symptoms, similar to that reported in adults.[10] Cardiac complications are well documented in adults with SpA, but reports of similar involvement in children are rare. One study in children reported that up to 8% have aortic regurgitation[11] and another reported that children with HLA-B27 positivity are prone to endo- and myocardial involvement.[12]

Axial disease is less prevalent in children than adults but may affect up to one-third within several years of disease onset.[13-15] In one study of unselected children with incident SpA, 20% had evidence of inflammatory sacroiliitis at diagnosis, 88% of whom also had evidence of erosion or sclerosis. Of these children only one-third reported a history of back pain or endorsed back pain during physical examination.[16]

In that study, there were no physical examination maneuvers that discriminated between those children with and without sacroiliitis, and back pain was actually more frequent in children with a normal MRI versus those with an MRI demonstrating sacroiliitis. Using predictive modeling, the estimated probability of having a positive pelvic MRI was 0.84 if the patient was HLA-B27 positive and had an elevated C-reactive protein.[16] This finding of high prevalence of "silent" sacroiliitis in children with SpA in that study corroborates with findings of Bollow and colleagues[13] and Stoll and colleagues.[14] In a pediatric Italian cohort, 28% of consecutive children with enthesitis-related arthritis had an MRI consistent with sacroiliitis a median of 15 months after disease onset.[15]

CLINICAL OUTCOMES

In a multicenter cross-sectional study by Gensler and colleagues,[17] juvenile-onset disease had a significantly higher association with total hip arthroplasty and lower radiographic spinal disease burden as measured by the Bath Ankylosing Spondylitis Radiology Index. In a study by Kim and colleagues,[18] juvenile-onset disease was associated with lower radiographic spinal disease, as measured by the modified stokes ankylosing spondylitis score (mSASSS), despite longer mean duration of disease. Kim and colleagues[18] also reported that radiographic progression, as measured by change over time in the mSASSS, was significantly lower in juvenile-onset disease. Studies that compare functional outcomes have shown worse,[5,19] equivalent,[17] and better outcomes[17] in juvenile-onset versus adult-onset disease. These disparities are likely secondary to differences in cohort inclusion criteria and outcomes measured.

PATHOGENESIS

Recent advances in the evaluation of the genetics of JIA support the notion that inflammatory arthritis is a continuum across the arbitrary cut-point of age 16 years for juvenile- versus adult-onset disease.[20] In one HLA association study based on 5000 children with JIA and 14,400 controls in whom bivariate analysis was done to identify genetic correlation, or lack thereof, between JIA categories.[21] Children with enthesitis-related arthritis were genetically distinct from the other categories of JIA. Not surprisingly, comparison of these findings to those from adult studies demonstrated that children with enthesitis-related arthritis closely resemble adults with ankylosing spondylitis genetically, specifically at *HLA-B27*. Additional work is needed to determine if differences in juvenile- versus adult-onset disease phenotypes are secondary to true pathologic differences or differences in immune function and perhaps the microbiome in the growing child.[20]

Alterations in microbiota are increasingly associated with SpA in both pediatric- and adult-onset disease. There are several studies that demonstrate similarities in microbiota alterations in both juvenile- and adult-onset disease. Similarities include depletion of the *Faecalibacterium prausnitzii*, which are bacteria with antiinflammatory effects.[22] Although adult-onset disease has been associated with increased frequency of *Bacteroides fragilis*,[23] pediatric studies have demonstrated the opposite[14]; the finding of decreased *Bacteroides* in juvenile-onset disease in is accordance with microbiota studies in other categories of JIA.[24] The investigators postulate these differences may cause altered immunologic priming in children and subsequent increased risk of autoimmune disease generally rather than inherent differences in SpA pathogenesis.[22]

IMAGING: THE ROLE OF MAGNETIC RESONANCE IMAGING IN EVALUATION OF JUVENILE SPONDYLOARTHRITIS

MRI is increasingly used for evaluation of suspected sacroiliitis in the pediatric population. Radiographs may still be performed to rule out other pathology or when requested by insurance companies in order to get approval for an MRI. In children the potential for misclassification for the presence or absence of sacroiliitis by radiograph, when MRI is used as the reference standard, is high thereby dampening enthusiasm for its use.[25,26] Standard evaluation by MRI is similar in pediatric and adult practice although the use of gadolinium remains controversial, despite evidence in both pediatric[27,28] and adult[29] studies that demonstrate the use of gadolinium adds little to no incremental value for the evaluation of sacroiliitis. In pediatrics, some still favor the use of gadolinium to confirm the presence of synovitis, if the differential includes tumor or infection, or if the hips or spine are being imaged concurrently.

Magnetic Resonance Evaluation of Axial Disease

Age-related changes can be seen in both pediatric- and adult-onset disease. In pediatric disease, these changes are primarily driven by marrow and cartilage maturation (**Fig. 1**), whereas in adults they are driven by degenerative change. Understanding the normal features of the maturing sacroiliac joint is critical to understand before inflammatory change can be accurately identified. Using images prospectively collected on 70 healthy children aged 8 to 18 years, Chauvin and colleagues[30] developed an ordinal system that grades the amount of subchondral signal in the maturing skeleton from I to IV, with type I demonstrating homogeneous bright subchondral signal extending along the sacral apophyses and type IV being essentially equivalent to no signal and what is typically seen in adults. Increased signal was present in most prepubertal children; by the time they approach skeletal maturity, subchondral signal was detectable in only a minority (**Fig. 2**). Importantly, in this healthy population, the metaphyseal-equivalent signal was homogeneous and symmetric. The use of diffusion-weighted imaging (DWI) may improve reliability of interpretation in cases of uncertainty. One study demonstrated the mean normalized apparent diffusion coefficient (nADC) is higher in skeletally immature patients with unfused sacral apophyses than in skeletally

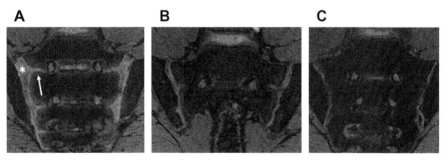

A   **B**   **C**

Fig. 1. Normal sacroiliac joint apophyseal cartilage development demonstrated on Dual Echo Steady State (DESS) sequences in a (*A*) 9-year-old girl, (*B*) 13-year-old boy, and (*C*) 17-year-old boy. In the young child (*A*), there is abundant hyperintense apophyseal cartilage (*asterisk*) seen along the sacroiliac joint as well as superior and inferior aspects of the segmental sacral apophyses (*arrow*). As the sacrum matures (*B*), the cartilage ossifies and becomes less apparent. In the older child (*C*), apophyseal cartilage is no longer present and just the articular cartilage is seen. (*Courtesy of* N. Chauvin, MD, Hershey, PA.)

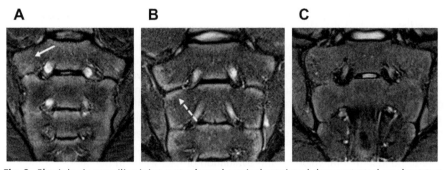

Fig. 2. Physiologic sacroiliac joint metaphyseal equivalent signal demonstrated on short tau inversion recovery (STIR) in a (A) 9-year-old girl, (B) 12-year-old girl, and (C) 16-year-old girl. In the young child (A) there is abundant hyperintense apophyseal and metaphyseal equivalent signals seen along the articular aspect of the sacrum as well as superior and inferior aspects of the segmental sacral apophyses (*arrow*) that can be mistaken for bone marrow edema. During maturation (B), the signal becomes thinner and less apparent (*dashed arrow*). In the older child (C), the metaphyseal equivalent hyperintense signal is minimal with progressive fusion of the sacral apophyses. (*Courtesy of* N. Chauvin, MD, Hershey, PA.)

mature patients.[31] A follow-up study demonstrated nADC can reliably and feasibly distinguish children with sacroiliitis from those with mechanical back pain.[31]

The Chauvin and colleagues'[30] study of 70 healthy children also evaluated the prevalence of cortical irregularities and found that cortical irregularities are common, occur most often along the ilium, and were most numerous in the peripubertal group. These findings correlate with a prior autopsy-based study,[32] which reported that the sacroiliac bony surfaces are smooth until puberty and thereafter often develop bony ridges and grooves, primarily on the ilium. This finding is different from that seen in adults, in whom irregularities may infer degenerative change, which we do not expect to see in the pediatric population. It is paramount to recognize these features as variations in normal anatomy so that they are not mistaken for erosions.

Magnetic Resonance Imaging Changes of Inflammatory Arthritis

There are no pediatric specific definitions of inflammatory or structural lesions in children, and most pediatric studies use the definitions provided by ASAS.[33] In one study of pediatric imaging in patients with SpA the adult ASAS criteria had low sensitivity when the radiologists' global assessment of sacroiliitis was used as the reference standard.[34] That study suggested that modifying the ASAS definition to include bone marrow edema on one slice only and inclusion of synovitis or capsulitis in the absence of bone marrow edema could improve the diagnostic utility in children. However, this is controversial, as other pediatric studies demonstrate that all cases of synovitis or capsulitis in children were in the presence of bone marrow edema.[27]

In children, the utility of routine MRI assessment of the spine for inflammatory lesions remains controversial. In one study apophyseal joint arthritis or end-plate edema, in accordance with the ASAS/Outcome Measures in Rheumatology (OMERACT) Study Group definitions, was identified in more than half of patients.[35] Most, but not all, children with lumbar spine inflammatory lesions had concomitant sacroiliitis. In a subsequent study apophyseal joint arthritis was uncommon in the absence of sacroiliitis.[36]

In children, MRI is also useful to evaluate pelvic enthesitis. In children, the most common sites of pelvic enthesitis are around the hip and the retroarticular interosseous ligaments.[37] Seventy-five percent of children with pelvic enthesitis also have findings consistent with sacroiliitis.

Magnetic Resonance Imaging Tools to Assess Disease Activity and Change over Time

Considerable strides have been made in the past few years to validate tools for the objective assessment of inflammation and damage in the axial joints. The Spondyloarthritis Research Consortium of Canada (SPARCC) sacroiliac joint inflammation score (SIS) assesses the site, size, and severity of sacroiliac joint inflammation. The total score ranges from 0 to 72, and the accepted minimally important change in total score is 2.5. This tool has been validated in adults and used in clinical trials to assess response to therapy.[38,39] Reliability and validity of the SPARCC SIS has also been evaluated in children.[40] The SPARCC sacroiliac structural score (SSS) assesses a spectrum of structural lesions, including erosion, fat metaplasia, backfill, and ankylosis; each domain is scored 0 to 20 or 0 to 40; there is no total score.[41] The SPARCC structural is also reliable for assessment of pediatric disease. The SSS was modified for the assessment of pediatric disease to include sclerosis because it is not easily confused with degenerative changes as in adults. There are pediatric- and adult-specific scoring training and calibration modules for both the SIS and SSS available through the CaRE Arthritis platform (CaREArthritis.com). There are also efforts underway to develop and validate a pediatric-specific sacroiliac joint scoring system (JIA MRI score, Juvenile Idiopathic Arthritis MRI Score) using the OMERACT consensus methodology. In the preliminary work 2 domains—inflammation and structural—were identified along with pediatric definitions for key inflammatory and structural lesions.[42]

Apparent diffusion coefficient (ADC) measures the magnitude of water molecule diffusion within tissue using MRI with DWI. ADC from DWI can distinguish active from inactive sacroiliitis and can be followed over time to assess response to treatment in adults.[43–47] In children, this technique holds promise as an objective imaging biomarker but also as a clinical tool when the distinction between immature structural bone and inflammation is unclear. In one small retrospective study of 10 adolescents with established sacroiliitis and 10 controls with mechanical back pain, the mean ADC values at the sacroiliac joints were significantly higher in subjects with sacroiliitis ($P<.001$).[31] A subsequent study demonstrated that normalized ADC change after tumour necrosis factor inhibitor therapy was greater for both radiographic (measured by change in SPARCC SIS) and clinical responders, although the differences were not statistically significant.[48]

THE ROLE OF ULTRASOUND IMAGING IN JUVENILE SPONDYLOARTHRITIS

Although MRI plays an important role in the imaging of the axial skeleton, most peripheral joints and the enthesis in particular are very accessible and reliably imaged with ultrasonography.[49] Ultrasonography has distinct advantages over MRI, being much less costly and time consuming.[50] In addition, it has a superior spatial resolution, which is especially important in the assessment of smaller entheses such as those of the extensor tendons and collateral ligaments of the fingers (**Fig.3**). Visualization of these structures has enhanced our understanding of the complexity of the musculoskeletal system in these areas including the associated pathology, for example, in dactylitis (see **Fig. 3**).[49] Several entheses can be assessed at the same time, and

A

B

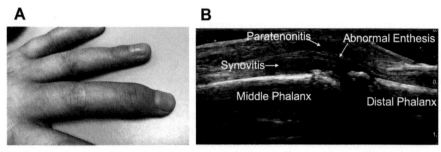

Paratenonitis   Abnormal Enthesis

Synovitis→

Middle Phalanx   Distal Phalanx

Fig. 3. Visualization of complex pathology clinically manifesting as dactylitis. (*A*) Clinical photo and (*B*) corresponding ultrasound image. (*B*) High spatial resolution allows visualization of detailed changes in the distal interphalangeal region including synovitis, paratenonitis, and abnormal enthesis of extensor tendon.

the examination can also be conducted in younger children without the need for sedation.[51,52] The real-time imaging capabilities enable the examiner to directly correlate imaging and clinical findings and also to demonstrate findings to the patient and parents. Finally, the lack of ionizing radiation is particularly important in children.[51,52]

Ultrasound Technique

The ultrasound modalities used in the assessment of children for pathology associated with SpA are no different than in adults. Structural findings are assessed using brightness-mode (B-mode) sonography. This technique uses the transmission and reflection of high-frequency longitudinal mechanical waves (ultrasonic waves). The image is generated by differing energy of waves reflected from surfaces of different tissues. The reflected "echoing" waves are analyzed and displayed by a computer, which creates a real-time display of tissues and structures being examined. The intensity of the brightness indicates the energy of the reflected sound waves.

Vascular anatomy can be assessed by combining B-mode sonography with Doppler sonography, which will detect blood flow. Synovial hyperemia, for example, leads to increased Doppler signals because of the increased blood flow. Both power- and color Doppler sonography can be used. In very young children smaller transducers, for example, hockey sticks, may have advantages and be used in more views compared with older children or adults.

The Need for the Use of Imaging in the Assessment of Juvenile Spondyloarthritis

There are several areas in which imaging can provide an enhancement of the clinical examination:

- *Detection of subclinical synovitis and enthesitis and clarification of equivocal findings:* the clinical signs of synovitis and enthesitis including swelling, limited range of motion, and pain can be unreliable because of the location of the joint or enthesis (hip, shoulder, etc.), the influence of body mass index, naturally occurring variability, and the age of the patient.[52] In the pediatric setting this also includes the clinical history, which, depending on the age of the child, may be highly unreliable emphasizing the need for additional measurement tools to assess the possible presence of pathology.Pediatric studies have consistently reported a rate of subclinical synovitis around 30% to 40% of joints,[53–55] with these subclinical findings being predictive of flare and therefore clinically relevant.[56] Doppler signals can also be seen in a high percentage of asymptomatic entheseal sites.

Weiss and colleagues[57] found that US-confirmed enthesitis is common in children with enthesitis-related arthritis, particularly at the insertions of the quadriceps, the common extensor, and the Achilles tendons.

- *Detailed assessment of relevant structures:* several entheses may be relevant in the disease process and accessible clinically, yet our understanding of pathologic changes and even the routine clinical assessment is limited. One example is a detailed assessment of the proximal gluteal enthesis carefully distinguishing findings in healthy children from pathology in order to allow a reliable assessment with ultrasonography.[58]
- *Detection and documentation of damage beyond cartilage/bone damage:* ultrasonography provides a very complete assessment of soft tissue structures as well as cartilage/bone in many locations. The functional relevance of damage to soft tissues such as tendons but also supporting structures such as the finger pulleys may be significant. **Fig. 4** shows the dislocation of a flexor tendon from its regular position due to damage to the A2 pulley in the case of tenosynovitis.
- *Resolution of discrepancies between patient perception and physician assessment:* disagreement between the physician and patient assessment of disease activity in secondary pain amplification can lead to over- or undertreatment and overall effects on the therapeutic relationship and compliance. The visual demonstration of findings can help to reach agreement and will overall strengthen the statements made by the physician based on the clinical examination.[59]
- *Patient/parent education:* the patient-physician relationship and compliance can further be strengthened by a better understanding of disease process through visual demonstration, as concepts such as inflammation or even the term "arthritis" or "enthesitis" may be relatively abstract and difficult to understand for many patients and their parents.[59]
- *Imaging-guided interventions:* interventions such as injections into joints, tendon sheaths, and perientheseal bursae continue to have a role in the therapeutic approach to patients with spondyl arthropathies, and the possibility to avoid the need for sedation through a faster and more direct access to the target structure as well as the increased reliability to target structures also in very young children support the role of ultrasonography to guide these interventions.

Synovitis

The assessment of synovitis through ultrasonography is well established, including the correlation of imaging findings with inflammation on histology,[60] clear definitions,[61] as

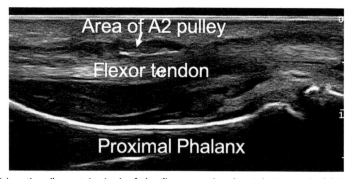

Fig. 4. Dislocation (bow-stringing) of the flexor tendon (straight instead of following the bone closely) of the finger at the level of the A2 pulley as a result of longstanding tenosynovitis and loosening of the A2 pulley.

well as scores for quantification.[62] Contrary to adults, the pediatric patient presents with a unique anatomy of incompletely ossified bones that serve as the basic structure when imaging a joint.[63] The changes associated with the incomplete ossification and subsequent maturation of bone need to be interpreted correctly, including blood flow detected through Doppler ultrasonography.[64] Physiologic blood flow, which may be very prevalent in the growing joint, needs to be carefully differentiated from pathologic findings.

Tenosynovitis and Paratendonitis

Ultrasonography has helped to remind (pediatric) rheumatologist that many tendons are surrounded by connective tissue lined with single-layer synovial cells called paratenon (eg, the Achilles tendon),[65] and other tendons have a double-layered synovial sheath.[65] The imaging appearance of pathology in both structures does not differ between children and adults.

Enthesis

The enthesis is a relatively complex structure consisting of several components including the tendon itself, various portions of fibrocartilage, subtendinous bursae, fat, and the insertion of tendon fibers into bone through fibrocartilage[66] **(Fig. 5)**. Histologic and molecular analyses suggest that all of these components may play important and distinct roles in the pathogenesis of enthesitis.[66] Imaging of the tendon insertion into bone through fibrocartilage and hyaline cartilage of the incompletely ossified bone can differ significantly from adults depending on the age. This is again related to the cartilage that is not ossified yet depending on the age of the child.

Knowledge of entheseal development in children as well as consideration of vascularization is important in order to differentiate pathologic from normal findings.[67–69]

In children, similar to adults, ultrasound findings in various entheses may show differences in specificity for their association with SpA as opposed to physiologic findings or other pathologies. For example, the tibial tuberosity has been demonstrated in children to be a site of frequent findings of physiologic Doppler signals.[69] Signals

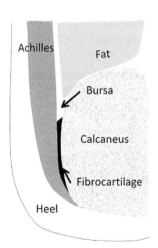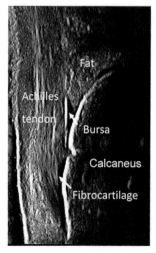

Fig. 5. Structures forming the entheseal complex shown schematically (*left*) and with the corresponding ultrasound image (*right*).

in this location may therefore not be very specific for pathology as part of SpA, and this location may also be often affected by apophysitis (see next paragraph). In contrast, findings in this region in adults were very important to distinguish patients with SpA from healthy controls.[70]

Differential Diagnosis Including Apophysitis

Children have distinct pathologies—different from adults—that need to be considered in the differential diagnosis of entheseal pathology in particular. Although in adults the body of the tendon (in addition to the enthesis) is often subject to mechanical/degenerative pathologies (tendonitis) the enthesis itself represents the weakest point in children and is prone to pathology including acute damage, for example, in avulsions of the tendon at the enthesis (as opposed to tendon ruptures in the adult), but also chronic changes such as apophysitis. Traction apophysitis is a term used to describe the occurrence of insertional tendinopathy at an apophyseal site and possible avulsion of osteochondralfragments.[71] It needs to be differentiated from enthesitis as a manifestation of juvenile SpA. The most common examples are Osgood-Schlatter disease at the site of the patellar tendon's insertion into the proximal tibia and Sever disease at the insertion of the Achilles tendon into the calcaneus. The inflammation and injury result from chronic repetitive traction exceeding the resistance to tensile forces at the insertion site of the tendon. It will typically occur during a period of rapid growth, especially in physically very active children. This period coincides with the ossification of the previously cartilaginous insertion of the tendon. The differentiation of apophysitis from enthesitis as in enthesitis-related arthritis can be achieved through history and clinical examinations well as the imaging characteristics.

Validation of Ultrasonography in the Assessment of Pathology in Juvenile Spondyloarthritis

Before any measurement tool can be used in clinical practice or research reliably it needs to be validated. Several processes can be followed for validation but the OMERACT initiative has established a very clear and structured framework for the development of core outcomes and the associated measurement tools for trials and observational studies in rheumatology.[72]

In adults, a significant amount of work on the ultrasound imaging of the synovium, the tendon, and the enthesis has been completed by various individual investigators, the OMERACT group, as well as the GRAPPA group.[72–74] There is still debate though whether entheseal changes in patients with predominantly axial SpA can be evaluated with ultrasonography the same way than those in patients with PsA even though both groups of patients belong to the same overall group of SpA.[73] Ultrasound imaging data suggest that damage and remodeling may be much more significant in patients with PsA than in those with axial SpA with entheseal involvement, and this may suggest relevant differences in pathogenesis revealed by ultrasound imaging but also the need to look at these 2 groups separately from an imaging and validation of imaging point of view. In terms of quantification of findings (scores) for the enthesis and for the synovial joint, various scores have been validated but no globally accepted ultrasound score has been established and existing scores vary widely in their metrics.

In pediatric rheumatology the validation process has been in part different from adults. It started with definitions for the ultrasound findings of the healthy joint[63] in order to acknowledge the impact of the pediatric anatomy on findings in B-mode and Doppler ultrasonography. Although this process has been completed for the synovial joint, it is not complete yet for the enthesis or the other properties of the tendon including tendon sheath and paratenon. It is likely that inflammatory changes may not differ so much in children for the enthesis and other properties of the tendon but structural lesions (calcifications, enthesophytes) have been observed much less in children compared with adults.[57]

The specificity of Doppler signals close to the enthesis for SpA needs to be further evaluated both in adult as well as pediatric SpA and is connected to the need to precisely define the various grades on semiquantitative scoring methods as well as the definition of a threshold suggesting pathologic Doppler signals. Rather than in cross-sectional assessments it may be beneficial to use Doppler sonography in longitudinal assessments. Tse and colleagues[75] demonstrated the ability of color Doppler sonography to show improvement in increased vascularity at the cortical bone insertion of enthesis and along the adjacent synovium in children with enthesitis-related arthritis.

SUMMARY

Key differences in nomenclature and classification criteria between children and adults with SpA are important for both families and physicians to comprehend. In comparison to adult-onset disease, juvenile-onset disease has a lower prevalence of HLA-B27 positivity and acute anterior uveitis, more peripheral arthritis and enthesitis, and less axial involvement. Most of the children have oligoarticular peripheral arthritis and at least 1 tender enthesis at presentation and up to one-third develop axial disease within a few years. As with adult-onset disease, MRI is the preferred modality for assessment of early axial disease; however, age-related maturation changes must be considered when assessing for pathology. Subchondral edema is common is pre- and peripubertal children and easily confused with bone marrow edema. Cortical irregularities are also present in more than 50% of normal healthy peripubertal sacroiliac joints, again easily confused with erosion for those unfamiliar with these expected age-related changes. Ultrasonography is the preferred imaging tool for assessment of peripheral joints and entheses. Knowledge of age-related changes in the cartilage are imperative for accurate interpretation of ultrasound results. Changes associated with the incomplete ossification and the maturation of bone need to be interpreted correctly, including increased blood flow detected through Doppler ultrasonography. In children, physiologic vascularization may be common at certain entheseal sites and in maturing joints—similar findings in adults would be considered pathologic. In conclusion, there are many similarities in the underlying disease process between juvenile- and adult-onset diseases, but there are also critical differences to be aware of in regard to clinical phenotype and interpretation of relevant imaging studies used to assess disease activity and progression.

DISCLOSURE

The authors have nothing to disclose.

REFERENCES

1. Petty RE, Southwood TR, Manners P, et al. International League of Associations for Rheumatology classification of juvenile idiopathic arthritis: second revision, Edmonton, 2001. J Rheumatol 2004;31(2):390–2.
2. Rudwaleit M, van der Heijde D, Landewe R, et al. The development of Assessment of SpondyloArthritis international Society classification criteria for axial spondyloarthritis (part II): validation and final selection. Ann Rheum Dis 2009; 68(6):777–83.

3. Taylor W, Gladman D, Helliwell P, et al. Classification criteria for psoriatic arthritis: development of new criteria from a large international study. Arthritis Rheum 2006;54(8):2665–73.
4. Weiss PF, Chauvin NA, Roth J. Imaging in Juvenile Spondyloarthritis. Curr Rheumatol Rep 2016;18(12):75.
5. Chen HA, Chen CH, Liao HT, et al. Clinical, functional, and radiographic differences among juvenile-onset, adult-onset, and late-onset ankylosing spondylitis. J Rheumatol 2012;39(5):1013–8.
6. O'Shea FD, Boyle E, Riarh R, et al. Comparison of clinical and radiographic severity of juvenile-onset versus adult-onset ankylosing spondylitis. Ann Rheum Dis 2009;68(9):1407–12.
7. Riley MJ, Ansell BM, Bywaters EG. Radiological manifestations of ankylosing spondylitis according to age at onset. Ann Rheum Dis 1971;30(2):138–48.
8. Jadon DR, Ramanan AV, Sengupta R. Juvenile versus adult-onset ankylosing spondylitis – clinical, radiographic, and social outcomes. a systematic review. J Rheumatol 2013;40(11):1797–805.
9. Gmuca S, Xiao R, Brandon TG, et al. Multicenter inception cohort of enthesitis-related arthritis: variation in disease characteristics and treatment approaches. Arthritis Res Ther 2017;19(1):84.
10. Mielants H, Veys EM, Goemaere S, et al. Gut inflammation in the spondyloarthropathies: clinical, radiologic, biologic and genetic features in relation to the type of histology. A prospective study. J Rheumatol 1991;18(10):1542–51.
11. Stamato T, Laxer RM, de Freitas C, et al. Prevalence of cardiac manifestations of juvenile ankylosing spondylitis. Am J Cardiol 1995;75(10):744–6.
12. Huppertz H, Voigt I, Muller-Scholden J, et al. Cardiac manifestations in patients with HLA B27-associated juvenile arthritis. Pediatr Cardiol 2000;21(2):141–7.
13. Bollow M, Braun J, Biedermann T, et al. Use of contrast-enhanced MR imaging to detect sacroiliitis in children. Skeletal Radiol 1998;27(11):606–16.
14. Stoll ML, Bhore R, Dempsey-Robertson M, et al. Spondyloarthritis in a pediatric population: risk factors for sacroiliitis. J Rheumatol 2010;37(11):2402–8.
15. Pagnini I, Savelli S, Matucci-Cerinic M, et al. Early predictors of juvenile sacroiliitis in enthesitis-related arthritis. J Rheumatol 2010;37(11):2395–401.
16. Weiss PF, Xiao R, Biko DM, et al. Assessment of sacroiliitis at diagnosis of juvenile spondyloarthritis by radiography, magnetic resonance imaging, and clinical examination. Arthritis Care Res (Hoboken) 2016;68(2):187–94.
17. Gensler LS, Ward MM, Reveille JD, et al. Clinical, radiographic and functional differences between juvenile-onset and adult-onset ankylosing spondylitis: results from the PSOAS cohort. Ann Rheum Dis 2008;67(2):233–7.
18. Kim TJ, Shin JH, Sung IH, et al. Comparison on radiographic progression for 5 years between juvenile onset ankylosing spondylitis and adult onset ankylosing spondylitis: an observational study of the Korean SpondyloArthropathy Registry (OSKAR) data. Clin Exp Rheumatol 2016;34(4):668–72.
19. Stone M, Warren RW, Bruckel J, et al. Juvenile-onset ankylosing spondylitis is associated with worse functional outcomes than adult-onset ankylosing spondylitis. Arthritis Rheum 2005;53(3):445–51.
20. Nigrovic PA, Martinez-Bonet M, Thompson SD. Implications of juvenile idiopathic arthritis genetic risk variants for disease pathogenesis and classification. Curr Opin Rheumatol 2019;31(5):401–10.
21. Hinks A, Bowes J, Cobb J, et al. Fine-mapping the MHC locus in juvenile idiopathic arthritis (JIA) reveals genetic heterogeneity corresponding to distinct adult inflammatory arthritic diseases. Ann Rheum Dis 2017;76(4):765–72.

22. Stoll ML, Weiss PF, Weiss JE, et al. Age and fecal microbial strain-specific differences in patients with spondyloarthritis. Arthritis Res Ther 2018;20(1):14.

23. Stebbings S, Munro K, Simon MA, et al. Comparison of the faecal microflora of patients with ankylosing spondylitis and controls using molecular methods of analysis. Rheumatology (Oxford) 2002;41(12):1395–401.

24. Tejesvi MV, Arvonen M, Kangas SM, et al. Faecal microbiome in new-onset juvenile idiopathic arthritis. Eur J Clin Microbiol Infect Dis 2016;35(3):363–70.

25. Weiss PF, Xiao R, Brandon TG, et al. Radiographs in screening for sacroiliitis in children: what is the value? Arthritis Res Ther 2018;20(1):141.

26. Jaremko JL, Liu L, Winn NJ, et al. Diagnostic utility of magnetic resonance imaging and radiography in juvenile spondyloarthritis: evaluation of the sacroiliac joints in controls and affected subjects. J Rheumatol 2014;41(5):963–70.

27. Weiss PF, Xiao R, Biko DM, et al. Detection of inflammatory sacroiliitis in children with magnetic resonance imaging: is gadolinium contrast enhancement necessary? Arthritis Rheumatol 2015;67(8):2250–6.

28. Herregods N, Jaremko JL, Baraliakos X, et al. Limited role of gadolinium to detect active sacroiliitis on MRI in juvenile spondyloarthritis. Skeletal Radiol 2015;44(11): 1637–46.

29. de Hooge M, van den Berg R, Navarro-Compan V, et al. Magnetic resonance imaging of the sacroiliac joints in the early detection of spondyloarthritis: no added value of gadolinium compared with short tau inversion recovery sequence. Rheumatology (Oxford) 2013;52(7):1220–4.

30. Chauvin NA, Xiao R, Brandon TG, et al. MRI of the sacroiliac joint in healthy children. AJR Am J Roentgenol 2019;1–7. https://doi.org/10.2214/AJR.18.20708.

31. Bray TJ, Vendhan K, Roberts J, et al. Association of the apparent diffusion coefficient with maturity in adolescent sacroiliac joints. J Magn Reson Imaging 2016; 44(3):556–64.

32. Vleeming A, Schuenke MD, Masi AT, et al. The sacroiliac joint: an overview of its anatomy, function and potential clinical implications. J Anat 2012;221(6):537–67.

33. Rudwaleit M, Jurik AG, Hermann KG, et al. Defining active sacroiliitis on magnetic resonance imaging (MRI) for classification of axial spondyloarthritis: a consensual approach by the ASAS/OMERACT MRI group. Ann Rheum Dis 2009; 68(10):1520–7.

34. Herregods N, Dehoorne J, Van den Bosch F, et al. ASAS definition for sacroiliitis on MRI in SpA: applicable to children? Pediatr Rheumatol Online J 2017;15(1):24.

35. Vendhan K, Sen D, Fisher C, et al. Inflammatory changes of the lumbar spine in children and adolescents with enthesitis-related arthritis: magnetic resonance imaging findings. Arthritis Care Res (Hoboken) 2014;66(1):40–6.

36. Bray TJ, Amies T, Vendhan K, et al. Discordant inflammatory changes in the apophyseal and sacroiliac joints: serial observations in enthesitis-related arthritis. Br J Radiol 2016;89(1065):20160353.

37. Herregods N, Dehoorne J, Pattyn E, et al. Diagnositic value of pelvic enthesitis on MRI of the sacroiliac joints in enthesitis related arthritis. Pediatr Rheumatol Online J 2015;13(1):46.

38. Maksymowych WP, Heijde DV, Baraliakos X, et al. Tofacitinib is associated with attainment of the minimally important reduction in axial magnetic resonance imaging inflammation in ankylosing spondylitis patients. Rheumatology (Oxford) 2018;57(8):1390–9.

39. van der Heijde D, Baraliakos X, Hermann KA, et al. Limited radiographic progression and sustained reductions in MRI inflammation in patients with axial

spondyloarthritis: 4-year imaging outcomes from the RAPID-axSpA phase III randomised trial. Ann Rheum Dis 2018;77(5):699–705.

40. Weiss PF, Maksymowych W, Lambert RG, et al. Feasibility and Reliability of the Spondyloarthritis Research Consortium of Canada Sacroiliac Joint Inflammation Score for Children with Spondyloarthritis. Arthritis Research & Therapy 2018 Mar 22;20(1):56. PMC5865339.

41. Maksymowych WP, Wichuk S, Chiowchanwisawakit P, et al. Development and preliminary validation of the spondyloarthritis research consortium of Canada magnetic resonance imaging sacroiliac joint structural score. J Rheumatol 2015;42(1):79–86.

42. Otobo TM, Conaghan PG, Maksymowych WP, et al. Preliminary definitions for sacroiliac joint pathologies in the OMERACT juvenile idiopathic arthritis magnetic resonance imaging score (OMERACT JAMRIS-SIJ). J Rheumatol 2019;46(9): 1192–7.

43. Bozgeyik Z, Ozgocmen S, Kocakoc E. Role of diffusion-weighted MRI in the detection of early active sacroiliitis. AJR Am J Roentgenol 2008;191(4):980–6.

44. Gaspersic N, Sersa I, Jevtic V, et al. Monitoring ankylosing spondylitis therapy by dynamic contrast-enhanced and diffusion-weighted magnetic resonance imaging. Skeletal Radiol 2008;37(2):123–31.

45. Gezmis E, Donmez FY, Agildere M. Diagnosis of early sacroiliitis in seronegative spondyloarthropathies by DWI and correlation of clinical and laboratory findings with ADC values. Eur J Radiol 2013;82(12):2316–21.

46. Pedersen SJ, Poddubnyy D, Sorensen IJ, et al. Course of MRI inflammation and structural lesions in the sacroiliac joints in a randomized double-blind placebo-controlled trial of adalimumab in patients with axial spondyloarthritis as assessed by the Berlin and SPARCC methods (the DANISH Study). Arthritis Rheumatol 2016;68(2):418–29.

47. Sieper J, van der Heijde D, Dougados M, et al. A randomized, double-blind, placebo-controlled, sixteen-week study of subcutaneous golimumab in patients with active nonradiographic axial spondyloarthritis. Arthritis Rheumatol 2015;67(10): 2702–12.

48. JPB T, Vendhan K, Ambrose N, et al. Diffusion-weighted imaging is a sensitive biomarker of response to biologic therapy in enthesitis-related arthritis. Rheumatology (Oxford) 2017;56(3):399–407.

49. Kaeley GS. Review of the use of ultrasound for the diagnosis and monitoring of enthesitis in psoriatic arthritis. Curr Rheumatol Rep 2011;13(4):338–45.

50. Damasio MB, Malattia C, Martini A, et al. Synovial and inflammatory diseases in childhood: role of new imaging modalities in the assessment of patients with juvenile idiopathic arthritis. Pediatr Radiol 2010;40(6):985–98.

51. Chauvin NA, Khwaja A. Imaging of inflammatory arthritis in children: status and perspectives on the use of ultrasound, radiographs, and magnetic resonance imaging. Rheum Dis Clin North Am 2016;42:587–606.

52. Malattia C, Tzaribachev N, van den Berg M, et al. Juvenile idiopathic arthritis - the role of imaging from a rheumatologist's perspective. Pediatr Radiol 2018;48: 785–91.

53. Rebollo-Polo M, Koujok K, Weisser C, et al. Ultrasound findings on patients with juvenile idiopathic arthritis in clinical remission. Arthritis Care Res 2011;63: 1013–9.

54. Breton S, Jousse-Joulin S, Cangemi C, et al. Comparison of clinical and ultrasonographic evaluations for peripheral synovitis in juvenile idiopathic arthritis. Semin Arthritis Rheum 2011;41:272–8.

55. Lanni S, van Dijkhuizen EHP, Vanoni F, et al. Ultrasound changes in synovial abnormalities induced by treatment in juvenile idiopathic arthritis. Clin Exp Rheumatol 2018;36:329–34.

56. De Lucia O, Ravagnani V, Pregnolato F, et al. Baseline ultrasound examination as possible predictor of relapse in patients affected by juvenile idiopathic arthritis (JIA). Ann Rheum Dis 2018;77(10):1426–31.

57. Weiss PF, Chauvin NA, Klink AJ, et al. Detection of enthesitis in children with enthesitis-related arthritis: dolorimetry compared to ultrasonography. Arthritis Rheumatol 2014;66(1):218–27.

58. Laurell L, Court-Payen M, Nielsen S, et al. Ultrasonography and color Doppler of proximal gluteal enthesitis in juvenile idiopathic arthritis: a descriptive study. Pediatr Rheumatol Online J 2011;9(1):22.

59. Favier LA, Ting TV, Modi AC. Feasibility of a musculoskeletal ultrasound intervention to improve adherence in juvenile idiopathic arthritis: a proof-of concept trial. Pediatr Rheumatol Online J 2018;16(1):75.

60. Walther M, Harms H, Krenn V, et al. Correlation of power Doppler sonography with vascularity of the synovial tissue of the knee joint in patients with osteoarthritis and rheumatoid arthritis. Arthritis Rheum 2001;44:331–8.

61. Roth J, Ravagnani V, Backhaus M, et al, OMERACT Ultrasound Group. Preliminary definitions for the sonographic features of synovitis in children. Arthritis Care Res 2017;69:1217–23.

62. Ting IV, Vega-Fernandez P, Oberle EJ, et al, CARRA JIA Ultrasound Workgroup. A novel ultra- sound image acquisition protocol and scoring system for the pediatric knee. Arthritis Care Res 2019;71(7):977–85.

63. Roth J, Jousse-Joulin S, Magni-Manzoni S, et al. Omeract definitions for the sonographic appearance of the normal pediatric joint. Arthritis Care Res 2015;67(1):136–42.

64. Windschall D, Collado P, Vojinovic J, et al. OMERACT paediatric ultrasound subtask force. Age-related vascularization and ossification of joints in children: an international pilot study to test multi-observer ultrasound reliability. Arthritis Care Res 2017. https://doi.org/10.1002/acr.23335.

65. Kannus P. Structure of the tendon connective tissue. Scand J Med Sci Sports 2000;10(6):312–20.

66. Benjamin M, Moriggl B, Brenner E. The "enthesis organ" concept: Why enthesopathies may not present as focal insertional disorders. Arthritis Rheum 2004;50:3306–13.

67. Jousse-Joulin S, Cangemi C, Gerard S, et al. Normal sonoanatomy of the paediatric entheses including echostructure and vascularisation changes during growth. Eur Radiol 2015;25(7):2143–52.

68. Chauvin NA, Ho-Fung V, Jaramillo D, et al. Ultrasound of the joints and entheses in healthy children. Pediatr Radiol 2015;45(9):1344–54.

69. Roth J, Stinson SE, Chan J, et al. Differential pattern of Doppler signals at lower-extremity entheses of healthy children. Pediatr Radiol 2019;49(10):1335–43.

70. Macchioni P, Salvarani C, Possemato N, et al. Ultrasonographic and clinical assessment of peripheral enthesitis in patients with psoriatic arthritis, psoriasis, and fibromyalgia syndrome — the ULISSE Study. J Rheumatol 2019;46:904–11.

71. Yanagisawa S, Osawa T, Saito K, et al. Assessment of Osgood-Schlatter disease and the skeletal maturation of the distal attachment of the patellar tendon in pre-adolescent males. Orthop J Sports Med 2014;2(7):2325.

72. Terslev L, Naredo E, Keen HI, et al. The OMERACT stepwise approach to select and develop imaging outcome measurement instruments: the musculoskeletal ultrasound example. J Rheumatol 2019;46(10):1394–400.
73. Tom S, Zhong Y, Cook R, et al. Development of a preliminary ultrasonographic enthesitis score in psoriatic arthritis - GRAPPA Ultrasound Working Group. J Rheumatol 2019;46(4):384–90.
74. Balint PV, Terslev L, Aegerter P, et al, OMERACT Ultrasound Task Force members. Reliability of a consensus-based ultrasound definition and scoring for enthesitis in spondyloarthritis and psoriatic arthritis: an OMERACT US initiative. Ann Rheum Dis 2018;77(12):1730–5.
75. Tse SM, Laxer R, Babyn P, et al. Radiologic improvement of juvenile idiopathic: arthritis-enthesitis-related arthritis following anti-tumor necrosis factor-alpha blockade with etanercept. J Rheumatol 2006;33:1186–8.

Referral/Diagnosis

Classification Criteria in Axial Spondyloarthritis

What Have We Learned; Where Are We Going?

Rhys J. Hayward[a,b], Pedro M. Machado, MD, PhD[a,c,d],*

KEYWORDS

- Axial spondyloarthritis • Ankylosing spondylitis • Classification • Diagnosis
- Back pain • Inflammation • Magnetic resonance imaging • Radiographs

KEY POINTS

- Axial spondyloarthritis (axSpA) is a chronic inflammatory condition that can present with either radiographic changes or without.
- Historically there was the requirement for radiographic changes, whereas the updated classifications incorporate clinical manifestations, family history, response to therapy, MRI, and genetic and laboratory findings.
- Classification criteria have progressed in line with scientific advances incorporating the utility of MRI to identify inflammatory changes to the sacroiliac joint before radiographic changes.
- The ASAS classification criteria are the most relevant criteria set that increase the scope and parameters. They have facilitated SpA research, including epidemiology, outcomes research, and treatment.
- Clinical judgment remains the mainstay for diagnosis of axSpA. Physicians should not misuse classification criteria, avoiding their use before a clinical diagnosis is made.

INTRODUCTION

Spondyloarthritis (SpA) is a generic term for a family of diseases, which can either have a predominantly axial (axial SpA [axSpA]; cardinal manifestation: chronic back pain) or a predominantly peripheral phenotype (peripheral SpA [pSpA]; cardinal manifestation(s): arthritis, enthesitis, or dactylitis). The range of clinical features of SpA is broad

[a] Department of Rheumatology, Northwick Park Hospital, London North West University Healthcare NHS Trust, Watford Road, Harrow, Middlesex HA1 3UJ, London, UK; [b] Department of Rheumatology, University College London Hospitals NHS Foundation Trust, 3rd Floor, 250 Euston Road, NW1 2PG, London, UK; [c] Department of Neuromuscular Diseases, University College London, 1st Floor, Russell Square House, 10-12 Russell Square, WC1B 5EH, London, UK; [d] Centre for Rheumatology, University College London, Room 415, 4th Floor, Rayne Institute, 5 University St, Bloomsbury, London WC1E 6JF
* Corresponding author. Centre for Rheumatology and Department of Neuromuscular Diseases, University College London, 1st Floor, Russell Square House, 10-12 Russell Square, London WC1B 5EH, UK.
E-mail address: p.machado@ucl.ac.uk

Rheum Dis Clin N Am 46 (2020) 263–278
https://doi.org/10.1016/j.rdc.2020.01.008
0889-857X/20/© 2020 Elsevier Inc. All rights reserved.
rheumatic.theclinics.com

and includes chronic (typically inflammatory) back pain, arthritis, enthesitis, dactylitis, as well as extra-articular manifestations (EAMs), such as psoriasis, uveitis, and inflammatory bowel disease (IBD). SpA is associated with the major histocompatibility complex class I human leukocyte antigen-B27 (HLA-B27)[1,2] and axSpA can be further divided into 2 subsets: axSpA with (radiographic axial SpA [r-axSpA] or ankylosing spondylitis [AS]) and without definite radiographic changes in the sacroiliac joints (SIJs) (nonradiographic axial SpA [nr-axSpA]).

SpA encompasses diseases historically designated as AS, psoriatic arthritis (PsA), enteropathic arthritis (IBD-related arthritis), reactive arthritis, arthritis related to uveitis, and a subgroup of juvenile idiopathic arthritis (enthesitis-related arthritis) (**Fig. 1**). For this article we will be focusing on the axial component of the disease. HLA-B27 is present in about 8% in populations of European descent, and the prevalence of axSpA mirrors the prevalence of HLA-B27 in a given population, ranging between 0.3% and 1.4%.[3] The aim of this article is to highlight how diagnosis is evolving and classification of axSpA has changed, including much of the terminology.

DIAGNOSIS AND CLASSIFICATION OF AXIAL SPONDYLOARTHRITIS

The diagnosis of axSpA should be a clinical exercise based on the recognition of a pattern of clinical, laboratory, and imaging features that, taken together, are suggestive of axSpA. This exercise includes the consideration of differential diagnosis. Classification criteria are mainly used for research purposes and intended to create homogenous groups of patients with a certain condition applying a standardized definition. **Fig. 2** gives an historical perspective of SpA classification criteria over time and landmark developments related to the development of new criteria; **Table 1** summarizes the various published criteria.

The modified New York (mNY) criteria for AS[2,4,5] required the presence of radiographic changes at the SIJ.[6] For a very long time, these were primary classification criteria for those patients with inflammatory back pain (IBP) or with limitation of spinal/chest mobility.[7] The main limitation of these criteria is the requirement of definite radiographic changes of the SIJs; the criteria were often applied as diagnostic criteria and this has the very real potential of causing a delay to diagnosis and ultimately treatment. It is known that it can take several years before there is progression from inflammation in the SIJs to clear evidence of radiographic changes. Moreover, a certain

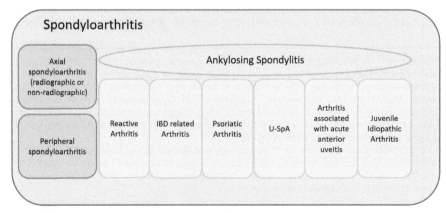

Fig. 1. The spondyloarthritis spectrum. IBD, inflammatory bowel disease; U-SpA, undifferentiated spondyloarthritis.

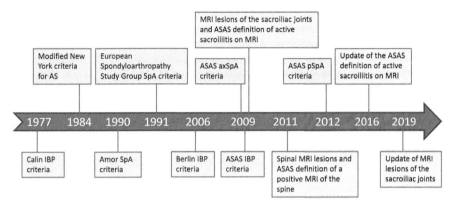

Fig. 2. Development of classification criteria for spondyloarthritis and inflammatory back pain and MRI definitions over time. AS, ankylosing spondylitis; ASAS, Assessment of Spondyloarthritis International Society; axSpA, axial spondyloarthritis; IBP, inflammatory back pain; pSpA, peripheral spondyloarthritis; SpA, spondyloarthritis. (*Data from* Refs.[7,9,10,12,19,20,68–73])

proportion of those with axSpA may never go onto develop definite radiographic damage and therefore, although unequivocally having the clinical characteristics of AS, may never fulfill these criteria.

AXIAL SPONDYLOARTHRITIS: AN HISTORICAL PERSPECTIVE

The mNY criteria for AS[7] were published in 1985. It was a body of work that standardized the classification of AS; the change was to include sacroiliitis grade ≥ 2 bilaterally or sacroiliitis grade 3 unilaterally to define the presence of radiographic sacroiliitis; this was mandatory and clinical presentations alone were not enough. This could be potentially detrimental as radiographic changes may not always be present; moreover, there is also the issue of discrepancies in interpretation of radiographs that can play a role in heterogeneity and further delay of diagnosis. The reliability of SIJ grading is poor, and training makes little impact on improving the reproducibility.[8] Equally the mNY clinical criteria do not take into account the peripheral and EAMs of the disease.

Subsequently, Amor and colleagues[9] developed their criteria. These criteria, however, aim to classify patients within the entirety of the SpA group and are not specific only to the axial disease. Therefore, for the purposes of classifying axSpA they help but are not enough. These criteria use a scoring system, with ≥ 6 being classifiable and ≥ 5 being probable of SpA. Adding a weighting structure is useful but can be seen as arduous. They use an imaging component but only with regard to a definite radiographic change (similar to the mNY criteria), which scores 3 points, the most attainable for a single component. The criteria then highlight a list of potential clinical components with associated scores being: lumbar or dorsal pain during the night, or morning stiffness of lumbar or dorsal spine (1 point); asymmetric oligoarthritis (2 points); buttock pain (1 point); if affecting alternately the right or left buttock (2 points); dactylitis (2 points); enthesitis (2 points); iritis (2 points); nongonococcal urethritis or cervicitis accompanying, or within 1 month before, the onset of arthritis (1 point); presence or history of psoriasis, balanitis, or IBD (2 points); good response to nonsteroidal anti-inflammatory drugs (NSAIDs) in less than 48 hours, or relapse of the pain in less than 48 hours if NSAIDs discontinued (2 points); presence of HLA-B27, of familial history of AS, Reiter syndrome, uveitis, psoriasis, or chronic enterocolopathies (2 points).

Then the European Spondyloarthropathy Study Group (ESSG) developed a criteria set. Their rationale was that there were areas of SpA that were being neglected in the classification, which, ultimately, could help to better categorize patients belonging to the SpA spectrum. They completed a multicenter Europe-wide study identifying the sensitivity and specificity of a wider criteria set. They started with 183 variables but this was narrowed down to 25, then further to the following 7 with the primary criteria being that a patient had to have either IBP or synovitis (asymmetric or predominately lower limbs) and at least 1 of the following, positive family history; IBD; urethritis; cervicitis or acute diarrhea $\leq$1 month before onset of symptoms; alternating buttock pain; enthesopathy; or radiographic sacroiliitis. It is important to note that these criteria can be used for both axSpA and pSpA and is therefore not specific to only axial disease. Diagnosis of sacroiliitis depends on radiographic changes but not inflammatory changes (only visible on MRI). These criteria do not include MRI inflammatory changes to the spine, or for that matter radiographic changes, which could be perceived as a limiting factor. Nevertheless the sensitivity and specificity was comparable with the criteria of Amor and colleagues, with sensitivity 86.7% and 84.8% and specificity 87% and 89.9%, respectively.[10]

In 2009 the term axSpA was created by the Assessment of Spondyloarthritis International Society (ASAS) who went on to create the ASAS classification criteria for axSpA.[11,12] This is the first classification criteria set developed after the introduction of MRI for axial disease.[13] Therefore, one can assume that this concept would reduce the likelihood of their being false negatives based on normal radiographic findings; the set equally increased the positive predictive value of axSpA to 93.3%.[14] As there have been no further developments or new introductions of other criteria, from here on we will look into the use of this criteria set in more detail. It is important to emphasize again at this stage that classification criteria are not diagnostic; clinical reasoning can and should always supersede fitting patients into a particular classification structure.[15] The gold standard for diagnosis would still fall on the clinician to incorporate all the patient information, including laboratory, imaging, and clinical findings to complete the diagnosis.[16]

The ASAS criteria have 2 arms from which a classification can be made, an imaging and a clinical arm. In the imaging arm, the presence of MRI inflammation, which plays an important role in the rheumatologist's judgment to make a diagnosis of axial SpA, is a prominent factor, together with the classical presence of radiographic sacroiliitis. However, not all patients with axSpA have sacroiliitis on imaging (eg, in the validation study of the ASAS criteria,[12] 25% of the patients did not have radiographic or MRI evidence of sacroiliitis), underscoring that in clinical practice the rheumatologist bases his decision also on many other clinical and laboratory features, and that a diagnosis of axSpA can be made in the absence of sacroiliitis on imaging, including MRI sacroiliitis/inflammation.[17] The clinical arm was intended for use where there was no imaging available (or where imaging is negative)[18] and one therefore cannot assume or prove radiographic or inflammatory changes of the SIJs. Because of the strong association of sacroiliitis with axSpA, and because of high sensitivity and specificity, if sacroiliitis is present on imaging, only 1 other SpA feature needs to be present to classify a patient as having axSpA according to the ASAS criteria, whereas 2 additional features are required in the HLA-B27/clinical arm.[12] The features and requirements of each arm are listed in **Table 1**.

The new criteria for axSpA can be applied in patients with back pain for longer than 3 months with an onset before the age of 45 years.[11,12] Of note, chronic back pain, not necessarily being IBP, is present as an entry criterion, reflecting that, in clinical practice, patients with noninflammatory chronic back pain may represent up to 20% to

Table 1
Published classification criteria for spondyloarthritis[a]

	Entry criterion:	Imaging criterion:	Clinical criteria:
mNY criteria for AS	Imaging criterion plus ≥1 clinical criterion	Radiographic sacroiliitis[b]	• Low back pain and stiffness for more than 3 mo that improves with exercise, but is not relieved by rest • Limitation of motion of the lumbar spine in the sagittal and frontal planes • Limitation of chest expansion relative to normal values correlated for age and sex
Amor[9] criteria for SpA	Sum of points of items below must be ≥6; a sum of points ≥5 classifies for probable SpA	Radiographic sacroiliitis[b] (3 points)	• Lumbar or dorsal pain during the night, or morning stiffness of lumbar or dorsal spine (1 point) • Asymmetric oligoarthritis (2 points) • Buttock pain (1 point), if affecting alternately the right or the left buttock (2 points) • Dactylitis (2 points) • Enthesitis (2 points) • Iritis (2 points) • Nongonococcal urethritis or cervicitis accompanying, or within 1 mo before, the onset of arthritis (1 point) • Acute diarrhea accompanying, or within 1 mo before, the onset of arthritis (1 point) • Presence or history of psoriasis, balanitis, or IBD (Crohn's/ulcerative colitis) (2 points) • Good response to NSAIDs in <48 h, or relapse of the pain in <48 h if NSAIDs discontinued (2 points) • Presence of HLA-B27, or familial history of AS, Reiter syndrome, uveitis, psoriasis, or chronic enterocolopathies (2 points)
ESSG criteria for SpA	IBP (modified Calin)[20] or synovitis (asymmetric or predominantly in the lower limbs), and ≥1 clinical or radiological criterion	Radiographic sacroiliitis[b]	• Buttock pain alternating between right and left gluteal areas • Urethritis, cervicitis, or acute diarrhea within 1 mo before arthritis • IBD • Psoriasis • Positive family history

(continued on next page)

Table 1
(continued)

ASCBPAS criteria for axSpA	CBP (≥3 mo) with an onset <45 y of age and:	(a) Imaging criterion plus >1 the clinical criteria or	Radiographic sacroiliitis[b] or MRI sacroiliitis[c]	• IBP (ASAS)[68] • Arthritis • Enthesitis (heel) • Uveitis • Dactylitis • Psoriasis • Crohn's/ulcerative colitis • Increased CRP • Good response to NSAIDs • Family history of SpA • HLA-B27
		(b) Positive HLA-B27 plus ≥2 other clinical criteria		
ASAS criteria for pSpA	Peripheral arthritis, enthesitis, or dactylitis and:	(a) Imaging criterion or ≥1 clinical SpA feature from group A or	Radiographic sacroiliitis[b] or MRI sacroiliitis[c]	Group A • Uveitis • Psoriasis • Crohn's/ulcerative colitis • Preceding infection • HLA-B27 Group B • Arthritis • Enthesitis • Dactylitis • IBP ever (ASAS)[68] • Family history for SpA
		(b) ≥2 other clinical SpA features from group B		

Abbreviations: AS, ankylosing spondylitis; ASAS, assessment of spondyloarthritis international society; axSpA, axial spondyloarthritis; CBP, chronic back pain; CRP, C-reactive protein; ESSG, European Spondyloarthropathy Study Group; HLA, human leukocyte antigen; IBD, inflammatory bowel disease; IBP, inflammatory back pain; mNY, modified New York; MRI, magnetic resonance imaging; NSAIDs, nonsteroidal anti-inflammatory drugs; pSpA, peripheral spondyloarthritis; SpA, spondyloarthritis.

[a] Please note that the definition of IBP and some SpA features varies between different criteria sets; for details please consult the original publications.

[b] Defined as radiographic sacroiliitis grade ≥2 bilaterally or grade 3 to 4 unilaterally: grade 0 = normal; grade 1 = suspicious changes; grade 2 = minimum abnormality (small localized areas with erosion or sclerosis, without alteration in the joint width); grade 3 = unequivocal abnormality (moderate or advanced sacroiliitis with erosions, evidence of sclerosis, widening, narrowing, or partial ankyloses); grade 4 = severe abnormality (total ankyloses).

[c] Defined as bone marrow edema (short tau inversion recovery sequence) or osteitis (T1 postgadolinium sequence) highly suggestive of SpA, clearly present and located in the typical anatomic areas (subchondral or periarticular bone marrow): if there is only one signal (lesion) per MRI slice suggesting active inflammation, the lesion should be present on at least 2 consecutive slices; if there is more than one signal (lesion) on a single slice, one slice may be sufficient.

Data from Refs.[9,20,68]

30% of patients with axSpA, whereas IBP can be observed in 20% to 25% of patients with noninflammatory (mechanical) causes of chronic back pain.[19–21] Detailed analysis in the ASAS axSpA validation study also demonstrated that IBP as an entry criterion did not perform better than chronic back pain.[12] However, the presence of IBP is an important symptom that should prompt further diagnostic tests for axSpA. Age is also an important factor in the entry criteria, reflecting that complaints associated with axSpA usually start in the second or third decade of life, and by the age of 45 years, more than 95% of patients are symptomatic.[22] Importantly, evidence suggests that disease activity, comorbidities, and treatment responses are similar for nr-axSpA and r-axSpA.[23]

A CRITICAL VIEW OF THE COMPONENTS OF THE ASSESSMENT OF SPONDYLOARTHRITIS INTERNATIONAL SOCIETY CLASSIFICATION CRITERIA FOR AXIAL SPONDYLOARTHRITIS

Under the imaging arm it is first prudent to consider the aspects of positivity. The primary issue being a low interrater and intrarater reliability of radiograph interpretation.[24] Within the skein of MRI interpretation it is important to consider the impact of mechanical elements on an interpretation of sacroiliitis suggestive of axSpA. Bone marrow edema (BMO)/osteitis is not unique to inflammatory conditions, it has been shown to be present in postpartum women (with and without pelvic pain), cleaning staff, long distance runners, soldiers, athletes, and healthy individuals.[25–28] However, differences in the level of BMO of the axSpA group compared with the mechanical group have been reported, with axSpA having a tendency to higher levels of inflammation and presence of erosions, ankylosis, and fat infiltration. The misinterpretation of inflammation has been explored further with extensive and intermediate inflammation having a higher odds ratio of developing erosions at the SIJ after 4 years,[29] leading to the conclusion that limited BMO may be due to transient mechanical force, but extensive BMO seems to have a higher correlation to pathologic changes. With extensive changes having more than 1 cm depth of inflammation.

The performance of MRI in the diagnosis of axSpA was recently systematically reviewed by Jones and colleagues.[30] The authors found that, at the SIJ level, BMO is the most sensitive and specific individual lesion. Structural lesions, including fat deposition, have moderate sensitivity and specificity, whereas erosions demonstrate good specificity but relatively poor sensitivity (with the caveat that some of the studies used high fixed specify values, which may have added a negative impact on sensitivity values). Combination of BMO and erosions, or BMO and fat deposition, yielded higher sensitivity and specificity than BMO alone. Predefined numbers of lesions or cutoffs have also been analyzed and suggest that BMO in ≥ 3 quadrants and erosions in ≥ 3 quadrants show high sensitivity and specificity and the presence of 3 to 5 fatty lesions also yield good sensitivity. However, further studies are required to validate these findings. In the spine, studies investigating the value of corner inflammatory lesions found moderate sensitivity and specificity, whereas spinal fatty lesions were found to have relatively poor sensitivity and specificity. Although the results suggest that spinal lesions alone are unlikely to have sufficient diagnostic performance for use in axSpA, these lesions might be useful in combination with features identified on SIJ MRI (an area that requires further research).

The systematic literature review by Jones and colleagues[30] served as evidence to support recommendations for acquisition and interpretation of MRI of the spine and SIJs in the assessment of patients with suspected axSpA,[31] including recommended sequences, anatomic coverage, acquisition parameters, and interpretation of active and structural MRI lesions. The full list of recommendations can be found in the article but 2 key messages should be highlighted (1) imaging cannot be viewed in isolation and needs to be interpreted in the context of clinical presentation and results of laboratory investigations and (2) the full range and combination of active and structural lesions of the SIJs and spine should be taken into account when deciding if the MRI scan is suggestive of axSpA or not (ie, contextual interpretation of active and structural lesions is key to enhancing diagnostic utility of MRI is patients with suspected axSpA).

HLA-B27 positivity is given a high level of weighting in the classification of axSpA according to ASAS; however, due to it requiring 2 SpA features and imaging only requiring 1 feature, imaging takes precedence. This is further reflected as there is also an increased prevalence of HLA-B27 in the r-axSpA group compared with the nr-axSpA group.[32,33] HLA-B27 is positive in 85% to 95% of patients with r-axSpA and in 75% to 85% of patients with nr-axSpA.[34–36]

One classification feature of SpA is a positive family history of the disease. The question here is what is the relevance? If we have further information already, such as HLA-B27 status, does a family history assist our diagnosis further? Which SpA feature is more relevant to a diagnosis of axSpA? Van Lunteren and colleagues[37] looked at 3 cohorts of patients with axSpA to identify if a family history was relevant if the HLA-B27 status was known. They found that there was no consensus across all 3 groups. A family history of AS was relevant in the ASAS cohort but not in the *DEvenir des Spondyloarthropathies Indifferenciees Recentes* ([DESIR] a longitudinal French cohort, including patients aged 18–50 years with IBP)[38] or the European SPondyloArthritis Caught Early ([SPACE] an inception cohort, including patients aged $\geq$16 years with chronic back pain from the Netherlands, Italy, Norway, or Sweden)[39] cohorts; equally, family history of acute anterior uveitis (AAU) was associated with a diagnosis in the SPACE cohort but not the ASAS or DESIR groups. This indicates that HLA-B27 has a greater relation to a positive diagnosis of axSpA than a positive family history does.

Further work into a positive family history has tried to identify which diagnosis in the SpA family has a greater probability of association with axSpA.[16] A positive correlation was seen between a family history of AS or anterior uveitis, when correlated with HLA-B27 status. Reactive arthritis, IBD, or psoriasis did not contribute to a diagnosis of axSpA. Therefore, when considering family history as a positive SpA feature to cement the patient's diagnosis, it would seem that there is a hierarchy to consider. There also seems to be some evidence that using HLA-B27 status, if known, is more useful.[16]

An increased C-reactive protein (CRP) is an important component. CRP can be increased in up to 40% of patients with axSpA, and is more frequently increased in patients with r-axSpA than in patients with nr-axSpA.[40] Therefore, its sensitivity in axSpA can be, and has been questioned.[34] However, a positive CRP is one of the associated risk factors for developing radiographic progression.[6] CRP is also a component of the Ankylosing Spondylitis Disease Activity Score, a composite measure of disease activity.[41–43] On the basis that there is less positivity in nr-axSpA than r-axSpA and a higher distribution of women in the nr-axSpA group than in the r-axSpA group,[18] is this a case where women with the disease tend to have lower CRP's than men? If so, it raises the question, when incorporating CRP in the classification criteria, that there will be a higher CRP in the r-axSpA group than in the nr-axSpA group.

Dactylitis is a component that can increase the susceptibility of axSpA and can occur as a peripheral manifestation. The ESPeranza cohort, a cohort of patients from Spain, assessed the frequency of dactylitis within the SpA group and found an incidence of 9.5%.[44] This is slightly higher than those found in the SPACE cohort.[39] Although dactylitis is associated with peripheral SpA it has been identified that 15% of all patients who had a diagnosis of dactylitis had axial and not peripheral SpA.[44]

Enthesitis is another peripheral manifestation that has been highlighted as an aspect contributing to classification; it is a straightforward component to assess in the clinic. The ASAS classification criteria only include enthesitis in the heel with their criteria, and do not include others; this has been further supported with work by Ozsoy-Unubol and Yagci[45] who completed ultrasound assessments on 9 enthesitis points in a range of patients with axSpA and mechanical back pain. Their assessment was of Achilles tendon; plantar fascia; patella tendon, distal and proximal; quadriceps; tibialis anterior; triceps; common flexor tendon, and the common extensor tendon. They identified that the most common site for power Doppler signal and calcification (a finding with diagnostic value[46]) was the Achilles and patella tendon, with actually the distal and proximal patella tendon having the highest incidence in the axSpA group. The issue, however, is that these patellar areas also showed the highest incidences in the mechanical back pain group, whereas enthesitis of the Achilles tendon was prevalent in 40% of the axSpA group but was only present in 6.7% of the mechanical back pain group. This highlights many things: primarily that enthesitis can be inflammatory or mechanical; therefore enthesitis in isolation should be viewed with caution because this could be a mechanical cause from changes in activity or exercise loads, and that enthesitis at the patella, as long as not mechanical, can add significance to the diagnosis of axSpA.

The other issue is one of concomitant fibromyalgia. Areas of enthesitis that are assessed in axSpA are similar to the pain point areas assessed when considering a diagnosis of fibromyalgia[47]; therefore, multiple positive "enthesitis" sites on a patient should be assessed with caution for what could be an underlying fibromyalgia, which can have similarities to the presentation of axSpA.[48–51] The use of ultrasonography for assessment of enthesitis may reduce the number of false positives of clinical identification of pain without a pathologic condition in the tendon.[52] However, it is recognized that not every facility will have access to an ultrasound assessment in clinic and instead will need to wait for a radiology review, which could further delay the diagnostic work up.

Uveitis is also an SpA feature, in this case an EAM; up to 33% of patients with axSpA will develop uveitis,[53] 50% of those who have suffered with uveitis will go onto develop recurrent disease.[54] Uveitis can be classified as infectious, noninfectious (associated with axSpA), or masquerade.[55] The standardization of uveitis is then descriptive of anatomic location being anterior, intermediate, posterior, or panuveitis.[56] It has been shown that 85% of uveitis in patients with SpA is anterior.[57] The other aspects to uveitis that make it so useful to assist with classification is that the age of onset is between 20 and 59 years[58]; although this is higher than that for axSpA it is similar and therefore one could assume that they can go together at both diagnosis and within the clinical follow-up setting. Interestingly, HLA-B27-positive uveitis presents as a nongranulomatous AAU[59]; this has led to the development of studies to identify those patients with AAU and HLA-B27 positivity to try and identify if they have an underlying axSpA.[60]

There is a close association between SpA and IBD. There is a growing body of evidence that suggests that the IBD profile and that of SpA are in fact one and the same.[61–63] The reason for this could be that the gut is the primary interaction site between the host immune system and microorganisms.[62] The "trigger" of axSpA could be that following inflammation in the gut there is a change to the adaptive immune system and that the new "normal" of antibody status has changed from that previously accepted, therefore triggering an autoimmune response.[64] Both diseases also share the HLA-B27 antigen, which is why 6.5% of SpA patients will develop IBD within 5 years from diagnosis, and 30% of patients with IBD will develop SpA.[64] In addition, synovial T cells could be developed from the gut because the same macrophages have been found in the gut as in the synovium.[63] Clearly these 2 conditions overlap a great deal and should each be taken into consideration when diagnosing and managing the other, particularly because 46.2% of patients with SpA without bowel symptoms or disease had inflammation in the bowel on colonoscopy.[65]

The link between psoriasis and the SpA spectrum is clear.[66] The question is the relevance of psoriasis in axial disease. Is it a different pathology to psoriatic spondylitis? Is axSpA the axial involvement one of the manifestations of a peripheral disease? There is currently no widely accepted definition of axial involvement in PsA. Although there might be differences in efficacy of certain drugs/mechanisms of action for peripheral and axial manifestations of the disease, ASAS and the Group for Research and Assessment of Psoriasis and Psoriatic Arthritis have agreed to develop a consensus definition of axial involvement in PsA to be used for research purposes. Such a definition will serve primarily as a classification tool to be applied to patients with clinically diagnosed PsA to build a homogeneous group of patients for inclusion in noninterventional or interventional studies.

THE CLASSIFICATION OF AXIAL SPONDYLOARTHRITIS INCEPTION COHORT STUDY

In October 2013, after a 2-day meeting of the Arthritis Advisory Committee, a panel of experts who make recommendations to the US Food and Drug Administration (FDA), the FDA rejected the application by 2 manufacturers of tumor necrosis factor blockers (adalimumab and certolizumab) for the treatment of nr-axSpA. One of the reasons was concern from the FDA regarding the specificity of the ASAS axSpA classification criteria when erroneously used for diagnostic purposes. This has led to a delay in US regulatory approval for nr-axSpA compared with the EMA (first EMA approval in 2012; first FDA approval in 2019, after the conduct of new phase 3 clinical trials for nr-axSpA recommended by the FDA).

In 2017, a meta-analysis showed that the ASAS axSpA criteria performed well in patients included in 7 cohorts from various geographic areas.[67] The meta-analysis included 4990 patients in total, generating a very high pooled sensitivity and specificity (82% and 87%, respectively) for the axSpA criteria, with little variation across studies. The pooled sensitivity of the imaging arm ($\pm$ clinical arm) and clinical arm ($\pm$ imaging arm) was 57% and 49%, respectively (26% and 23% when considering patients fulfilling each arm exclusively). High estimates of pooled specificity were found for both arms, irrespective of the definition (range, 92%–97%). However, the positive likelihood ratio of the imaging arm only was higher when compared with the clinical arm only (9.6 vs 3.6). It should be noted that the criteria's performance also depends on the prevalence of SpA in the underlying population (pretest probability).

Despite these results, the validity of the ASAS axSpA criteria has been questioned. Hence, there has been the development of the classification of axial spondyloarthritis inception cohort study (NCT03993847). This is aimed at identifying the current sensitivity and specificity of the classification criteria worldwide. This longitudinal study is aiming to recruit 500 patients from North America (a minimum of 300 from the United States) and 500 from outside North America. It is an inception cohort wherein those patients referred to rheumatology with undiagnosed back pain of $\geq$3 months duration with onset $\leq$45 years will be recruited. The primary objective of the trial is to validate the performance of the current ASAS classification criteria; if a specificity of $\geq$90% and a sensitivity of ≥75% of the original ASAS criteria will be found in the study, the ASAS criteria will be considered validated and no further analyses will be done. Only if the primary objective is not met, will refinements of the criteria be made and tested. A secondary objective is to identify confidence in ascertainment of (active) sacroiliitis by MRI. The tertiary outcome is to determine the predictive value of the criteria over a 5-year follow-up period.

SUMMARY

This review aimed to highlight issues about the diagnosis and classification of axSpA, namely the issue of over diagnosis; how mechanical factors can play a large role in altered imaging on MRI that could alter the outcome of the imaging arm. In addition, we have highlighted that caution should be used when considering certain components of the criteria to classify the disease, especially under the clinical arm. For example, although clearly enthesitis has its place and, when used appropriately, it can alter the clinician's decision, it has been shown that the exact weighting of this should be carefully considered.

We are working in a time when medical advances mean that both assessment and treatment are continually progressing. If one treatment is not efficacious there are a wider range of alternative treatment options and less barriers, as these become more financially competitive. Therefore, we must be clear that the correct diagnosis has been made and that we, as clinicians, are not "jumping" to an incorrect diagnosis through poorly understood or misinterpreted findings as diagnostics. This is a time to be excited about, but also cautious with, the progress in identifying and diagnosing, this complex and often missed spectrum of diseases, particularly in a time when there are more Allied Health Professionals (AHPs) working in primary and secondary care and will be instrumental in the diagnosis of such conditions.

In the future in this condition, work should be carried out to further educate health care providers about SpA and its features, and how the specificity of imaging can impact diagnosis and what role EAMs play in this. The diagnosis of axSpA is a clinical diagnosis and classification criteria are not aimed to be diagnostic tools. The split between r-axSpA and nr-axSpA is artificial and we should move toward the unifying concept of axSpA. Our understanding of genetics, biomarkers, and immunopathophenotypes will drive further refinement of axSpA classification criteria.

It is important that we diagnose this potentially disabling condition early. What should be developed is a way to stratify these patients into the correct diagnosis. That could, and should, include further identification of the susceptibility of the condition within the broader hospital setting and those clinicians assessing and diagnosing those patients with SpA features, such as dermatology, gastroenterology, and ophthalmology, to have a lower threshold for referring their patients for an opinion from rheumatology if they present with chronic spinal/buttock pain. Equally in primary care more attention should be sought to identify those patients with other clinical manifestations and raising awareness to their care providers; whether this be General Practitioners or the ever growing and developing role of AHPs fulfilling these roles in the community.

ACKNOWLEDGMENTS

P.M. Machado is supported by the National Institute for Health Research (NIHR) University College London Hospitals NHS Foundation Trust (UCLH) Biomedical Research Centre (BRC). The views expressed are those of the authors and not necessarily those of the (UK) National Health Service (NHS), the NIHR, or the (UK) Department of Health.

DISCLOSURE

R.J. Hayward has nothing to disclose. P.M. Machado has received consulting/speaker's fees from Abbvie, BMS, Celgene, Eli Lilly, Janssen, MSD, Novartis, Pfizer, Roche, and UCB.

REFERENCES

1. Sieper J, Poddubnyy D. Axial spondyloarthritis. Lancet 2017;390(10089):73–84.
2. van Tubergen A, Weber U. Diagnosis and classification in spondyloarthritis: identifying a chameleon. Nat Rev Rheumatol 2012;8(5):253–61.
3. Stolwijk C, van Onna M, Boonen A, et al. Global prevalence of spondyloarthritis: a systematic review and meta-regression analysis. Arthritis Care Res (Hoboken) 2016;68(9):1320–31.
4. Dubreuil M, Deodhar AA. Axial spondyloarthritis classification criteria: the debate continues. Curr Opin Rheumatol 2017;29(4):317–22.
5. Proft F, Poddubnyy D. Ankylosing spondylitis and axial spondyloarthritis: recent insights and impact of new classification criteria. Ther Adv Musculoskelet Dis 2018;10(5–6):129–39.
6. Malaviya AN, Rawat R, Agrawal N, et al. The nonradiographic axial spondyloarthritis, the radiographic axial spondyloarthritis, and ankylosing spondylitis: the tangled skein of rheumatology. Int J Rheumatol 2017;2017:1824794.
7. van der Linden S, Valkenburg HA, Cats A. Evaluation of diagnostic criteria for ankylosing spondylitis. A proposal for modification of the New York criteria. Arthritis Rheum 1984;27(4):361–8.
8. van Tubergen A, Heuft-Dorenbosch L, Schulpen G, et al. Radiographic assessment of sacroiliitis by radiologists and rheumatologists: does training improve quality? Ann Rheum Dis 2003;62(6):519–25.
9. Amor B, Dougados M, Mijiyawa M. Criteria of the classification of spondylarthropathies. Rev Rhum Mal Osteoartic 1990;57(2):85–9 [in French].
10. Dougados M, van der Linden S, Juhlin R, et al. The European Spondylarthropathy Study Group preliminary criteria for the classification of spondylarthropathy. Arthritis Rheum 1991;34(10):1218–27.
11. Rudwaleit M, Landewé R, van der Heijde D, et al. The development of Assessment of SpondyloArthritis International Society classification criteria for axial spondyloarthritis (part I): classification of paper patients by expert opinion including uncertainty appraisal. Ann Rheum Dis 2009;68(6):770–6.
12. Rudwaleit M, van der Heijde D, Landewé R, et al. The development of Assessment of SpondyloArthritis International Society classification criteria for axial spondyloarthritis (part II): validation and final selection. Ann Rheum Dis 2009; 68(6):777–83.
13. Bakker P, Molto A, Etcheto A, et al. The performance of different classification criteria sets for spondyloarthritis in the worldwide ASAS-COMOSPA study. Arthritis Res Ther 2017;19(1):96.
14. Sepriano A, Landewé R, van der Heijde D, et al. Predictive validity of the ASAS classification criteria for axial and peripheral spondyloarthritis after follow-up in the ASAS cohort: a final analysis. Ann Rheum Dis 2016;75(6):1034–42.

15. Deodhar A, Strand V, Kay J, et al. The term 'non-radiographic axial spondyloar- thritis' is much more important to classify than to diagnose patients with axial spondyloarthritis. Ann Rheum Dis 2016;75(5):791–4.

16. Ez-Zaitouni Z, Hilkens A, Gossec L, et al. Is the current ASAS expert definition of a positive family history useful in identifying axial spondyloarthritis? Results from the SPACE and DESIR cohorts. Arthritis Res Ther 2017;19(1):118.

17. van der Heijde D, Rudwaleit M, Landewe RB, et al. Justification for including MRI as a tool in the diagnosis of axial SpA. Nat Rev Rheumatol 2010;6(11):670–2.

18. Ghosh N, Ruderman EM. Nonradiographic axial spondyloarthritis: clinical and therapeutic relevance. Arthritis Res Ther 2017;19(1):286.

19. Rudwaleit M, Metter A, Listing J, et al. Inflammatory back pain in ankylosing spondylitis: a reassessment of the clinical history for application as classification and diagnostic criteria. Arthritis Rheum 2006;54(2):569–78.

20. Calin A, Porta J, Fries JF, et al. Clinical history as a screening test for ankylosing spondylitis. JAMA 1977;237(24):2613–4.

21. Rudwaleit M, van der Heijde D, Khan MA, et al. How to diagnose axial spondy- loarthritis early. Ann Rheum Dis 2004;63(5):535–43.

22. van den Berg R, van der Heijde DM. How should we diagnose spondyloarthritis according to the ASAS classification criteria: a guide for practicing physicians. Pol Arch Med Wewn 2010;120(11):452–7.

23. Zhao SS, Ermann J, Xu C, et al. Comparison of comorbidities and treatment be- tween ankylosing spondylitis and non-radiographic axial spondyloarthritis in the United States. Rheumatology (Oxford) 2019;58(11):2025–30.

24. Molto A, Gossec L, Lefèvre-Colau MM, et al. Evaluation of the performances of 'typical' imaging abnormalities of axial spondyloarthritis: results of the cross- sectional ILOS-DESIR study. RMD Open 2019;5(1):e000918.

25. Seven S, Østergaard M, Morsel-Carlsen L, et al. MRI lesions in the sacroiliac joints for differentiation of patients with axial spondyloarthritis from postpartum women, patients with disc herniation, cleaning staff, long distance runners and healthy persons—a prospective cross-sectional study of 204 participants. Arthritis Rheumatol 2019;71(12):2034–46.

26. de Winter J, de Hooge M, van de Sande M, et al. Magnetic resonance imaging of the sacroiliac joints indicating sacroiliitis according to the assessment of spondy- loarthritis international society definition in healthy individuals, runners, and women with postpartum back pain. Arthritis Rheumatol 2018;70(7):1042–8.

27. Varkas G, de Hooge M, Renson T, et al. Effect of mechanical stress on magnetic resonance imaging of the sacroiliac joints: assessment of military recruits by magnetic resonance imaging study. Rheumatology (Oxford) 2018;57(3):588.

28. Weber U, Jurik AG, Zejden A, et al. Frequency and anatomic distribution of mag- netic resonance imaging features in the sacroiliac joints of young athletes: exploring "background noise" toward a data-driven definition of sacroiliitis in early spondyloarthritis. Arthritis Rheumatol 2018;70(5):736–45.

29. Arnbak B, Jensen TS, Schiottz-Christensen B, et al. What level of inflammation leads to structural damage in the sacroiliac joints? A four-year magnetic reso- nance imaging follow-up study of low back pain patients. Arthritis Rheumatol 2019;71(12):2027–33.

30. Jones A, Bray TJP, Mandl P, et al. Performance of magnetic resonance imaging in the diagnosis of axial spondyloarthritis: a systematic literature review. Rheuma- tology (Oxford) 2019;58(11):1955–65.

31. Bray TJP, Jones A, Bennett AN, et al. Recommendations for acquisition and interpretation of MRI of the spine and sacroiliac joints in the diagnosis of axial spondyloarthritis in the UK. Rheumatology (Oxford) 2019;58(10):1831–8.

32. Song IH, Weiß A, Hermann KG, et al. Similar response rates in patients with ankylosing spondylitis and non-radiographic axial spondyloarthritis after 1 year of treatment with etanercept: results from the ESTHER trial. Ann Rheum Dis 2013; 72(6):823–5.

33. Chimenti MS, Conigliaro P, Navarini L, et al. Demographic and clinical differences between ankylosing spondylitis and non-radiographic axial spondyloarthritis: results from a multicentre retrospective study in the Lazio region of Italy. Clin Exp Rheumatol 2019;38(1):88–93.

34. Kiltz U, Baraliakos X, Karakostas P, et al. Do patients with non-radiographic axial spondylarthritis differ from patients with ankylosing spondylitis? Arthritis Care Res (Hoboken) 2012;64(9):1415–22.

35. Mathieu A, Paladini F, Vacca A, et al. The interplay between the geographic distribution of HLA-B27 alleles and their role in infectious and autoimmune diseases: a unifying hypothesis. Autoimmun Rev 2009;8(5):420–5.

36. Sieper J, van der Heijde D. Review: Nonradiographic axial spondyloarthritis: new definition of an old disease? Arthritis Rheum 2013;65(3):543–51.

37. van Lunteren M, van der Heijde D, Sepriano A, et al. Is a positive family history of spondyloarthritis relevant for diagnosing axial spondyloarthritis once HLA-B27 status is known? Rheumatology (Oxford) 2019;58(9):1649–54.

38. Dougados M, d'Agostino MA, Benessiano J, et al. The DESIR cohort: a 10-year follow-up of early inflammatory back pain in France: study design and baseline characteristics of the 708 recruited patients. Joint Bone Spine 2011;78(6): 598–603.

39. van den Berg R, de Hooge M, van Gaalen F, et al. Percentage of patients with spondyloarthritis in patients referred because of chronic back pain and performance of classification criteria: experience from the Spondyloarthritis Caught Early (SPACE) cohort. Rheumatology (Oxford) 2013;52(8):1492–9.

40. Rudwaleit M, Haibel H, Baraliakos X, et al. The early disease stage in axial spondylarthritis: results from the German Spondyloarthritis Inception Cohort. Arthritis Rheum 2009;60(3):717–27.

41. Machado PM, Landewe R, Heijde DV. Assessment of SpondyloArthritis international S. Ankylosing Spondylitis Disease Activity Score (ASDAS): 2018 update of the nomenclature for disease activity states. Ann Rheum Dis 2018;77(10): 1539–40.

42. Machado P, Landewe R. Spondyloarthritis: is it time to replace BASDAI with ASDAS? Nat Rev Rheumatol 2013;9(7):388–90.

43. Machado P, Landewe R, Lie E, et al. Ankylosing Spondylitis Disease Activity Score (ASDAS): defining cut-off values for disease activity states and improvement scores. Ann Rheum Dis 2011;70(1):47–53.

44. Tévar-Sánchez MI, Navarro-Compán V, Aznar JJ, et al. Prevalence and characteristics associated with dactylitis in patients with early spondyloarthritis: results from the ESPeranza cohort. Clin Exp Rheumatol 2018;36(5):879–83.

45. Ozsoy-Unubol T, Yagci I. Is ultrasonographic enthesitis evaluation helpful for diagnosis of non-radiographic axial spondyloarthritis? Rheumatol Int 2018; 38(11):2053–61.

46. Eder L, Barzilai M, Peled N, et al. The use of ultrasound for the assessment of enthesitis in patients with spondyloarthritis. Clin Radiol 2013;68(3):219–23.

47. Wolfe F, Clauw DJ, Fitzcharles MA, et al. 2016 revisions to the 2010/2011 fibromy-algia diagnostic criteria. Semin Arthritis Rheum 2016;46(3):319–29.

48. Almodovar R, Carmona L, Zarco P, et al. Fibromyalgia in patients with ankylosing spondylitis: prevalence and utility of the measures of activity, function and radio-logical damage. Clin Exp Rheumatol 2010;28(6 Suppl 63):S33–9.

49. Roussou E, Ciurtin C. Clinical overlap between fibromyalgia tender points and en-thesitis sites in patients with spondyloarthritis who present with inflammatory back pain. Clin Exp Rheumatol 2012;30(6 Suppl 74):24–30.

50. Salaffi F, De Angelis R, Carotti M, et al. Fibromyalgia in patients with axial spon-dyloarthritis: epidemiological profile and effect on measures of disease activity. Rheumatol Int 2014;34(8):1103–10.

51. Dougados M, Logeart I, Szumski A, et al. Evaluation of whether extremely high enthesitis or Bath Ankylosing Spondylitis Disease Activity Index (BASDAI) scores suggest fibromyalgia and confound the anti-TNF response in early non-radiographic axial spondyloarthritis. Clin Exp Rheumatol 2017;35:50–3. Suppl 105(3).

52. Gandjbakhch F, Terslev L, Joshua F, et al. Ultrasound in the evaluation of enthe-sitis: status and perspectives. Arthritis Res Ther 2011;13(6):R188.

53. Bacchiega ABS, Balbi GGM, Ochtrop MLG, et al. Ocular involvement in patients with spondyloarthritis. Rheumatology (Oxford) 2017;56(12):2060–7.

54. Zeboulon N, Dougados M, Gossec L. Prevalence and characteristics of uveitis in the spondyloarthropathies: a systematic literature review. Ann Rheum Dis 2008; 67(7):955–9.

55. Okada AA, Jabs DA. The standardization of uveitis nomenclature project: the future is here. JAMA Ophthalmol 2013;131(6):787–9.

56. Jabs DA, Nussenblatt RB, Rosenbaum JT, et al. Standardization of uveitis nomen-clature for reporting clinical data. Results of the First International Workshop. Am J Ophthalmol 2005;140(3):509–16.

57. Gritz DC, Wong IG. Incidence and prevalence of uveitis in Northern California; the Northern California Epidemiology of Uveitis Study. Ophthalmology 2004;111(3): 491–500 [discussion: 500].

58. Pasadhika S, Rosenbaum JT. Update on the use of systemic biologic agents in the treatment of noninfectious uveitis. Biologics 2014;8:67–81.

59. Biggioggero M, Crotti C, Becciolini A, et al. The management of acute anterior uveitis complicating spondyloarthritis: present and future. Biomed Res Int 2018;2018:9460187.

60. O'Rourke M, Haroon M, Alfarasy S, et al. The effect of anterior uveitis and previ-ously undiagnosed spondyloarthritis: results from the DUET cohort. J Rheumatol 2017;44(9):1347–54.

61. Scarpa R, del Puente A, D'Arienzo A, et al. The arthritis of ulcerative colitis: clin-ical and genetic aspects. J Rheumatol 1992;19(3):373–7.

62. Round JL, Mazmanian SK. The gut microbiota shapes intestinal immune re-sponses during health and disease. Nat Rev Immunol 2009;9(5):313–23.

63. Baeten D, Demetter P, Cuvelier CA, et al. Macrophages expressing the scav-enger receptor CD163: a link between immune alterations of the gut and synovial inflammation in spondyloarthropathy. J Pathol 2002;196(3):343–50.

64. Asquith M, Elewaut D, Lin P, et al. The role of the gut and microbes in the path-ogenesis of spondyloarthritis. Best Pract Res Clin Rheumatol 2014;28(5): 687–702.

65. Van Praet L, Van den Bosch FE, Jacques P, et al. Microscopic gut inflammation in axial spondyloarthritis: a multiparametric predictive model. Ann Rheum Dis 2013; 72(3):414–7.
66. Leung YY, Ogdie A, Orbai AM, et al. Classification and outcome measures for psoriatic arthritis. Front Med (Lausanne) 2018;5:246.
67. Sepriano A, Rubio R, Ramiro S, et al. Performance of the ASAS classification criteria for axial and peripheral spondyloarthritis: a systematic literature review and meta-analysis. Ann Rheum Dis 2017;76(5):886–90.
68. Sieper J, van der Heijde D, Landewe R, et al. New criteria for inflammatory back pain in patients with chronic back pain: a real patient exercise by experts from the Assessment of SpondyloArthritis international Society (ASAS). Ann Rheum Dis 2009;68(6):784–8.
69. Rudwaleit M, van der Heijde D, Landewe R, et al. The Assessment of SpondyloArthritis International Society classification criteria for peripheral spondyloarthritis and for spondyloarthritis in general. Ann Rheum Dis 2011;70(1):25–31.
70. Rudwaleit M, Jurik AG, Hermann KG, et al. Defining active sacroiliitis on magnetic resonance imaging (MRI) for classification of axial spondyloarthritis: a consensual approach by the ASAS/OMERACT MRI group. Ann Rheum Dis 2009; 68(10):1520–7.
71. Lambert RG, Bakker PA, van der Heijde D, et al. Defining active sacroiliitis on MRI for classification of axial spondyloarthritis: update by the ASAS MRI working group. Ann Rheum Dis 2016;75(11):1958–63.
72. Hermann KG, Baraliakos X, van der Heijde DM, et al. Descriptions of spinal MRI lesions and definition of a positive MRI of the spine in axial spondyloarthritis: a consensual approach by the ASAS/OMERACT MRI study group. Ann Rheum Dis 2012;71(8):1278–88.
73. Maksymowych WP, Lambert RG, Ostergaard M, et al. MRI lesions in the sacroiliac joints of patients with spondyloarthritis: an update of definitions and validation by the ASAS MRI working group. Ann Rheum Dis 2019;78(11):1550–8.

EAMs

Approach to the Patient with Axial Spondyloarthritis and Suspected Inflammatory Bowel Disease

Sebastián Eduardo Ibáñez Vodnizza, MD[a,b,c,*],
María Paz Poblete De La Fuente, MD[c,d],
Elisa Catalina Parra Cancino, MD[c,e,f]

KEYWORDS

- Axial spondyloarthritis • Inflammatory bowel disease • Digestive system
- Gastrointestinal diseases • Ankylosing spondylitis

KEY POINTS

- The evaluation of gastrointestinal symptoms in patients with axial spondyloarthritis requires careful evaluation, taking into account the increased risk of inflammatory bowel disease but not forgetting other causes, such as infections.
- Endoscopic studies remain fundamental in the diagnostic process.
- The available fecal and serologic markers do not allow, by themselves, a good distinction between the possible causes of intestinal inflammation.
- The treatment should be evaluated considering both the articular and intestinal manifestations and without forgetting the interactions and adverse effects of the different immunosuppressants available.

INTRODUCTION

Axial spondyloarthritis (axSpA) and inflammatory bowel diseases (IBD) share common genetic and pathogenic mechanisms, with an estimated prevalence of IBD in axSpA patients between 4.1% and 6.4%.[1]

[a] Rheumatology Department, Clínica Alemana de Santiago, Chile; [b] Rheumatology Department, Padre Hurtado Hospital, Santiago, Chile; [c] Medicine Faculty Clínica Alemana de Santiago, Universidad del Desarrollo, Santiago, Chile; [d] Internal Medicine Department, Padre Hurtado Hospital, Secretaría de medicina interna, 4° piso, Esperanza 2150, San Ramón, Santiago 8860000, Chile; [e] Gastroenterology Department, Clínica Alemana de Santiago, Chile; [f] Gastroenterology Department, Padre Hurtado Hospital, Secretaría de medicina interna, 4° piso, Esperanza 2150, San Ramón, Santiago 8860000, Chile
* Corresponding author. Clínica Alemana de Santiago, Av. Manquehue Norte 1410, piso 7°, Vitacura, Santiago 7650567, Chile.
E-mail address: sibanez@alemana.cl
Twitter: @manos81cl (S.E.I.V.)

Rheum Dis Clin N Am 46 (2020) 279–290
https://doi.org/10.1016/j.rdc.2020.01.004
0889-857X/20/© 2020 Elsevier Inc. All rights reserved.

The incidence of IBD after the diagnosis of axSpA is estimated at 0.6% per year,[2] and the diagnosis is more frequent near the initial diagnosis of axSpA, in younger patients,[3] in women,[4] in those with a higher body mass index,[5] and in those with greater disease activity, worse functionality and worse evaluation of baseline well-being.[2] It might be more frequent in populations of higher socioeconomic status, but the evidence is not definitive in this regard.[6]

To adequately and efficiently evaluate patients with gastrointestinal symptoms in the context of axSpA can be difficult, considering that many of these patients suffer from chronic pain, present high inflammatory parameters, and use drugs with possible gastrointestinal adverse effects. In addition, the immunosuppressive treatments that these patients can receive make it necessary to always consider infections within the differential diagnoses of IBD.

In this article, we propose a practical approach to patients diagnosed with axSpA and suspected IBD (**Table 1**).

IN WHICH PATIENTS WITH AXIAL SPONDYLOARTHRITIS SHOULD WE SUSPECT THE PRESENCE OF INFLAMMATORY BOWEL DISEASE?

Recently, screening criteria have been postulated.[7] They suggest that a patient who presents with one of the following symptoms should be evaluated by the gastroenterologist: rectal bleeding without an evident cause: chronic diarrhea (>4 weeks) with

Table 1 Approach to the patient with axSpA and suspected IBD	
Suspicion	Symptoms: rectal bleeding, chronic diarrhea, perianal disease, chronic abdominal pain, fever, weight loss, extraintestinal manifestations of IBD[a] Laboratory: Iron deficiency, leukocytosis, hypokalemia, hypoalbuminemia, high ESR or CRP, not explained by joint disease. Family history of IBD.
Evaluation	Endoscopic study if high clinical suspicion (always biopsy if possible). Fecal calprotectin >150 μg/g: consider additional tests (do not forget infections). Endoscopic capsule in selected cases (suspected IBD with normal colonoscopy). Extension study if IBD is confirmed (CT, MRI of small intestine; pelvic floor study).
Treatment	Stop smoking, lower body fat. NSAIDs and corticosteroids only if no better treatment available csDMARDs. No clear benefit for axial disease, consider if it is not possible to use biologicals. Biologics: adalimumab and infliximab useful for UC and CD, and joint involvement.
Colorectal cancer screening	From 8–10 y after onset of IBD symptoms, unless risk factors for early CRC are present. Surveillance frequency according to risk estimation (personal and family history, biopsy result). Biologicals: possible protective effect.

Abbreviations: CD, Crohn's disease; CRC, colorectal cancer; CRP, C-reactive protein; csDMARDs, conventional synthetic disease-modifying drugs; CT, computed tomography; ESR, erythrocyte sedimentation rate; NSAIDs, nonsteroidal anti-inflammatory drugs; UC, ulcerative colitis.
[a] Erythema nodosum, pyoderma gangrenosum, oral thrush, and cholangitis.

characteristics that suggest organicity (watery, wakes up the patient at night, or with accompanying symptoms such as weight loss, fever, signs of malabsorption, or extraintestinal symptoms such as erythema nodosum, pyoderma gangrenosum, oral thrush, cholangitis), and perianal disease (fissures, fistulas, abscesses, skin tags, and maceration or ulceration).

If the patient does not present any of those symptoms but has 2 of the following, a referral is also needed: chronic abdominal pain (>4 weeks, persistent or recurrent), iron deficiency with or without anemia, extraintestinal manifestations (mentioned within the major criteria), fever without apparent origin of more than a week of evolution, not explainable weight loss, or a family history of IBD.

These screening criteria for referral have the advantage of being based on the patient's clinical presentation and not relying on laboratory tests, except for the presence of iron deficiency. Although these criteria need to be validated, and their specificity and sensitivity evaluated, they reflect in a good way the clinic of patients who may present IBD.

HOW SHOULD A PATIENT DIAGNOSED WITH AXIAL SPONDYLOARTHRITIS AND SUSPECTED INFLAMMATORY BOWEL DISEASE BE STUDIED?

For the diagnosis of IBD, there is no definitive diagnostic test; rather, a combination of elements, compatible history, and laboratory tests (deposition study, endoscopy, histology, and images) are required.

Within the laboratory, the presence of anemia, thrombocytosis, erythrocyte sedimentation rate elevation, leukocytosis, hypokalemia, hypoalbuminemia, and C-reactive protein elevation help us to diagnose and to evaluate the severity of the condition. The microbiological study in stool is mandatory to rule out infections.[8]

a. Fecal and serologic markers
   i. Fecal calprotectin is a cytosolic protein derived from neutrophils. There is a very good correlation between its values and inflammatory activity in the intestinal mucosa. Although a value of 50 μg/g or greater may be considered abnormal, an optimal cut-off for distinguishing IBD from other entities, like infections, has not been fully determined,[9] hence the importance of associating it with a microbiological study of feces.[10] Another factor that can raise the levels of fecal calprotectin is the use of nonsteroidal anti-inflammatory drugs (NSAIDs),[11] which is common in the treatment of axSpA. In contrast, higher levels of fecal calprotectin are associated with greater severity of axSpA, in patients without gastrointestinal symptoms.[12] Therefore, the current role of calprotectin in the diagnosis of IBD in patients with axSpA with high disease activity is not clear. Some experts recommend that invasive studies should not be performed in patients with gastrointestinal symptoms if the value is less than 100 μg/g, to repeat the fecal calprotectin if the value is between 100 and 150 μg/g, and consider additional tests if it is greater than 150 μg/g.[13] In patients with IBD, the elevation of calprotectin may precede clinical symptoms by up to 3 months, being a very good noninvasive follow-up parameter, because it has a good correlation with the endoscopic indexes of inflammation, and its progressive decrease is one of the best markers of response to treatment.[13] Serum calprotectin, less used in clinical practice, has been associated with subclinical microscopic colitis in patients with axSpA and elevated C-reactive protein.[14]
   ii. Lactoferrin, a protein found in neutrophil granules, acts inhibiting bacterial proliferation by binding iron. Like calprotectin, it is resistant to degradation and proteolysis, and has a sensitivity of 67% to 80% and a specificity of 65% to 82% to

identify patients with IBD. Fecal lactoferrin has been correlated with active inflammation seen in endoscopy, and with clinical symptoms, but its use is less standardized than that of fecal calprotectin.[10]

iii. Serologic markers such as antineutrophil cytoplasm and anti-*Saccharomyces cerevisiae* antibodies can be used to support the diagnosis, but they have low sensitivity and specificity, and do not allow distinguishing between ulcerative colitis (UC) and Crohn's disease (CD). The additional diagnostic value of anticarbohydrate antibodies like antimannobioside, antilaminaribioside, or antichitobioside antibodies, and of antimicrobials antibodies against the *Escherichia coli* outer membrane porin C, flagellin, and *Pseudomonas fluorescens*–associated sequence I-2, is minimal.[15]

b. Colonoscopy and endoscopic capsule

i. In the case of suspected IBD, a colonoscopy should be performed, always with ileal intubation, and biopsies should be taken of all segments, both healthy and those with an inflammatory appearance. Ileocolonoscopy can confirm the diagnostic suspicion, evaluate the extent and degree of involvement, and identify complications (fistulas, stenosis, and neoplasms). A frequent mistake is to biopsy only from macroscopic inflamed segments, being that there may be a microscopic intestinal compromise, and it will be the latter that determines the extent of the disease.[16] In UC the affectation is only colonic, always continuous from rectum to proximal, with a clear boundary between healthy and diseased mucosa. Depending on the severity, the findings could be edema and loss of the submucosal vascular pattern; friable, erythematous mucosa, with superficial erosions; and ulceration with exudate and spontaneous bleeding.[8] In CD the affectation can exist from mouth to anus, with a patched pattern. The degree of affectation can go from isolated scars to deep ulcers, with geographic or serpiginous aspect, with a cobblestone pattern, complicated with stenosis or fistulas, or with scars that retract the mucosa. It is possible to present only ileal involvement, so ileal evaluation is always necessary.[16] Colonoscopy is not recommended as a test for IBD screening in patients with axSpA without digestive complaints, but it should be noted that, in this group, ileocolonoscopy has revealed inflammatory lesions in up to one-third of patients.[17,18]

ii. The endoscopic capsule has been shown to be superior to colonoscopy in detecting inflammatory lesions compatible with CD in patients with axSpA, observing inflammation of the small intestine in 42.2% versus 10.7% of patients, respectively.[19] Interestingly, the positive results were not associated with gastrointestinal symptoms but with high levels of fecal calprotectin, which has also been observed in other studies.[20] Further studies are required to assess whether studying these asymptomatic patients modifies the long-term results of the disease. In patients with suspected IBD, mainly CD, with elevated C-reactive protein, unexplained iron deficiency anemia, high fecal calprotectin, and normal colonoscopy, the endoscopic capsule is a sensitive tool to detect abnormalities in the mucosa of the small intestine with a diagnostic performance comparable with other modalities (magnetic resonance enterography, MRI, ultrasound examination with contrast of the small intestine), and it seems to be superior in the evaluation of the proximal small intestine. The presence of at least 3 ulcers in the small intestine is considered as a diagnosis of CD, provided that the patient has not used NSAIDs for at least 1 month before. It should be kept in mind that its use is contraindicated in patients with swallowing disorders and in suspected stenosis and/or intestinal obstruction given the risk of impaction.[21,22]

c. Other studies
  i. Gastroduodenoscopy is only recommended when IBD is suspected in pediatric patients. In adults, it is only performed in CD when the symptoms justify its use, because there may be compromise of the upper digestive tract (part of the extension study).[23]
  ii. Images are fundamental for the extension study, being much more important in CD than in UC. At the time of diagnosis of CD, the small intestine should be evaluated with a noninvasive test to define the extent and phenotype of the disease. Computed tomography or MRI enterography can evaluate the small intestine with similar sensitivity and specificity.[24] Both techniques allow the determination of the extent of the disease, the presence of fistulas or stenosis, and the degree of inflammatory activity, based on the thickness of the wall and the increased intravenous contrast uptake.[25] MRI can reduce the radiation exposure, especially in young patients, and allows the differentiation between inflammation and residual fibrostenosis, relevant information for treatment.
  iii. A pelvic floor study (MRI, endosonography, evaluation under anesthesia) should also be carried out on suspicion of perianal disease involvement.

WHAT RESULTS SHOULD BE CONSIDERED DIAGNOSTIC IN THE BIOPSY?

a. *UC:* Histology in UC characteristically presents alterations of the histoarchitecture with branching and shortening of the crypts. The presence of cryptic microabscesses is related to the activity of the disease, although this alteration is also present in infectious conditions, so it is not diagnostic of UC by itself. In initial UC, the presence of diffuse or focal plasma cell clusters can be observed and may be the earliest feature.[8]
b. *CD:* In CD, the histology is more varied, the affectation is transmural, so the biopsy, being more superficial (mucosa), can be normal or with minimal alterations. The presence of granulomas is the pathognomonic lesion, found in about 10% of biopsies. Distortion of crypts, increase in plasma cells, and accumulation of eosinophils may be present. The presence of abnormalities between normal areas supports the diagnosis.[8]

WHAT IS THE ROLE OF NONSTEROIDAL ANTI-INFLAMMATORY DRUGS, CORTICOSTEROIDS AND CONVENTIONAL SYNTHETIC DISEASE-MODIFYING DRUGS IN TREATMENT?

a. *NSAIDs:* In clinical practice, the relationship between IBD reactivation and the use of NSAIDs is recognized, although a recent meta-analysis did not find a consistent association between its use and the risk of flair.[26] Causality is difficult to demonstrate because patients with active disease seem to use more NSAIDs.[27,28] Some experts suggest that, in nonactive IBD, using celecoxib or etoricoxib for short periods is acceptable,[29–32] but further research is still needed.
b. *Corticosteroids:* The usefulness of corticosteroids in axSpA is controversial,[33,34] but in patients with active IBD, in whom it is desired to avoid the use of NSAIDs, who present flares of their axSpA, corticosteroids may be an option, especially in patients without access to biologics.[35]
c. *Conventional synthetic disease-modifying drugs:* There is no clear benefit of sulfasalazine in the axial symptoms of axSpA,[36] and the evidence is worse for mesalazine, azathioprine,[37] and methotrexate.[38] In cases with active IBD and axSpA, with no possibility of biologic use, where it is decided to use any of these disease-modifying drugs, adverse effects, and possible drug interactions, should be carefully considered given the lack of proven efficacy.

WHICH BIOLOGICAL CAN BE USED?

Within the approved biologicals, with proven efficacy in axSpA, only some have usefulness in IBD. Infliximab and adalimumab are the best studied tumor necrosis factor-α blockers with approval for use in CD, UC, and axSpA.[39,40] Certolizumab has proven usefulness for CD,[41] and is being studied in UC,[42] with efficacy reports already published.[43] Golimumab is currently approved only for UC,[44] although there are usefulness reports in CD.[45,46] Etanercept has no proven usefulness in IBD.[47]

Secukinumab, a monoclonal antibody against IL-17, has proven usefulness in axSpA, but, despite the fact that, owing to its mechanism of action, a good response was expected, the results have been negative in IBD,[48] and there was a concern of increased incidence of IBD in patients starting treatment. In a retrospective analysis of 7355 patients, incident cases were uncommon[49]; however, some groups still recommend caution and monitoring of digestive symptoms.[50]

Although ustekinumab is useful in CD,[51] it failed to demonstrate efficacy in axSpA.[52] Vedolizumab has demonstrated efficacy in CD and UC,[53] but there is concern that it may be related to the appearance of arthritis,[54,55] although a recent post hoc analysis showed the opposite.[56]

IS THERE EVIDENCE FOR THE USE OF JANUS KINASE INHIBITORS?

Tofacitinib has no proven usefulness in CD,[57] but it has proven action in UC[58] and its usefulness in axSpA is being studied.[59,60] Filgotinib looks promising in CD[61] and in axSpA.[62]

WHAT IS THE ROLE OF SMOKING AND BODY COMPOSITION?
Smoking

Quitting smoking has a demonstrated benefit in patients with CD and should be established as an important treatment goal.[63] It has been reported that smoking is protective against UC, but its causality has not been clarified.[64] The rather modest benefits of transdermal nicotine replacement suggest that more research is required in this area.[63] A recent study showed that nonsmokers seem to have a lesser risk of developing IBD.[65] Similarly, smoking is associated with a worse disease profile in patients with axSpA.[66]

Body Composition

Body fat decreases with higher disease severity, and fat-free mass decreases with longer disease duration in CD, UC and axSpA.[67,68] Higher fat mass content has been associated with worse response to tumor necrosis factor-α blockers.[69]

WHAT IS THE RISK OF COLORECTAL CANCER?

a. *Start of monitoring:* Long-term UC and CD are associated with an increased risk of colorectal cancer (CRC), with different estimates between studies.[70,71] Current guidelines recommend monitoring for CRC from 8 to 10 years after the start of IBD symptoms. However, the incidence within 8 to 10 years from the onset of IBD varies from 12% to 42%, and the risk factors predictive of early CRC are onset of IBD at 28 years or older and active tobacco smoking.[72] These patients should be considered for earlier screening.

b. *Surveillance frequency:* Because the scientific data available for patients with CD are more limited,[73] the same surveillance schedules apply as for patients with UC,[8] for an early detection of dysplasia and prevention of the development of

CRC. Patients with low risk (active endoscopic or histologic inflammation, left colitis or affecting <50% colon) should be scoped every 5 years, those with intermediate risk (mild active endoscopic or histologic inflammation, postinflammatory polyps, first-degree family history of CRC after age 50) should have a colonoscopy every 2 to 3 years, and those with high risk (moderate or severe endoscopic or histologic active inflammation, first-degree relative with CRC before age 50, history of primary sclerosing cholangitis, stenosis in the last 5 years, biopsy with dysplasia in the last 5 years in a patient who refused surgery) should undergo annual colonoscopy.[70,74,75]

c. *Biologicals:* There is a lack of data and experience to estimate the impact of biologic therapy on the risk of CRC in patients with axSpA and IBD, but it seems that the risk does not increase and that there may be a chemopreventive effect in controlling the inflammation of the mucosa.[76]

ARE THERE CLINICAL SCALES FOR MONITORING THE ACTIVITY OF INFLAMMATORY BOWEL DISEASE IN PATIENTS WITH AXIAL SPONDYLOARTHRITIS?

In the Netherlands, the use of the Dudley Inflammatory Bowel Symptom Questionnaire (DISQ) in patients with spondyloarthritis was validated. This consists of 15 questions that are scored from 0 to 4, and a higher score is related to worse gastrointestinal symptoms.[77] It must be validated in other populations but can be considered as a useful tool for monitoring the disease.

SUMMARY

IBD can be found frequently in axSpA. The diagnostic study should be performed carefully, considering the differential diagnoses and the limitations of the different diagnostic test. There are good therapeutic options, although biological therapies can be difficult to access in some parts of the world.

DISCLOSURE

The authors have no commercial or financial conflicts of interest to disclose, and no funding sources to report.

REFERENCES

1. de Winter JJ, van Mens LJ, van der Heijde D, et al. Prevalence of peripheral and extra-articular disease in ankylosing spondylitis versus non-radiographic axial spondyloarthritis: a meta-analysis. Arthritis Res Ther 2016;18(1):196.
2. Essers I, Ramiro S, Stolwijk C, et al. Characteristics associated with the presence and development of extra-articular manifestations in ankylosing spondylitis: 12-year results from OASIS. Rheumatology (Oxford) 2015;54(4):633–40.
3. Stolwijk C, Essers I, van Tubergen A, et al. The epidemiology of extra-articular manifestations in ankylosing spondylitis: a population-based matched cohort study. Ann Rheum Dis 2015;74(7):1373–8.
4. Rusman T, van Vollenhoven RF, van der Horst-Bruinsma IE. Gender differences in axial spondyloarthritis: women are not so lucky. Curr Rheumatol Rep 2018;20(6). https://doi.org/10.1007/s11926-018-0744-2.
5. Rahmani J, Kord-Varkaneh H, Hekmatdoost A, et al. Body mass index and risk of inflammatory bowel disease: a systematic review and dose-response meta-analysis of cohort studies of over a million participants. Obes Rev 2019. https://doi.org/10.1111/obr.12875.

6. Abegunde AT, Muhammad BH, Bhatti O, et al. Environmental risk factors for inflammatory bowel diseases: evidence based literature review. World J Gastroenterol 2016;22(27):6296–317.

7. Sanz Sanz J, Juanola Roura X, Seoane-Mato D, et al. Screening of inflammatory bowel disease and spondyloarthritis for referring patients between rheumatology and gastroenterology. Rheumatol Clin 2018;14(2):68–74.

8. Maaser C, Sturm A, Vavricka SR, et al. ECCO-ESGAR guideline for diagnostic assessment in IBD part 1: initial diagnosis, monitoring of known IBD, detection of complications. J Crohns Colitis 2019;13(2):144–64. Oxford Academic. Available at: https://academic.oup.com/ecco-jcc/article/13/2/144/5078195. Accessed June 26, 2019.

9. Benítez JM, García-Sánchez V. Faecal calprotectin: management in inflammatory bowel disease. World J Gastrointest Pathophysiol 2015;6(4):203–9.

10. Lehmann FS, Burri E, Beglinger C. The role and utility of faecal markers in inflammatory bowel disease. Ther Adv Gastroenterol 2015;8(1):23–36.

11. Klingberg E, Carlsten H, Hilme E, et al. Calprotectin in ankylosing spondylitis–frequently elevated in feces, but normal in serum. Scand J Gastroenterol 2012;47(4):435–44.

12. Duran A, Kobak S, Sen N, et al. Fecal calprotectin is associated with disease activity in patients with ankylosing spondylitis. Bosn J Basic Med Sci 2016;16(1):71–4.

13. Guardiola J, Lobatón T, Cerrillo E, et al. Recommendations of the Spanish Working Group on Crohn's Disease and Ulcerative Colitis (GETECCU) on the utility of the determination of faecal calprotectin in inflammatory bowel disease. Gastroenterol Hepatol 2018;41(8):514–29.

14. Cypers H, Varkas G, Beeckman S, et al. Elevated calprotectin levels reveal bowel inflammation in spondyloarthritis. Ann Rheum Dis 2016;75(7):1357–62.

15. Soubières AA, Poullis A. Emerging biomarkers for the diagnosis and monitoring of inflammatory bowel diseases. Inflamm Bowel Dis 2016;22(8):2016–22.

16. Feuerstein JD, Cheifetz AS. Crohn disease: epidemiology, diagnosis, and management. Mayo Clin Proc 2017;92(7):1088–103.

17. Mielants H, Veys EM, Cuvelier C, et al. Subclinical involvement of the gut in undifferentiated spondylarthropathies. Clin Exp Rheumatol 1989;7(5):499–504.

18. Leirisalo-Repo M, Turunen U, Stenman S, et al. High frequency of silent inflammatory bowel disease in spondylarthropathy. Arthritis Rheum 1994;37(1):23–31.

19. Kopylov U, Starr M, Watts C, et al. Detection of Crohn disease in patients with spondyloarthropathy: the SpACE capsule study. J Rheumatol 2018;45(4):498–505.

20. Simioni J, Skare TL, Campos APB, et al. Fecal calprotectin, gut inflammation and spondyloarthritis. Arch Med Res 2019;50(1):41–6.

21. Song HJ, Moon JS, Jeon SR, et al. Diagnostic yield and clinical impact of video capsule endoscopy in patients with chronic diarrhea: a Korean multicenter CAPENTRY study. Gut Liver 2017;11(2):253–60.

22. Jensen MD, Brodersen JB, Kjeldsen J. Capsule endoscopy for the diagnosis and follow up of Crohn's disease: a comprehensive review of current status. Ann Gastroenterol 2017;30(2):168–78.

23. Upper gastrointestinal involvement of Crohn's disease: a prospective study on the role of upper endoscopy in the diagnostic work-up. Available at: https://www.ncbi.nlm.nih.gov/pubmed/22350786. Accessed July 2, 2019.

24. Systematic review with meta-analysis: magnetic resonance enterography vs. computed tomography enterography for evaluating disease activity in small.

Available at: https://www.ncbi.nlm.nih.gov/pubmed/24912799. Accessed July 8, 2019.

25. Puylaert CAJ, Tielbeek JAW, Bipat S, et al. Grading of Crohn's disease activity using CT, MRI, US and scintigraphy: a meta-analysis. Eur Radiol 2015;25(11): 3295–313.

26. Moninuola OO, Milligan W, Lochhead P, et al. Systematic review with meta-analysis: association between acetaminophen and nonsteroidal anti-inflammatory drugs (NSAIDs) and risk of Crohn's disease and ulcerative colitis exacerbation. Aliment Pharmacol Ther 2018;47(11):1428–39.

27. Long MD, Kappelman MD, Martin CF, et al. Role of nonsteroidal anti-inflammatory drugs in exacerbations of inflammatory bowel disease. J Clin Gastroenterol 2016; 50(2):152–6.

28. Kvasnovsky CL, Aujla U, Bjarnason I. Nonsteroidal anti-inflammatory drugs and exacerbations of inflammatory bowel disease. Scand J Gastroenterol 2015; 50(3):255–63.

29. Olivieri I, Cantini F, Castiglione F, et al. Italian expert panel on the management of patients with coexisting spondyloarthritis and inflammatory bowel disease. Autoimmun Rev 2014;13(8):822–30.

30. Sandborn WJ, Stenson WF, Brynskov J, et al. Safety of celecoxib in patients with ulcerative colitis in remission: a randomized, placebo-controlled, pilot study. Clin Gastroenterol Hepatol 2006;4(2):203–11.

31. El Miedany Y, Youssef S, Ahmed I, et al. The gastrointestinal safety and effect on disease activity of etoricoxib, a selective cox-2 inhibitor in inflammatory bowel diseases. Am J Gastroenterol 2006;101(2):311–7.

32. Miao X-P, Li J-S, Ouyang Q, et al. Tolerability of selective cyclooxygenase 2 inhibitors used for the treatment of rheumatological manifestations of inflammatory bowel disease. Cochrane Database Syst Rev 2014;(10):CD007744.

33. Bandinelli F, Scazzariello F, Pimenta da Fonseca E, et al. Low-dose modified-release prednisone in axial spondyloarthritis: 3-month efficacy and tolerability. Drug Des Devel Ther 2016;10:3717–24.

34. Haibel H, Fendler C, Listing J, et al. Efficacy of oral prednisolone in active ankylosing spondylitis: results of a double-blind, randomised, placebo-controlled short-term trial. Ann Rheum Dis 2014;73(1):243–6.

35. Padovan M, Castellino G, Govoni M, et al. The treatment of the rheumatological manifestations of the inflammatory bowel diseases. Rheumatol Int 2006;26(11): 953–8.

36. Chen J, Liu C. Sulfasalazine for ankylosing spondylitis. Cochrane Database Syst Rev 2005;(2):CD004800.

37. Dougados M, Dijkmans B, Khan M, et al. Conventional treatments for ankylosing spondylitis. Ann Rheum Dis 2002;61(Suppl 3):iii40–50.

38. Chen J, Veras MMS, Liu C, et al. Methotrexate for ankylosing spondylitis. Cochrane Database Syst Rev 2013;(2):CD004524.

39. Fragoulis GE, Liava C, Daoussis D, et al. Inflammatory bowel diseases and spondyloarthropathies: from pathogenesis to treatment. World J Gastroenterol 2019; 25(18):2162–76.

40. Pouillon L, Bossuyt P, Vanderstukken J, et al. Management of patients with inflammatory bowel disease and spondyloarthritis. Expert Rev Clin Pharmacol 2017; 10(12):1363–74.

41. Goel N, Stephens S. Certolizumab pegol. MAbs 2010;2(2):137–47.

42. Study of cimzia for the treatment of ulcerative colitis - full text view - ClinicalTrials.-gov. Available at: https://clinicaltrials.gov/ct2/show/NCT01090154. Accessed July 6, 2019.

43. Osterman MT, Clark-Snustad KD, Singla A, et al. P136 certolizumab pegol is effective in the maintenance of response in moderate-severe ulcerative colitis: an open-label maintenance study. Gastroenterology 2018;154(1):S71.

44. Flamant M, Paul S, Roblin X. Golimumab for the treatment of ulcerative colitis. Expert Opin Biol Ther 2017;17(7):879–86.

45. Russi L, Scharl M, Rogler G, et al. The efficacy and safety of golimumab as third- or fourth-line anti-TNF therapy in patients with refractory Crohn's disease: a case series. Inflamm Intest Dis 2017;2(2):131–8.

46. Martineau C, Flourié B, Wils P, et al. Efficacy and safety of golimumab in Crohn's disease: a French national retrospective study. Aliment Pharmacol Ther 2017; 46(11–12):1077–84.

47. Sandborn WJ, Hanauer SB, Katz S, et al. Etanercept for active Crohn's disease: a randomized, double-blind, placebo-controlled trial. Gastroenterology 2001; 121(5):1088–94.

48. Hueber W, Sands BE, Lewitzky S, et al. Secukinumab, a human anti-IL-17A mono-clonal antibody, for moderate to severe Crohn's disease: unexpected results of a randomised, double-blind placebo-controlled trial. Gut 2012;61(12):1693–700.

49. Schreiber S, Colombel J-F, Feagan BG, et al. Incidence rates of inflammatory bowel disease in patients with psoriasis, psoriatic arthritis and ankylosing spon-dylitis treated with secukinumab: a retrospective analysis of pooled data from 21 clinical trials. Ann Rheum Dis 2019;78(4):473–9.

50. Fries W, Belvedere A, Cappello M, et al. Inflammatory bowel disease onset during secukinumab treatment: real concern or just an expression of dysregulated im-mune response? Clin Drug Investig 2019. https://doi.org/10.1007/s40261-019-00803-7.

51. Kotze PG, Ma C, Almutairdi A, et al. Clinical utility of ustekinumab in Crohn's dis-ease. J Inflamm Res 2018;11:35–47.

52. Deodhar A, Gensler LS, Sieper J, et al. Three multicenter, randomized, double-blind, placebo-controlled studies evaluating the efficacy and safety of ustekinu-mab in axial spondyloarthritis. Arthritis Rheumatol 2019;71(2):258–70.

53. Scribano ML. Vedolizumab for inflammatory bowel disease: from randomized controlled trials to real-life evidence. World J Gastroenterol 2018;24(23):2457–67.

54. Tadbiri S, Peyrin-Biroulet L, Serrero M, et al. Impact of vedolizumab therapy on extra-intestinal manifestations in patients with inflammatory bowel disease: a mul-ticentre cohort study nested in the OBSERV-IBD cohort. Aliment Pharmacol Ther 2018;47(4):485–93.

55. Varkas G, Thevissen K, Brabanter GD, et al. An induction or flare of arthritis and/or sacroiliitis by vedolizumab in inflammatory bowel disease: a case series. Ann Rheum Dis 2017;76(5):878–81.

56. Feagan BG, Sandborn WJ, Colombel J-F, et al. Incidence of arthritis/arthralgia in inflammatory bowel disease with long-term vedolizumab treatment: post hoc an-alyses of the GEMINI trials. J Crohns Colitis 2019;13(1):50–7.

57. Panés J, Sandborn WJ, Schreiber S, et al. Tofacitinib for induction and mainte-nance therapy of Crohn's disease: results of two phase IIb randomised placebo-controlled trials. Gut 2017;66(6):1049–59.

58. Sandborn WJ, Su C, Sands BE, et al. Tofacitinib as induction and maintenance therapy for ulcerative colitis. N Engl J Med 2017;376(18):1723–36.

59. van der Heijde D, Deodhar A, Wei JC, et al. Tofacitinib in patients with ankylosing spondylitis: a phase II, 16-week, randomised, placebo-controlled, dose-ranging study. Ann Rheum Dis 2017;76(8):1340–7.

60. Maksymowych WP, van der Heijde D, Baraliakos X, et al. Tofacitinib is associated with attainment of the minimally important reduction in axial magnetic resonance imaging inflammation in ankylosing spondylitis patients. Rheumatology (Oxford) 2018;57(8):1390–9.

61. Vermeire S, Schreiber S, Petryka R, et al. Clinical remission in patients with moderate-to-severe Crohn's disease treated with filgotinib (the FITZROY study): results from a phase 2, double-blind, randomised, placebo-controlled trial. Lancet 2017;389(10066):266–75.

62. van der Heijde D, Baraliakos X, Gensler LS, et al. Efficacy and safety of filgotinib, a selective Janus kinase 1 inhibitor, in patients with active ankylosing spondylitis (TORTUGA): results from a randomised, placebo-controlled, phase 2 trial. Lancet 2018;392(10162):2378–87.

63. Parkes GC, Whelan K, Lindsay JO. Smoking in inflammatory bowel disease: impact on disease course and insights into the aetiology of its effect. J Crohns Colitis 2014;8(8):717–25.

64. Matsuoka K, Kobayashi T, Ueno F, et al. Evidence-based clinical practice guidelines for inflammatory bowel disease. J Gastroenterol 2018;53(3):305–53.

65. Salih A, Widbom L, Hultdin J, et al. Smoking is associated with risk for developing inflammatory bowel disease including late onset ulcerative colitis: a prospective study. Scand J Gastroenterol 2018;53(2):173–8.

66. Zhao S, Jones GT, Macfarlane GJ, et al. Associations between smoking and extra-axial manifestations and disease severity in axial spondyloarthritis: results from the BSR Biologics Register for Ankylosing Spondylitis (BSRBR-AS). Rheumatology (Oxford) 2018. https://doi.org/10.1093/rheumatology/key371.

67. Yadav DP, Kedia S, Madhusudhan KS, et al. Body composition in Crohn's disease and ulcerative colitis: correlation with disease severity and duration. Can J Gastroenterol Hepatol 2017;2017. https://doi.org/10.1155/2017/1215035.

68. Ibáñez Vodnizza S, Visman IM, van Denderen C, et al. Muscle wasting in male TNF-α blocker naïve ankylosing spondylitis patients: a comparison of gender differences in body composition. Rheumatology (Oxford) 2017;56(9):1566–72.

69. Ibáñez Vodnizza SE, Nurmohamed MT, Visman IM, et al. Fat mass lowers the response to tumor necrosis factor-α blockers in patients with ankylosing spondylitis. J Rheumatol 2017;44(9):1355–61.

70. Magro F, Gionchetti P, Eliakim R, et al. Third European evidence-based consensus on diagnosis and management of ulcerative colitis. part 1: definitions, diagnosis, extra-intestinal manifestations, pregnancy, cancer surveillance, surgery, and ileo-anal pouch disorders. J Crohns Colitis 2017;11(6):649–70.

71. Andersen NN, Jess T. Has the risk of colorectal cancer in inflammatory bowel disease decreased? World J Gastroenterol 2013;19(43):7561–8.

72. Cohen-Mekelburg S, Schneider Y, Gold S, et al. Risk of early colorectal cancers needs to be considered in inflammatory bowel disease care. Dig Dis Sci 2019. https://doi.org/10.1007/s10620-019-05554-1.

73. Panés J, Bouzas R, Chaparro M, et al. Systematic review: the use of ultrasonography, computed tomography and magnetic resonance imaging for the diagnosis, assessment of activity and abdominal complications of Crohn's disease. Aliment Pharmacol Ther 2011;34(2):125–45.

74. Cairns SR, Scholefield JH, Steele RJ, et al. Guidelines for colorectal cancer screening and surveillance in moderate and high risk groups (update from 2002). Gut 2010;59(5):666–89.
75. Keller DS, Windsor A, Cohen R, et al. Colorectal cancer in inflammatory bowel disease: review of the evidence. Tech Coloproctol 2019;23(1):3–13.
76. Stidham RW, Higgins PDR. Colorectal cancer in inflammatory bowel disease. Clin Colon Rectal Surg 2018;31(3):168–78.
77. Stebbings S, Jenks K, Treharne GJ, et al. Validation of the Dudley inflammatory bowel symptom questionnaire for the assessment of bowel symptoms in axial SpA: prevalence of clinically relevant bowel symptoms and association with disease activity. Rheumatology (Oxford) 2012;51(5):858–65.

Imaging

Emerging Imaging Techniques in Spondyloarthritis

Dual-Energy Computed Tomography and New MRI Sequences

Min Chen, MD[a], Paul Bird, PhD, GradDipMRI, FRACP[b],
Lennart Jans, MD, PhD[a],*

KEYWORDS

- Spondyloarthritis • Dual-energy computed tomography • MRI • Sacroiliac joints

KEY POINTS

- Imaging of the sacroiliac joint is important for axial spondyloarthritis. Bone marrow edema and erosions are key imaging features of sacroiliitis.
- Dual-energy computed tomography (CT) can detect inflammatory bone marrow edema in the sacroiliac joints and provides an alternative choice for patients in whom MRI is contraindicated.
- Three-dimensional MRI sequences improve the visualization of erosions on MRI.
- BoneMRI is a new MRI sequence that allows radiographlike and CT-like images to be generated based on magnetic resonance (MR) images using a deep-learning method, bringing MR the potential to be a 1-stop imaging modality for spondyloarthritis.

INTRODUCTION

Axial spondyloarthritis (SpA) is a group of chronic inflammatory diseases predominantly affecting the axial skeleton.[1] The inflammation typically affects the sacroiliac joints (SIJs) and spine, with sacroiliitis playing a key role in the classification of the disease. As objective evidence for SpA, imaging of the SIJs is an important focus in rheumatology and radiology journals.[2] Imaging features of sacroiliitis can be classified into active inflammatory lesions, of which bone marrow edema (BME) is the hallmark of disease activity,[3] and structural changes, including erosions, sclerosis, ankylosis, backfill, and fat metaplasia, characterizing structural aspects of progressive disease.[3] In clinical practice, the state-of-the-art imaging modality for detection of BME is

[a] Department of Radiology, Ghent University Hospital, Corneel Heymanslaan 10, 9000 Ghent, Belgium; [b] University of New South Wales, Randwick, New South Wales 2031, Australia
* Corresponding author.
E-mail address: lennart.jans@ugent.be

Rheum Dis Clin N Am 46 (2020) 291–300
https://doi.org/10.1016/j.rdc.2020.01.010
0889-857X/20/© 2020 Elsevier Inc. All rights reserved.

rheumatic.theclinics.com

fat-suppressed MRI sequences such as the short tau inversion recovery (STIR) sequence, and, although structural MRI scores exist, radiography still serves as the reference for grading structural lesions.[4]

In the last decade, numerous studies have focused on new techniques for improving lesion visualization and evaluation in SIJs, including both BME and structural lesions (**Fig. 1**). This article presents an overview of the emerging imaging techniques and provides an insight into the future application of these methods.

EMERGING IMAGING TECHNIQUES FOR BONE MARROW EDEMA
New MRI Techniques

Fluid-sensitive MRI sequences (STIR, T2-weighted sequence with fat suppression [T2-FS]) have been widely used for the detection of BME in SpA for many years and are an important component of the Assessment of Spondyloarthritis International Society (ASAS) classification criteria.[2] Recently, Greese and colleagues[5] proposed that T2-FS may have a better image quality as well as better detection of BME compared with STIR sequences. On T2-FS images, more patients were classified as positive MRI using ASAS criteria than on STIR images.[5] Magnetic resonance (MR) sequences using other fat saturation techniques have also been explored in SIJs, including spectral attenuated inversion recovery (SPAIR) T2-weighted sequence (hybrid fat saturation technique, which combines an inversion recovery pulse with an adiabatic radiofrequency pulse)[6] and T2-weighted multipoint Dixon sequence (fat suppression based on chemical shift).[7] These sequences have shorter scan time or better image quality than STIR/T2-FS, and provide alternatives for BME detection in patients with axial SpA.

A novel MRI technique for BME detection is diffusion-weighted imaging (DWI). DWI is based on the signal attenuation caused by the incoherent thermal motion of water molecules.[8,9] Edema in bone marrow may lead to an increase of extracellular water and yield high signal on DWI.[9–11] Furthermore, bone marrow changes can be quantitatively evaluated using apparent diffusion coefficient (ADC) values calculated from DWI images (**Fig. 2**). Patients with axial SpA may have increased ADC values despite the appearances on routine MRI sequences still being normal.[10] ADC values have been shown to be related to disease activity,[12] are sensitive to therapeutic response,[13] and may improve the specificity in detecting sacroiliitis.[14] However, an important

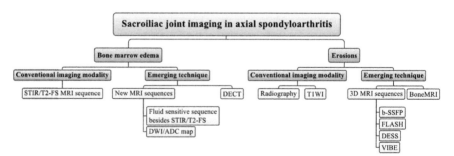

Fig. 1. Imaging modalities for SIJ in axial spondyloarthritis. 3D, three-dimensional; ADC, apparent diffusion coefficient; b-SSFP, balanced steady-state free precession sequence; DECT, dual-energy computed tomography; DESS, double excitation in the steady-state sequence; DWI, diffusion-weighted imaging; FLASH, fast low-angle shot; GRE, gradient echo; T1WI, T1-weighted imaging; T2-FS, T2-weighted fat suppression; VIBE, volume-interpolated breath-hold examination.

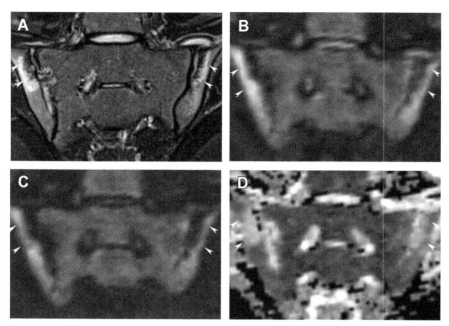

Fig. 2. MRI of a 17-year-old girl with sacroiliitis. (*A*) MR STIR image shows BME in both SIJs (*arrowheads*). (*B*) Diffusion-weighted MR image (b = 500 s/mm^2) and (*C*) diffusion-weighted MR image (b = 1000 s/mm^2) show high signal of the bone marrow edema (*arrowheads*). (*D*) ADC map shows increased ADC values of bone marrow edema (*arrowheads*).

caveat is that the spatial resolution of DWI images is not optimal. Visual analysis on DWI does not provide additional value to T2-FS images in inflammatory BME detection in SIJs.[11] Recently, Kucybala and colleagues[15] showed that visual analysis on DWI and ADC maps alone yielded a low specificity (54.0%) for BME detection using STIR images as a reference in 49 patients suspected for SpA. In addition, the postprocessing time and the variability of ADC value measurements among different readers and MR units remain a challenge preventing widespread technique application. For these reasons, debate continues as to the value of DWI in SpA.[16]

Dual-Energy Computed Tomography

Although it is widely used for BME detection, the cost of MRI is high and the acquisition time is long. Furthermore, MRI has been the only technique for BME visualization in vivo for a considerable period. In a proportion of patients, MRI is contraindicated. The emerging technique of dual-energy computed tomography (DECT) provides an innovative alternative for BME detection in SpA.

The main difference between DECT and conventional computed tomography (CT) is that DECT involves the acquisition of images at 2 different energy levels (typically at 80 and 140 kV). DECT can therefore differentiate between elements with a high atomic number, such as iodine, xenon, and calcium, and most of human body tissues with low atomic numbers, including carbon, oxygen, hydrogen, and nitrogen.[17] CT images equivalent to conventional 120-kV CT can be derived from the original datasets. Meanwhile, the radiation dose of DECT is equal to standard CT because it is divided between the 2 energy levels.[18] For rheumatic diseases, DECT has been applied in gout (urate detection[19]), rheumatic arthritis (BME detection[20] and iodine mapping[21]), psoriatic arthritis (iodine mapping[22]), and for other crystal arthropathies such as calcium pyrophosphate deposition disease.[23]

BME can be detected by DECT through a virtual noncalcium (VNCa) technique.[24] Using an algorithm based on the x-ray absorption features of bone mineral, yellow bone marrow, and red bone marrow, calcium can be subtracted. Bone marrow can be visualized and displayed on a color-coded map (**Fig. 3**). Color coding ranged from blue (fat/yellow bone marrow), green (water/BME), to yellow/red (increasing red marrow/blood content). An increase of water content in bone marrow can be evaluated both visually and quantitatively through the measurements of CT numbers.[24–27] In addition, the overlay of VNCa images on CT images allows the simultaneous assessment of bone marrow and bone. The feasibility of DECT for detecting inflammatory BME in the SIJs has been shown by Wu and colleagues[27] in a group of 47 patients with SpA. Compared with MRI, DECT showed good sensitivity and specificity for inflammatory BME in SIJs by different readers, with a range of 87% to 93% and 91% to 94%, respectively.[27]

Several limitations should be noted for the application of DECT for BME detection in SpA. BME of the subcortical area (within 2–3 mm from the cortical bone) cannot be accurately detected,[24,25,27] although this limitation has the potential to be overcome with further improvement of the technique. Moreover, red bone marrow and sclerotic areas may mimic BME lesions on VNCa images, and inexperienced readers may misinterpret these findings.[24]

In summary, although further validation is needed, DECT is useful for sacroiliac BME evaluation, especially in patients with SpA with contraindications to MRI.

EMERGING IMAGING TECHNIQUES FOR STRUCTURAL LESIONS IN SPONDYLOARTHRITIS

As another focus of research, erosion plays the most important role of all structural lesions in SpA.[28] As the traditional imaging method of choice, the role of radiography (**Fig. 4**A) has been challenged.[29] CT of the SIJs can provide the best representation of osseous lesions (**Fig. 4**B, E); however, it is not routinely used in clinical practice because of high radiation dose.[30] On MRI, the T1-weighted spin-echo (T1SE) sequence (**Fig. 4**C, F) is the most commonly used for detecting erosions in SpA, and is more reliable and accurate than radiography.[31–33] The interreader reliability of erosion detection on T1SE is comparable with BME detection on STIR (κ value 0.72 vs 0.61).[34] Using CT as a gold standard, the reported sensitivity and specificity of T1SE in erosion detection are 61% to 79% and 88% to 95%, respectively.[32,33,35]

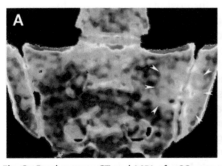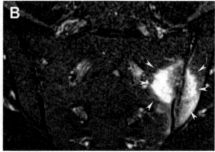

Fig. 3. Dual-energy CT and MRI of a 28-year-old man with sacroiliitis. BME (*arrowheads*) of the left SIJ is displayed as bright green areas with yellow and red spots on the dual-energy CT image (*A*), corresponding with the high signal on the MR STIR image (*B*).

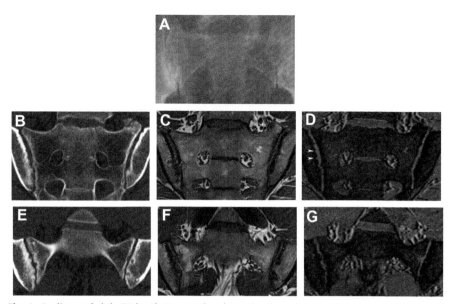

Fig. 4. Radiograph (*A*), CT (*B*, *E*), T1-weighted MRI (*C*, *F*), and VIBE MR images (*D*, *G*) of a 30-year old man with erosions in both SIJs. With reference to CT, erosions are better depicted on VIBE images than on T1-weighted MR images and on radiograph, especially the small erosions in the upper iliac side of the right SIJ (*arrowheads*).

There are still limitations of routine T1-weighted imaging (T1WI) sequences. The partial volume effect, limited contrast between cortical bone and joint space, as well as the unclear boundaries between erosions and subcortical bone marrow[32] decrease the accuracy of erosion detection. Thus, new MRI sequences and techniques have been studied to improve the visualization of erosions on MRI.

Three-Dimensional Magnetic Resonance Sequences (High-Resolution Sequences)

Three-dimensional (3D) MRI sequences or high-resolution sequences have the advantage of higher spatial resolution, lower partial volume effects, and multiplanar reconstruction.[36] In the last decade, several 3D sequences have been studied for the detection of erosions in axial SpA. These techniques include 3D fast low-angle shot (FLASH),[37] 3D double excitation in the steady-state sequence (DESS),[37] 3D water-suppressed balanced steady-state free precession sequence (b-WS-SSFP),[32] and 3D volume-interpolated breath-hold examination (VIBE)[35,38] sequences. Besides the high spatial resolution, the applied sequences are gradient echo (GRE) sequences intrinsically, thus can potentially better depict erosions of SIJs by virtue of their high contrast between joint cavity, cartilage and cortical bone.[39]

Among the 3D MRI sequences, the 3D VIBE sequence has been of most interest in recent years (**Fig. 4**D, E). The VIBE sequence affords short acquisition times without reducing image quality and allows generation of T1-weighted images with fat suppression.[40] The 3D VIBE sequence has shown a higher sensitivity and interreader reliability for detecting erosions than T1WI, with reference to CT. Diekhoff and colleagues[38] found a patient-level sensitivity of 95% and specificity of 93% for erosion detection using 3D VIBE sequences on 3.0-T MRI in 110 patients suspected for SpA and 18 healthy controls. The sensitivity and specificity of T1WI for erosion detection in the same cohort were 79% and 93% respectively. Higher sensitivity and similar specificity of VIBE compared with T1WI were also found by Baraliakos and colleagues[35] in another cohort of 109 patients with SpA, on a 1.5-T MR scanner. In addition, VIBE images tend to display more erosions than CT,[35,38] which might indicate that a higher sensitivity benefits from the better visualization of cartilage. Because VIBE sequences may be subject to more artifacts than routine spin-echo T1WI, including intravoxel dephasing and susceptibility to paramagnetic effects, the higher sensitivity of VIBE than CT could also be attributed to a higher rate of false-positive findings caused by paramagnetic artifacts.[35] Further studies are needed to validate the diagnostic value of 3D VIBE sequences in SpA classification.

Despite the limited number of studies, 3D MRI sequences showed promising results in the detection of erosions in SIJ. It is worth noting that all the examined 3D sequences are fat suppressed and cannot be used for evaluating fat deposition in SIJs, which is another lesion of interest in SpA.[41] The 3D MRI sequences cannot yet substitute for routine T1WI.

BoneMRI

Apart from 3D GRE sequences, a novel MR technique, BoneMRI images, has been developed thanks to the rapid advancement of artificial intelligence techniques. Bone-MRI involves radiodensity contrast mapping optimized from MRI to CT based on 3D T1-weighted multiple gradient echo (T1w-MGE) MRI, using a deep learning–based approach.[42] With the BoneMRI technique, radiographlike and CT-like images can be acquired without ionizing radiation. Radiodensity contrast of osseous structures can thus be visualized on MR images. The BoneMRI technique has been successfully applied in the SIJs (**Fig. 5**). These images were acquired through a deep-learning training process using CT and T1w-MGE of the SIJs in 25 patients suspected for SpA. Studies on the image quality and diagnostic accuracy for osseous structural lesions of BoneMRI are ongoing.

The BoneMRI technique is a new horizon for evaluation of osseous structural lesions in SpA. More details of osseous structures in SIJs can be visualized on BoneMRI images, facilitating MRI to become a 1-stop modality for imaging of axial SpA. For future research, the value of BoneMRI should be tested in larger cohorts of patients with or

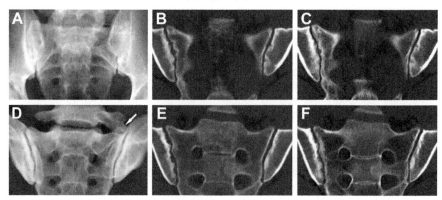

Fig. 5. Radiographlike images (A, D), CT-like images (B, E) acquired using BoneMRI technique, and CT images (C, F) of the same patient as in **Fig. 4**. The CT-like BoneMRI images have a high similarity to CT images. The osseous SIJs and erosions are well depicted on CT-like BoneMRI images. On the tilted view of the radiographlike image (D), the partial sacralization of L5 is more clearly shown (arrow).

Table 1
Summary of emerging imaging techniques in axial spondyloarthritis

Lesions of SIJ	Modality	Imaging Technique	Benefits	Limitations
BME	MRI	Fat-suppressed sequences: T2-SPAIR and T2-weighted multipoint Dixon sequence	Better image quality compared with STIR Shorter scan time	Reliability needs further validation
	MRI	DWI with ADC maps	Quantitative evaluation of disease activity May improve specificity for spondyloarthritis	Time consuming for quantitative analysis Questionable reliability
	CT	Dual-energy CT	Quantitative evaluation Provides an alternative for BME detection, especially for patients not accessible to MRI	Ionizing radiation Limited in detecting BME close to cortical bone Low accuracy in sclerotic areas
Erosions	MRI	3D GRE MRI (FLASH, DESS, b-WS-SSFP, VIBE)	High contrast between cartilage and cortical bone High spatial resolution and lower partial volume effects Applicable for multiplanar reconstruction	More subject to artifacts Reliability need further validation
	MRI	BoneMRI	Get radiographlike and CT-like images from MR scans Excellent depiction of osseous structures	Not yet commercially available

suspected for SpA. The diagnostic accuracy of BoneMRI images should also be compared with existing MR sequences for evaluation of structural lesions, including routine T1WI and 3D MRI sequences, as mentioned earlier.

SUMMARY

Imaging of the SIJs is one of the cornerstones in the diagnosis and monitoring of SpA. Evaluation of BME and structural lesions are both important for understanding the disease procedure. DECT provides an extra choice for imaging of BME in SIJs, whereas 3D MRI and BoneMRI techniques can better depict osseous structural lesions than routine MRI sequences. These emerging imaging techniques (summarized in **Table 1**) provide novel techniques that will enhance the characterizations of lesions in patients with axial spondyloarthropathy.

DISCLOSURE

The authors have nothing to disclose.

REFERENCES

1. Sieper J, Poddubnyy D. Axial spondyloarthritis. Lancet 2017;390:73–84.
2. Sieper J, Rudwaleit M, Baraliakos X, et al. The assessment of spondyloarthritis international Society (ASAS) handbook: a guide to assess spondyloarthritis. Ann Rheum Dis 2009;68(Suppl 2):ii1–44.
3. Rudwaleit M, Jurik AG, Hermann KGA, et al. Defining active sacroiliitis on magnetic resonance imaging (MRI) for classification of axial spondyloarthritis: a consensual approach by the ASAS/OMERACT MRI group. Ann Rheum Dis 2009;68:1520–7.
4. Mandl P, Navarro-Compan V, Terslev L, et al. EULAR recommendations for the use of imaging in the diagnosis and management of spondyloarthritis in clinical practice. Ann Rheum Dis 2015;74:1327–39.
5. Greese J, Diekhoff T, Sieper J, et al. Detection of sacroiliitis by short-tau inversion recovery and T2-weighted turbo spin echo sequences: results from the SIMACT study. J Rheumatol 2019;46:376–83.
6. Dalto VF, Assad RL, Crema MD, et al. MRI assessment of bone marrow oedema in the sacroiliac joints of patients with spondyloarthritis: is the SPAIR T2w technique comparable to STIR? Eur Radiol 2017;27:3669–76.
7. Ozgen A. The value of the T2-weighted multipoint dixon sequence in MRI of sacroiliac joints for the diagnosis of active and chronic sacroiliitis. Am J Roentgenol 2017;208:603–8.
8. Eshed I, Hermann KG. Novel imaging modalities in spondyloarthritis. Curr Opin Rheumatol 2015;27:333–42.
9. Raya JG, Dietrich O, Reiser MF, et al. Methods and applications of diffusion imaging of vertebral bone marrow. J Magn Reson Imaging 2006;24:1207–20.
10. Gezmis E, Donmez FY, Agildere M. Diagnosis of early sacroiliitis in seronegative spondyloarthropathies by DWI and correlation of clinical and laboratory findings with ADC values. Eur J Radiol 2013;82:2316–21.
11. Boy FN, Kayhan A, Karakas HM, et al. The role of multi-parametric MR imaging in the detection of early inflammatory sacroiliitis according to ASAS criteria. Eur J Radiol 2014;83:989–96.
12. Ren C, Zhu Q, Yuan H. Mono-exponential and bi-exponential model-based diffusion-weighted MR imaging and IDEAL-IQ sequence for quantitative evaluation of sacroiliitis in patients with ankylosing spondylitis. Clin Rheumatol 2018;37:3069–76.
13. Bray TJP, Vendhan K, Ambrose N, et al. Diffusion-weighted imaging is a sensitive biomarker of response to biologic therapy in enthesitis-related arthritis. Rheumatology 2017;56:399–407.
14. Beltran LS, Samim M, Gyftopoulos S, et al. Does the addition of DWI to fluid-sensitive conventional MRI of the sacroiliac joints improve the diagnosis of sacroiliitis? Am J Roentgenol 2018;210:1309–16.
15. Kucybala I, Ciuk S, Urbanik A, et al. The usefulness of diffusion-weighted imaging (DWI) and dynamic contrast-enhanced (DCE) sequences visual assessment in the early diagnosis of axial spondyloarthritis. Rheumatol Int 2019;39(9):1559–65.
16. Lambert RG, Maksymowych WP. Diffusion-weighted imaging in axial spondyloarthritis: a measure of effusion or does it elicit confusion? J Rheumatol 2018;45:729–30.

17. Mallinson PI, Coupal TM, McLaughlin PD, et al. Dual-energy CT for the musculo-skeletal system. Radiology 2016;281:690–707.

18. Yu L, Christner JA, Leng S, et al. Virtual monochromatic imaging in dual-source dual-energy CT: radiation dose and image quality. Med Phys 2011;38:6371–9.

19. Goo HW, Goo JM. Dual-energy CT: new horizon in medical imaging. Korean J Radiol 2017;18:555–69.

20. Jans L, De Kock I, Herregods N, et al. Dual-energy CT: a new imaging modality for bone marrow oedema in rheumatoid arthritis. Ann Rheum Dis 2018;77:958–60.

21. Fukuda T, Umezawa Y, Asahina A, et al. Dual energy CT iodine map for delineating inflammation of inflammatory arthritis. Eur Radiol 2017;27:5034–40.

22. Fukuda T, Umezawa Y, Tojo S, et al. Initial experience of using dual-energy CT with an iodine overlay image for hand psoriatic arthritis: comparison study with contrast-enhanced MR imaging. Radiology 2017;284:134–42.

23. Pascart T, Norberciak L, Legrand J, et al. Dual-energy computed tomography in calcium pyrophosphate deposition: initial clinical experience. Osteoarthritis Cartilage 2019;27(9):1309–14.

24. Pache G, Krauss B, Strohm P, et al. Dual-energy CT virtual noncalcium technique: detecting posttraumatic bone marrow lesions–feasibility study. Radiology 2010; 256:617–24.

25. Guggenberger R, Gnannt R, Hodler J, et al. Diagnostic performance of dual-energy CT for the detection of traumatic bone marrow lesions in the ankle: comparison with MR imaging. Radiology 2012;264:164–73.

26. Foti G, Catania M, Caia S, et al. Identification of bone marrow edema of the ankle: diagnostic accuracy of dual-energy CT in comparison with MRI. Radiol Med 2019;124(10):1028–36.

27. Wu H, Zhang G, Shi L, et al. Axial spondyloarthritis: dual-energy virtual noncalcium CT in the detection of bone marrow edema in the sacroiliac joints. Radiology 2019;290:157–64.

28. Weber U, Lambert RG, Ostergaard M, et al. The diagnostic utility of magnetic resonance imaging in spondylarthritis: an international multicenter evaluation of one hundred eighty-seven subjects. Arthritis Rheum 2010;62:3048–58.

29. Christiansen AA, Hendricks O, Kuettel D, et al. Limited reliability of radiographic assessment of sacroiliac joints in patients with suspected early spondyloarthritis. J Rheumatol 2017;44:70–7.

30. Redberg RF. Cancer risks and radiation exposure from computed tomographic scans how can we be sure that the benefits outweigh the risks? Arch Intern Med 2009;169:2049–50.

31. Poddubnyy D, Gaydukova I, Hermann KG, et al. Magnetic resonance imaging compared to conventional radiographs for detection of chronic structural changes in sacroiliac joints in axial spondyloarthritis. J Rheumatol 2013;40: 1557–65.

32. Hu L, Huang Z, Zhang X, et al. The performance of MRI in detecting subarticular bone erosion of sacroiliac joint in patients with spondyloarthropathy: a comparison with X-ray and CT. Eur J Radiol 2014;83:2058–64.

33. Diekhoff T, Hermann KG, Greese J, et al. Comparison of MRI with radiography for detecting structural lesions of the sacroiliac joint using CT as standard of reference: results from the SIMACT study. Ann Rheum Dis 2017;76:1502–8.

34. Weber U, Pedersen SJ, Ostergaard M, et al. Can erosions on MRI of the sacroiliac joints be reliably detected in patients with ankylosing spondylitis? - A cross-sectional study. Arthritis Res Ther 2012;14:R124.

35. Baraliakos X, Hoffmann F, Deng X, et al. Detection of erosions in the sacroiliac joints of patients with axial spondyloarthritis using the magnetic resonance imaging VIBE technique. J Rheumatol 2019;46(11):1445–9.

36. Abdulaal OM, Rainford L, MacMahon P, et al. 3T MRI of the knee with optimised isotropic 3D sequences: accurate delineation of intra-articular pathology without prolonged acquisition times. Eur Radiol 2017;27:4563–70.

37. Algin O, Gokalp G, Ocakoglu G. Evaluation of bone cortex and cartilage of spondyloarthropathic sacroiliac joint: efficiency of different fat-saturated MRI sequences (T1-weighted, 3D-FLASH, and 3D-DESS). Acad Radiol 2010;17:1292–8.

38. Diekhoff T, Greese J, Sieper J, et al. Improved detection of erosions in the sacroiliac joints on MRI with volumetric interpolated breath-hold examination (VIBE): results from the SIMACT study. Ann Rheum Dis 2018;77:1585–9.

39. Krohn M, Braum LS, Sieper J, et al. Erosions and fatty lesions of sacroiliac joints in patients with axial spondyloarthritis: evaluation of different MRI techniques and two scoring methods. J Rheumatol 2014;41:473–80.

40. Kataoka M, Ueda H, Koyama T, et al. Contrast-enhanced volumetric interpolated breath-hold examination compared with spin-echo T1-weighted imaging of head and neck tumors. Am J Roentgenol 2005;184:313–9.

41. Maksymowych WP, Wichuk S, Chiowchanwisawakit P, et al. Fat metaplasia on MRI of the sacroiliac joints increases the propensity for disease progression in the spine of patients with spondyloarthritis. RMD Open 2017;3:e000399.

42. van der Kolk B, van Stralen M, Podlogar M, et al. Reconstruction of osseous structures in MRI scans of the cervical spine with BoneMRI: a quantitative analysis. Poster in: ASNR 57th Annual Meeting. Boston, May 18-23, 2019.

The Future of Imaging in Axial Spondyloarthritis

Manouk de Hooge, PhD[a,b,*]

KEYWORDS

- Axial spondyloarthritis • Imaging • MRI • Conventional radiography
- Immunoscintigraphy • Low-dose CT

KEY POINTS

- MRI and conventional radiography are recommended imaging techniques in axial spondyloarthritis (axSpA) but are not the only options for diagnosing patients with axSpA.
- Studies report a minimal effect on the performance of the Assessment of Spondyloarthritis International Society classification criteria when adding structural MRI–sacroiliac (MRI-SI) lesions or spinal MRI lesions to the definition of a positive MRI.
- Despite several disadvantages, nuclear imaging methods should not be ruled out in the individual diagnostic process and evaluation of patients with axSpA.
- Taking into account the limited and contradicting data currently available, further investigation on the morphology and location of MRI-SI lesions is needed to distinguish MRI lesions in patients with axSpA from spondyloarthritis-like lesions.

THE CURRENT POSITION OF IMAGING IN AXIAL SPONDYLOARTHRITIS

With the lack of an appropriate gold standard and the absence of a pathognomonic feature, the recognition and diagnosis of axial spondyloarthritis (axSpA), especially in the early stages, is still a time-consuming process. AxSpA is considered to have a heterogeneous clinical presentation. In daily practice, patients suspected to have axSpA therefore often go through an extensive diagnostic work-up involving clinical assessment, laboratory tests, and imaging to identify illustrative features so that a diagnosis can be made. There are 2 important imaging techniques used for diagnostic purpose in axSpA. For late diagnosis, conventional radiography is often used. Patients with axSpA with severe disease, ankylosing spondylitis (AS), are characterized by the presence and development of syndesmophytes and radiographic sacroiliitis. Spinal structural damage is measured most accurately with the modified Stoke Ankylosis Spondylitis Spine Score (mSASSS), whereas the modified New York (mNY) criteria are preferred to assess radiographic sacroiliitis.[1] For early recognition of axSpA, MRI is the main tool. Unlike conventional radiography, MRI can visualize inflammation and

a Department of Rheumatology, Ghent University Hospital, Ghent, Belgium; b VIB Center of Inflammation Research, Ghent University, Ghent, Belgium
* Corneel Heymanslaan 10, 9000 Ghent, Belgium
E-mail address: msmdehooge@gmail.com

Rheum Dis Clin N Am 46 (2020) 301–313
https://doi.org/10.1016/j.rdc.2020.01.005
0889-857X/20/© 2020 Elsevier Inc. All rights reserved.

rheumatic.theclinics.com

is therefore used in addition to identify patients with axSpA in an early stage. Rheumatologists worldwide prefer imaging, especially MRI, rather than human leukocyte antigen (HLA) B27 testing in the diagnostic process.[2,3] Although imaging results play an important role in the diagnostic considerations of rheumatologists and increase the confidence in a diagnosis regardless of a positive or negative imaging outcome, physicians do not explicitly find imaging crucial in the diagnostic process of axSpA.[4,5] Besides the involvement in the diagnostic process, imaging is used for the classification of axSpA. In the Assessment of SpondyloArthritis International Society (ASAS) classification criteria for axSpA, the importance of imaging is evident because there is a clear role for radiography and MRI. Unlike in the diagnostic process, imaging in these criteria is limited to sacroiliitis, which can either refer to radiographic sacroiliitis, according to the mNY criteria, or to the presence of inflammation on MRI of the sacroiliac (SI) joints (MRI-SI); that is, a positive MRI-SI according to the ASAS definition.[6] Following this definition, a positive MRI-SI shows 1 or more inflammatory lesion highly suggestive of axSpA and visible on 2 or more consecutive slices, or more inflammatory lesions on the same slice. The sole presence of synovitis, capsulitis, or enthesitis is insufficient for a positive MRI-SI.[7,8] For diagnosis as well as classification of axSpA, MRI and radiography are the imaging techniques most commonly used, which is reflected in the European League Against Rheumatism (EULAR) recommendations for the use of imaging in axSpA.[9] Therefore the focus here is on radiography and MRI.

CHALLENGES AND AREAS OF DEVELOPMENT

With the development of the ASAS classification criteria, and therewith the official introduction of MRI in classifying patients with axSpA, there has been substantial improvement in the understanding and early recognition of axSpA. However, there are still areas that need attention, and several unmet needs remain.

Reliability of Reading Assessments

The interobserver and intraobserver reliability for imaging in axSpA has been a constant topic of discussion. In particular, the agreement on radiographic sacroiliitis is considered low and does not seem to improve with education or training.[10,11] The agreement on sacroiliitis on MRI according to the ASAS definition shows more potential (kappa = 0.73) but still 7.9% of patients with inflammatory back pain change classification criteria fulfillment solely based on different imaging assessment between readers.[12] When focusing on spinal lesions, there is a disappointing agreement between local and central (calibrated) readers in both radiographs (kappa = 0.26) as well as MRI scans (kappa = 0.27), in which local observers overestimate spinal lesions on imaging in the context of axSpA. The agreement between central readers seems to be good (kappa = 0.79) for radiographic spinal lesions, moderate (kappa = 0.58) for inflammation, and poor (kappa = 0.19) for syndesmophytes on MRI of the spine.[13,14] These data support the use of radiographic and MRI consensus scores determined by calibrated central readers rather than local readers, with the notion that spinal structural MRI lesions are also challenging for calibrated readers. For clinical trials and cohort studies, using central reader scores is an appropriate choice; however, obtaining central reader scores to use in daily practice seems less feasible.

Differentiation Between Axial Spondyloarthritis Lesions and Spondyloarthritis-like Lesions

A recent rapidly developing field of interest is focusing on the presence of MRI lesions found in the population at large that have similar characteristics to axSpA MRI lesions.

Alarmingly, several studies report on SpA-like bone marrow edema (BME) on MRI-SI in study populations of postpartum women,[15,16] runners,[16] military recruits,[17] athletes,[18] and in healthy people.[19,20] The ASAS definition of positive MRI-SI was met in a substantial percentage of patients throughout these studies. In addition, 1 study also reported an extremely high presence of inflammatory MRI-spine lesions (in 88.6% of male and 84.6% of female subjects) in healthy subjects.[20] The reason for frequently reported BME on MRI in healthy individuals is not known. A potential explanation is that it can be caused by mechanical stress. However, this is not certain, because conflicting data have been published on inflammation caused by mechanical involvement in axSpA.[17,21]

Now that it is evident that inflammatory SpA-like lesions are present in healthy people, the obvious question is: how can the axSpA be separated from the SpA-like lesions? Weber and colleagues[18] suggest that the location of BME lesions can be a distinctive feature. They found the posterior lower iliac bone to be the most affected SI joint region in athletes. In contrast, another study compared patients with chronic back pain to patients with axSpA, and found the lower posterior iliac region to be the most affected area with BME in patients with axSpA. The upper anterior sacral region was the most affected area for BME in the non-SpA patient group.[22] Another characteristic that should be evaluated to a larger extent is extensive inflammatory MRI lesions. According to de Winter and colleagues,[16] the extensiveness of BME MRI-SI lesions may contribute to the distinction between patients with axSpA and healthy persons, because deep (extensive) lesions are reported almost exclusively in patients with axSpA.

Final conclusions cannot be drawn yet, but these studies on possible background noise findings and the typical characteristics show an interesting area for gaining insights on MRI lesions representative for axSpA.

Defining a Positive MRI Scan

Another recurring topic of discussion is the comprehensiveness of the current definition of a positive MRI scan, as mentioned in the ASAS classification criteria for axSpA. There is some evidence that the structural MRI-SI abnormalities of fatty lesions and erosions may contribute to the usefulness of MRI in axSpA classification, although this is not the case for sclerosis and ankylosis.[23] Cutoffs of greater than or equal to 3 erosions, greater than or equal to 3 fatty lesions, and greater than or equal to 5 erosions and/or fatty lesions were found to be specific for axSpA ($\geq$95% specificity).[24] These cutoffs were subsequently used to assess the impact of structural MRI-SI lesions on the classification of patients with axSpA. Investigators concluded that adding structural MRI-SI lesions to the definition of sacroiliitis on imaging as well as replacing radiographic sacroiliitis by structural MRI-SI lesions has little impact on the classification of patients with axSpA. Most patients change from one subcategory to another but most (80.6%–95.5%, depending on the reader) do not change fulfillment of the ASAS classification criteria.[25]

At the time of developing the ASAS criteria, spinal MRI lesions were discarded for inclusion in the definition of a positive MRI because of limited evidence on the added value of these lesions in the classification of axSpA. Recently a study was published tackling this query. Ez-Zaitouni and colleagues[26] showed that, in patients with chronic back pain (SPACE cohort) and inflammatory back pain (DESIR cohort) with symptom onset less than 3 years, including positive MRI-spine as an imaging feature in the ASAS axSpA classification criteria yields few newly classified patients. Also, the number of patients with positive MRI-spine but negative MRI-SI was 1% and 7%, respectively. This finding is in line with previously published data in patients with long-standing disease.[27]

The definitions of MRI-SI lesions have recently been updated by the ASAS,[28] but no changes have been made to the classification criteria. Literature on the added utility of spinal MRI and structural MRI-SI lesions is present but is too limited to be a basis for radical changes in the definition of positive MRI. The few studies that investigate the added value of either structural MRI-SI or spinal MRI lesions show only marginal impact when added to the criteria. These findings all argue in favor of keeping the current definition of a positive MRI scan in the ASAS classification criteria.

The Natural Course of Disease

Until now there has not been a full understanding of the pathologic pathway of axSpA, but it is proposed that inflammation precedes structural damage. Inflammation on MRI-SI at baseline is highly predictive of radiographic SI progression after 5 years in HLA-B27-positive (odds ratio [OR], 5.4; 95% confidence interval [CI], 3.3–8.9) and HLA-B27–negative patients (OR, 2.2; 95% CI, 1.0–4.5).[29] This group also reported that, in 5 years, inflammation in 1 SI quadrant leads to sclerosis (OR, 1.7; 95% CI, 1.0–3.2), erosions (OR, 2.0; 95% CI, 1.5–2.5), or fatty lesions (OR, 1.7; 95% CI, 1.2–2.5) in the same quadrant.[30] In the spine, this association is less clear-cut; vertebral corner inflammation and fat deposition on MRI slightly increases the chance of new syndesmophyte forming at the same level but does not predict growth of existing syndesmophytes over 2 years. Nevertheless, most new syndesmophytes developed without preceding inflammation.[31,32]

These findings emphasize the pathophysiologic implications of inflammation in axSpA. They also suggest the presence of noninflammatory pathways, especially in the spine. However, the natural progression of lesions over a longer period remains unknown. Cohort studies that could offer insights currently exist, but longer follow-up is the key factor so it will take some time before there are answers.

Is There a Role for Posterior Elements?

Lesions in the posterior structures of the spine (pedicles, facet joints, spinous and transverse processes, and soft tissue) are often overlooked but may be of clinical significance because inflammation of the facet joints may lead to longer disease duration, higher disease activity, and functional impairment. In addition, it is suggested that the development of syndesmophytes is preceded by facet joint ankylosis.[33–35] So, do posterior elements of the spine play a role in the diagnostic process of axSpA? The number of studies investigating this topic is limited. A study group showed that including radiographic damage of the cervical facet joints in the assessment of spinal structural damage increases the sensitivity of the mSASSS method in patients with AS on anti-tumor necrosis factor (TNF) treatment, without introducing more measurement errors.[36] When focusing on MRI inflammation in the posterior elements, a high percentage (87.5%) of patients with AS with greater than or equal to 1 inflammatory posterior element lesion anywhere in the spine has been reported. The extent of inflammatory lesions was slightly lower in the posterior elements (6.7 ± 5.3 spinal levels) compared with inflammation in the vertebral body (8.4 ± 6.7 spinal levels) but still evidently present.[37] In line with those findings, another study reported inflammatory lesions in the posterior elements in patients with AS but to a lesser extent (3.7 ± 5.3), likely because the investigators only took facet joints into account.[38] Although studies show the presence of posterior inflammatory lesions in patients with axSpA, they also show a concordant presence with BME in the vertebra in AS,[39] nonradiographic axSpA,[39,40] and HLA-B27–positive patients with SpA.[41] However, all these studies lack a control group. Studies reporting on the added value of posterior element inflammation in early axSpA recognition including a proper control group (eg, patients with non-specific back pain) have yet to be performed.

With the complex anatomy of the facet joints, it is difficult to properly display damage in these structures. In addition, it is extremely challenging to evaluate the thoracic facet joints on plain radiographs because of overprojection of other structures such as the costotransverse and costovertebral joints. The advantage of MRI is that anatomic structures are visualized throughout the whole structure and therefore a three-dimensional image can be made. However, to our knowledge, there have not been any studies related to axSpA reporting on structural MRI lesions in the posterior elements. A reason may be that with MRI it is also difficult to accurately evaluate posterior elements, because they are only visible on 1 or 2 slices in the sagittal plane (the recommended MRI-spine scan protocol for axSpA lesions). For reasons mentioned earlier, it is likely that the involvement of structural damage of the facet joints in axSpA is currently underrated, but this may change in the near future. Recently there have been a few studies using computed tomography (CT) imaging techniques for assessing facet joint lesions. Tan and colleagues[42] showed 51 out 55 patients with AS with greater than or equal to 1 facet joint fusion on thoracolumbar CT scans. However, as with inflammatory lesions in the posterior elements and the vertebral body, ankylosis of the facet joints is often seen concordant with syndesmophytes in the vertebra; in 89.9% of the patients there is overlap. Another (low-dose) CT study including patients with AS with greater than or equal to 1 syndesmophyte on conventional radiographs covered the whole spine (C2 to S1) and found lesions in the cervical (means of 2.3–2.0), thoracic (means of 5.9–6.8), and lumbar (means of 1.0–1.8) segments assessed by 2 readers independently.[43] In the same cohort, the reliability of state and changes scores was measured and found to be good in all segments excluding the lumbar spine, where, in general, limited progression was seen. This study showed that low-dose CT is an appropriate imaging technique to evaluate progression of facet joint ankylosis in patients with AS.[44] Although the diagnostic utility of facet joint ankylosis in axSpA is still unclear, it is positive to have identified an imaging technique that depicts facet ankylosis well.

For lesions in the posterior elements, it seems that MRI best shows inflammation, whereas CT is promising for structural lesions. However, research on the precise involvement of these lesions is limited and studies with control groups are missing. Therefore, no conclusive verdict can be given on the utility of posterior element lesions in axSpA.

OUT OF THE COMFORT ZONE

Radiography and MRI are currently the preferred imaging techniques in axSpA.[9] Nonetheless, other techniques can be used to diagnose axSpA. Looking beyond the 2 common imaging techniques, there are alternative options that could counter the disadvantages of conventional radiography and/or MRI. Dual-energy CT scanning is discussed earlier in Min Chen and colleagues' article, "Emerging Imaging Techniques in Spondyloarthritis: Dual-Energy CT and New MRI Sequences," in this issue, as well as several new MRI sequences, other than the short-tau inversion recovery and T1-weighted sequences that are generally used in axSpA for MRI assessment. Therefore, these techniques are not repeated here. In addition, ultrasonography is not discussed further because this technique is useful for depicting small, peripheral joints but is not preferred for the joints involved in axSpA. The focus here is on the additional value of different nuclear imaging techniques to diagnose patients with axSpA.

Bone Scintigraphy

With this technique, the radionuclide technetium-99m (Tc-99m) is chemically attached to a ligand that is preferentially taken up by bone. The tracer uptake is increased in areas with a high bone turnover, such as inflamed sites, which makes it possible to visualize, for example, inflammation in the SI joints. Several decades ago, the results of studies using bone scintigraphy to identify sacroiliitis were promising. However, in 2008, an systematic literature review on the performance of scintigraphy concluded there was very low diagnostic value for this imaging technique axSpA.[45] In 2010 Song and colleagues[46] reported a moderate performance (sensitivity 64.9%/specificity 50.5%) of conventional bone scintigraphy using Tc-99m labeled methylene diphosphate in 207 chronic back pain patients. Instead of using MRI as an external standard as previous studies did, this study more accurately used the diagnosis of the rheumatologist (axSpA or no axSpA) to test the performance of scintigraphy scanning. Interestingly, when reporting on isolated unilateral sacroiliitis, specificity increased to 92.8% because false-positive rates decreased enormously. However, sensitivity decreased to 24.7%, which also showed the diminished diagnostic value of scintigraphy in axSpA. More recently, there have been some studies using anti–TNF alpha antibodies with radionuclides as a tracer in scintigraphy scanning. These studies report some use for scintigraphy in axSpA, but the scintigraphy never outperforms the MRI.[47,48] In a follow-up report, Carron and colleagues[49] found a strong correlation between tracer uptake on the immunoscintigraphy with Tc-99m–radiolabeled certolizumab and BME on MRI-SI in the same quadrant in patients with axSpA. There was a high correlation between tracer uptake and deep inflammatory MRI lesions (extended $\geq$1 cm from the articular surface of the SI joints into the bone, defined according to the SPARCC definition). This correlation was not found with so-called intense lesions. Although the number of patients in this study was limited, this finding has potential interest and touches on a reoccurring topic of the possible relevance of extensive (deep) inflammatory lesions in patients with axSpA.

There is limited added value in using bone scintigraphy the as imaging method in diagnosing patients with axSpA. Although immunoscintigraphy, using labeled monoclonal antibodies, does not outperform MRI this technique may provide more insight into the pathophysiologic course of disease at different stages. Moreover, in daily practice, finding the correct diagnosis and treatment requires an individualized approach and conventional scintigraphy or immunoscintigraphy can play a role in this process. Nevertheless, the high radiation burden is a disadvantage that should carefully be taken into account when considering this imaging technique.

^{18}F-Fluorodeoxyglucose PET/Computed Tomography

Another nuclear imaging method that is, of interest to present abnormal bone activity is ^{18}F-fluorodeoxyglucose (FDG) PET/CT. The diagnostic potential of PET imaging has been investigated in several studies. The concordance between inflammatory MRI-SI lesions and tracer uptake on ^{18}F-FDG-PET/CT scans was good, but there was no full overlap within the same quadrant in patients with either radiographic or nonradiographic axSpA.[50,51] The correlation between PET imaging and structural lesions is less straightforward. Strobel and colleagues[52] showed a low sensitivity of PET in patients with AS with sacroiliitis grade 2 or 3. Other studies reported poor agreements with erosions, sclerosis, and ankylosis on MRI-SI of patients with active SpA.[53,54] Nevertheless, not all structural MRI-SI lesions were badly correlated with tracer uptake on FDG-PET/CT scans. Particularly areas with both inflammatory as well as fatty lesions, but also areas with less inflammatory activity but where bone turnover is more prominent, such as areas with (postinflammatory) fatty lesions, correlate well with tracer uptake.[55,56] A better association between tracer uptake and BME and/or fatty lesions compared with only BME lesions was seen in both SI and spine; however, it is more explicit in the spine, with an increase in percentage agreement of 26.3%.[54] High levels of tracer uptake are therefore reported in areas with high BME MRI lesions as well as areas with low BME but high fatty MRI lesions, and lower levels of tracer uptake are reported in areas with more established MRI lesions (eg, erosions). Therefore, it can be suggested that FDG-PET/CT reflects areas with osteoblastic activity rather than pure inflammation in patients with axSpA. If this is the case, FDG-PET/CT scans might preferably be chosen for monitoring the course of disease because FDG-PET/CT scans can give a meaningful contribution to the prediction of structural damage. However, the credibility of that theory has yet to be proved. Proper studies on the utility of FDG-PET/CT scans are still missing because most studies currently available have a small study population and lack a control group. As with scintigraphy, PET/CT scans also have a very high radiation dose, which is a major disadvantage and makes both techniques less appropriate for daily care.

Low-Dose Computed Tomography

In 2015, a EULAR taskforce published recommendations for the use of imaging in axSpA. By these recommendations, conventional radiography and MRI are endorsed. Other imaging techniques are generally not recommended, with the exception of CT. With the conventional CT imaging technique, it is not possible to visualize inflammatory signs in addition to joint destruction. However, this technique may provide a contribution to the visualization of structural damage under conditions in which the radiographs are negative, it is not possible to perform MRI, and there is still a valid suspicion of axSpA.[9] Although recommended by EULAR, the value of MRI in detecting structural lesions is still under debate, and some literature even suggests CT instead of MRI as the gold standard to evaluate structural damage in SI joints.[57,58] Literature also shows that CT is much more sensitive than MRI for the detection and 2-year change in scores of syndesmophytes.[59] In addition, CT imaging proves to be more sensitive in detecting syndesmophytes than conventional radiography, which at the moment is still the recommended method to identify and assess syndesmophytes in patients with axSpA. The superiority of CT was most explicit in the detection of already existing syndesmophytes that grew over time, but CT also detected more new syndesmophytes.[60,61]

The argument that CT imaging comes with inherent risk factors because it has a high radiation exposure has been refuted with the development of the low-dose CT (ldCT) imaging technique in axSpA. With ldCT, the exposure to radiation is similar to that of radiography with the advantage of properly displaying three-dimensional structures such as the SI joints. However, it is understandable that MRI is given preference in clinical practice and classification of axSpA, because it is impossible to visualize either inflammatory or fatty lesions with conventional and low-dose CT.

SUMMARY

This article focuses mainly on the role of imaging for diagnostic and classification purposes. Besides these, imaging can be used to monitor disease and can play a part in predicting treatment response. The next article in this issue concentrates on these topics.

Several unmet needs and challenges with the common goal to increase the understanding and improve the recognition of axSpA have been discussed. There are difficulties in obtaining high agreement for readers assessing conventional radiography or MRI lesions typical of axSpA. In addition, SpA-like lesions are frequently recorded in healthy people. A part of the answer to how to overcome these difficulties may lie in the morphology of lesions, because deep MRI-SI lesions seem to be characteristic for axSpA. This area of research needs further exploration. Although there is a belief that the current definition of a positive MRI scan would improve when extended, studies investigating this all report that adding either structural MRI-SI lesions or spinal MRI lesions seems to yield a minimal effect on the utility of the ASAS classification criteria. Perhaps involving the posterior elements could give additional value to the classification and even the diagnosis of axSpA as well as the further understanding of the course of disease. Current literature cannot give a conclusive answer yet; however, it shows that this is a relevant field for future research.

Conventional radiography and MRI are the endorsed imaging techniques in axSpA. In addition to these techniques, this article discusses several studies using nuclear imaging techniques. The current studies on scintigraphy and FDG-PET/CT imaging techniques have limitations that must be taken into account. Most studies have small sample sizes and often miss a valid control group to test the performance of these techniques. The techniques themselves also have disadvantages. First, these techniques come with a high radiation burden. These methods are invasive because there is an administration of tracer into the body. Patients often experience this as unpleasant. Second, it is time consuming because it may take 1 hour to several hours for the body to take up the tracer. There is also a limitation in the assessment of the lesions. There are standardized scoring approaches for inflammation or structural damage on neither the scintigraphy nor the FDG-PET scan. The scoring methods are often semiquantitative and never validated, which makes the comparison with lesion scores on conventional radiographs or MRI ambivalent. This problem in contrast with the ldCT imaging technique, which has a low radiation dose and for which 2 scoring methods have been proved valid.[60,62] Despite several disadvantages, nuclear imaging methods should not be ruled out in the individual diagnostic process and evaluation of patients with axSpA. Especially for patients with medical implants or other nonremovable bodily metal and patients who may not be able to undergo an MRI examination safely for other reasons, these alternative imaging techniques can be used.

In addition, MRI and conventional radiography are powerful imaging techniques but are not the sole means of diagnosing patients with axSpA. Diagnosing a patient with axSpA is about recognizing patterns, a process in which the rheumatologist should acquire a clear view of the probability of the disease. This view is only obtained when taking imaging, as well as the patient's medical history, results from physical examination and laboratory tests into consideration.

DISCLOSURE

The author has nothing to disclose.

REFERENCES

1. van der Heijde D, Landewé R. Selection of a method for scoring radiographs for ankylosing spondylitis clinical trials, by the Assessment in Ankylosing Spondylitis Working Group and OMERACT. J Rheumatol 2005;32(10):2048–9.

2. van der Heijde D, Sieper J, Elewaut D, et al. Referral patterns, diagnosis, and disease management of patients with axial spondyloarthritis: results of an International survey. J Clin Rheumatol 2014;20:411–7.

3. Ez-Zaitouni Z, Bakker P, Van Lunteren M, et al. Presence of multiple spondyloarthritis (SpA) features is important but not sufficient for a diagnosis of axial spondyloarthritis: Data from the SPondyloArthritis Caught Early (SPACE) cohort. Ann Rheum Dis 2017;76:1086–92.

4. Ez-Zaitouni Z, Landewé R, van Lunteren M, et al. Imaging of the sacroiliac joints is important for diagnosing early axial spondyloarthritis but not all-decisive. Rheumatology (Oxford) 2018;57:1173–9.

5. van den Berg R, de Hooge M, van Gaalen F, et al. Percentage of patients with spondyloarthritis in patients referred because of chronic back pain and performance of classification criteria: Experience from the spondyloarthritis caught early (SPACE) cohort. Rheumatology (Oxford) 2013;52:1492–9.

6. Rudwaleit M, Jurik A, Hermann K, et al. Defining active sacroiliitis on magnetic resonance imaging (MRI) for classification of axial spondyloarthritis: a consensual approach by the ASAS/OMERACT MRI group. Ann Rheum Dis 2009;68:1520–7.

7. Sieper J, Rudwaleit M, Baraliakos X, et al. The Assessment of SpondyloArthritis international Society (ASAS) handbook: a guide to assess spondyloarthritis. Ann Rheum Dis 2009;68(suppl 2):ii1–44.

8. Lambert RGW, Bakker P, van der Heijde D, et al. Defining active sacroiliitis on MRI for classification of axial spondyloarthritis: Update by the ASAS MRI working group. Ann Rheum Dis 2016;75:1958–63.

9. Mandl P, Navarro-Compán V, Terslev L, et al. EULAR recommendations for the use of imaging in the diagnosis and management of spondyloarthritis in clinical practice. Ann Rheum Dis 2015;74:1327–39.

10. van Tubergen A, Heuft-Dorenbosch L, Schulpen G, et al. Radiographic assessment of sacroiliitis by radiologists and rheumatologists: does training improve quality? Ann Rheum Dis 2003;62:519–25.

11. van den Berg R, Lenczner G, Feydy A, et al. Agreement between clinical practice and trained central reading in reading of sacroiliac joints on plain pelvic radiographs: results from the DESIR cohort. Arthritis Rheumatol 2014;66:2403–11.

12. van den Berg R, Lenczner G, Thévenin F, et al. Classification of axial SpA based on positive imaging (radiographs and/or MRI of the sacroiliac joints) by local rheumatologists or radiologists versus central trained readers in the DESIR cohort. Ann Rheum Dis 2015;74:2016–21.

13. Claudepierre P, de Hooge M, Feydy A, et al. Reliability of mSASSS scoring in everyday practice in DESIR-cohort study centres: Cross-sectional study of agreement with trained readers. Ann Rheum Dis 2016;75:2213–4.

14. de Hooge M, Pialat JB, Reijnierse M, et al. Assessment of typical SpA lesions on MRI of the spine: do local readers and central readers agree in the DESIR-cohort at baseline? Clin Rheumatol 2017;36:1551–9.

15. Renson T, De Craemer A-S, Depicker A, et al. High prevalence of sacroiliac bone marrow edema on mri in postpartum women: a temporary phenomenon. Ann Rheum Dis 2019;78(suppl. 2):A89.

16. de Winter J, de Hooge M, van de Sande M, et al. Magnetic resonance imaging of the sacroiliac joints indicating sacroiliitis according to the assessment of spondyloarthritis international society definition in healthy individuals, runners, and women with postpartum back pain. Arthritis Rheumatol 2018;70:1042–8.

17. Varkas G, De Hooge M, Renson T, et al. Effect of mechanical stress on magnetic resonance imaging of the sacroiliac joints: assessment of military recruits by magnetic resonance imaging study. Rheumatology (Oxford) 2018;57:508–13.
18. Weber U, Jurik AG, Zejden A, et al. Frequency and anatomic distribution of magnetic resonance imaging features in the sacroiliac joints of young athletes: exploring "background noise" toward a data-driven definition of sacroiliitis in early spondyloarthritis. Arthritis Rheumatol 2018;70:736–45.
19. Marzo-Ortega H, McGonagle D, O'Connor P, et al. Baseline and 1-year magnetic resonance imaging of the sacroiliac joint and lumbar spine in very early inflammatory back pain. Relationship between symptoms, HLA-B27 and disease extent and persistence. Ann Rheum Dis 2009;68:1721–7.
20. Baraliakos X, Feldmann D, Ott A, et al. Prevalence of inflammatory and chronic changes suggestive of axial spondyloarthritis in magnetic resonance images of the axial skeleton in individuals <45 years in the general population as part of a large community study (SHIP). Ann Rheum Dis 2018;77(suppl. 2):170.
21. Lovell G, Galloway H, Hopkins W, et al. Osteitis pubis and assessment of bone marrow edema at the pubic symphysis with MRI in an elite junior male soccer squad. Clin J Sport Med 2006;16:117–22.
22. Baraliakos X, Thomaschoff J, Fruth M, et al. Localization and morphology of magnetic resonance imaging features of pathologic changes in the sacroiliac joints suggestive of axial spondyloarthritis – a systematic comparison of patients and controls with chronic back pain. Ann Rheum Dis 2019;78(suppl. 2):A85.
23. Weber U, Lambert RGW, Pedersen SJ, et al. Assessment of structural lesions in sacroiliac joints enhances diagnostic utility of magnetic resonance imaging in early spondylarthritis. Arthritis Care Res (Hoboken) 2010;62:1763–71.
24. de Hooge M, van den Berg R, Navarro-Compán V, et al. Patients with chronic back pain of short duration from the SPACE cohort: which MRI structural lesions in the sacroiliac joints and inflammatory and structural lesions in the spine are most specific for axial spondyloarthritis? Ann Rheum Dis 2016;75(7):1308–14.
25. Bakker P, van den Berg R, Lenczner G, et al. Can we use structural lesions seen on MRI of the sacroiliac joints reliably for the classification of patients according to the ASAS axial spondyloarthritis criteria? Data from the DESIR cohort. Ann Rheum Dis 2017;76:392–8.
26. Ez-Zaitouni Z, Bakker P, Van Lunteren M, et al. The yield of a positive MRI of the spine as imaging criterion in the ASAS classification criteria for axial spondyloarthritis: results from the SPACE and DESIR cohorts. Ann Rheum Dis 2017;76: 1731–6.
27. Weber U, Zubler V, Zhao Z, et al. Does spinal MRI add incremental diagnostic value to MRI of the sacroiliac joints alone in patients with non-radiographic axial spondyloarthritis? Ann Rheum Dis 2014;1–8. https://doi.org/10.1136/annrheumdis-2013-203887.
28. Maksymowych WP, Lambert RG, Østergaard M, et al. MRI lesions in the sacroiliac joints of patients with spondyloarthritis: an update of definitions and validation by the ASAS MRI working group. Ann Rheum Dis 2019;78(11):1550–8.
29. Dougados M, Sepriano A, Molto A, et al. Sacroiliac radiographic progression in recent onset axial spondyloarthritis: the 5-year data of the DESIR cohort. Ann Rheum Dis 2017;76:1823–8.
30. Rodrigues-Manica S, Sepriano A, Ramiro S, et al. Association between bone marrow edema and structural progression in the same quadrant in axial spondyloarthritis – 5-year data from the desir cohort. Ann Rheum Dis 2019;78(suppl. 2):A88.

31. van der Heijde D, Machado P, Braun J, et al. MRI inflammation at the vertebral unit only marginally predicts new syndesmophyte formation: a multilevel analysis in patients with ankylosing spondylitis. Ann Rheum Dis 2012;71:369–73.

32. Machado PM, Baraliakos X, van der Heijde D, et al. MRI vertebral corner inflammation followed by fat deposition is the strongest contributor to the development of new bone at the same vertebral corner: a multilevel longitudinal analysis in patients with ankylosing spondylitis. Ann Rheum Dis 2016;75:1486–93.

33. De Vlam K, Mielants H, Verstraete KL, et al. The zygapophyseal joint determines morphology of the enthesophyte. J Rheumatol 2000;27:1732–9.

34. De Vlam K, Mielants H, Veys EM. Involvement of the zygapophyseal joint in ankylosing spondylitis: relation to the bridging syndesmophyte. J Rheumatol 1999;26:1738–45.

35. Maas F, Spoorenberg A, Brouwer E, et al. Radiographic damage and progression of the cervical spine in ankylosing spondylitis patients treated with TNF-α inhibitors: facet joints vs. vertebral bodies. Semin Arthritis Rheum 2017;46:562–8.

36. Maas F, Arends S, Brouwer E, et al. Incorporating assessment of the cervical facet joints in the modified Stoke ankylosing spondylitis spine score is of additional value in the evaluation of spinal radiographic outcome in ankylosing spondylitis. Arthritis Res Ther 2017;19:77.

37. Maksymowych W, Crowther S, Dhillon S, et al. Systematic assessment of inflammation by magnetic resonance imaging in the posterior elements of the spine in ankylosing spondylitis. Arthritis Care Res 2010;62:4–10.

38. Lee S, Lee J, Hwang J, et al. Clinical importance of inflammatory facet joints of the spine in ankylosing spondylitis: a magnetic resonance imaging study. Scand J Rheumatol 2016;45:491–8.

39. Krabbe S, Sørensen IJ, Jensen B, et al. Inflammatory and structural changes in vertebral bodies and posterior elements of the spine in axial spondyloarthritis: Construct validity, responsiveness and discriminatory ability of the anatomy-based CANDEN scoring system in a randomised placebo-contro. RMD Open 2018;4(1):e000624.

40. Althoff CE, Sieper J, Song I, et al. Active inflammation and structural change in early active axial spondyloarthritis as detected by whole-body MRI. Ann Rheum Dis 2013;72:967–73.

41. Larbi A, Fourneret B, Lukas C, et al. Prevalence and topographic distribution of spinal inflammation on MR imaging in patients recently diagnosed with axial spondyloarthritis. Diagn Interv Imaging 2017;98:347–53.

42. Tan S, Yao J, Flynn JA, et al. Zygapophyseal joint fusion in ankylosing spondylitis assessed by computed tomography: associations with syndesmophytes and spinal motion. J Rheumatol 2017;44:1004–10.

43. Stal R, van Gaalen F, Sepriano A, et al. Detection of facet joint ankylosis on whole spine low-dose ct in radiographic axial spondyloarthritis: data from the sensitive imaging of axial spondyloarthritis (SIAS) cohort. Ann Rheum Dis 2019;78(suppl. 2):A1355.

44. Stal R, van Gaalen F, Sepriano A, et al. Two-year progression of facet joint ankylosis on whole spine low-dose ct in patients with radiographic axial spondyloarthritis: data from the sensitive imaging of axial spondyloarthritis (SIAS) cohort. Ann Rheum Dis 2019;78(suppl. 2):A1356.

45. Song IH, Carrasco-Fernández J, Rudwaleit M, et al. The diagnostic value of scintigraphy in assessing sacroiliitis in ankylosing spondylitis: a systematic literature research. Ann Rheum Dis 2008;67:1535–40.

46. Song IH, Brandt H, Rudwaleit M, et al. Limited diagnostic value of unilateral sacroiliitis in scintigraphy in assessing axial spondyloarthritis. J Rheumatol 2010;37: 1200–2.

47. Carron P, Lambert B, De Vos F, et al. Scintigraphic detection of TNFα with a radio-labeled anti-TNFα in patients with active peripheral spondyloarthritis and rheumatoid arthritis. Arthritis Rheum 2013;65:S472.

48. de Andrade Alexandre D, de Souza S, Moraes do Carmo C, et al. Use of 99mTc-anti-TNF-α scintigraphy in a patient with non-radiographic axial spondyloarthritis. Ann Nucl Med 2014;28:936–9.

49. Carron P, de Hooge M, Renson T, et al. Immunoscintigraphy of sacroiliac joints shows very good agreement with inflammation on MRI in axial Spondyloarthritis patients. Ann Rheum Dis 2019;78(suppl 2):A1354.

50. Ouichka R, Bouderraoui F, Raynal M, et al. Performance of 18 F-sodium fluoride positron emission tomography with computed tomography to assess inflammatory and structural sacroiliitis on magnetic resonance imaging in axial spondyloarthritis. Clin Exp Rheumatol 2019;37:19–25.

51. Toussirot É, Caoduro C, Ungureanu C, et al. ^{18}F-fluoride PET/CT assessment in patients fulfilling the clinical arm of the ASAS criteria for axial spondyloarthritis. A comparative study with ankylosing spondylitis. Clin Exp Rheumatol 2015; 33:588.

52. Strobel K, Fischer DR, Tamborrini G, et al. 18F-Fluoride PET/CT for detection of sacroiliitis in ankylosing spondylitis. Eur J Nucl Med Mol Imaging 2010;37: 1760–5.

53. Raynal M, Remy O, Melchior J, et al. Performance of 18fluoride sodium positron emission tomography with computed tomography to assess inflammatory and structural sacroiliitis respectively on magnetic resonance imaging and computed tomography in axial spondyloarthritis. Arthritis Res Ther 2019;21:119.

54. Buchbender C, Ostendorf B, Ruhlmann V, et al. Hybrid 18f-labeled fluoride positron emission tomography/Magnetic Resonance (MR) imaging of the sacroiliac joints and the spine in patients with axial spondyloarthritis: A pilot study exploring the link of MR bone pathologies and increased osteoblastic ac. J Rheumatol 2015;42:1631–7.

55. Baraliakos X, Buchbender C, Ostendorf B, et al. Conventional magnetic resonance imaging (MR), hybrid 18f-fluoride positron emission tomography MRI (18f-f- PET/MRI) and computer tomography of the spine – A detailed description of pathologic signals in patients with active ankylosing spondylitis. Ann Rheum Dis 2014;73:79.

56. Bruijnen STG, van der Weijden MAC, Klein JP, et al. Bone formation rather than inflammation reflects Ankylosing Spondylitis activity on PET-CT: a pilot study. Arthritis Res Ther 2012;14:R71.

57. Baraliakos X, Braun J. Outcome assessment in axial spondyloarthritis-imaging techniques, their relation to outcomes and their use in clinical trials. Indian J Rheumatol 2013;8:S38–43.

58. Diekhoff T, Hermann KGA, Greese J, et al. Comparison of MRI with radiography for detecting structural lesions of the sacroiliac joint using CT as standard of reference: results from the SIMACT study. Ann Rheum Dis 2017;76:1502–8.

59. Tan S, Yao J, Flynn JA, et al. Quantitative syndesmophyte measurement in ankylosing spondylitis using CT: longitudinal validity and sensitivity to change over 2 years. Ann Rheum Dis 2015;74:437–47.

60. Tan S, Yao J, Flynn JA, et al. Quantitative measurement of syndesmophyte volume and height in ankylosing spondylitis using CT. Ann Rheum Dis 2014;73: 544–50.
61. de Koning A, de Bruin F, van den Berg R, et al. Low-dose CT detects more progression of bone formation in comparison to conventional radiography in patients with ankylosing spondylitis: Results from the SIAS cohort. Ann Rheum Dis 2018; 77:293–9.
62. de Bruin F, de Koning A, van den Berg R, et al. Development of the CT Syndesmophyte Score (CTSS) in patients with ankylosing spondylitis: data from the SIAS cohort. Ann Rheum Dis 2018;77:371–7.

Can Imaging Be a Proxy for Remission in Axial Spondyloarthritis?

Krystel Aouad, MD[a,b], Ann-Sophie De Craemer, MD[c,d],
Philippe Carron, MD, PhD[c,d],*

KEYWORDS

- Spondyloarthritis • Imaging • Remission • Monitoring

KEY POINTS

- Imaging plays an important role in the diagnosis of axial spondyloarthritis and is a surrogate marker for disease activity, just as many other parameters to guide treatment decisions.
- Monitoring of patients on treatment with sequential MRI has shown considerable reduction of inflammation with better treatment response in patients with objective signs of inflammation at baseline.
- Treating-to-target based on imaging remission has not yet proven its efficacy in axial spondyloarthritis.
- Emerging imaging tools, such as whole-body MRI and ^{18}F-fluoride PET-CT, have shown some evidence in monitoring of disease activity in clinical trials.

INTRODUCTION

Clinical remission is now a major target for the treatment of spondyloarthritis (SpA). The 2017 updated EULAR recommendations for axial SpA (axSpA) and psoriatic arthritis (PsA) focus on a treat-to-target (T2T) strategy.[1] They indicate that T2T should be the standard and general approach to care of SpA. The targets to be achieved within 3 to 6 months of starting therapy are defined as remission or, alternatively, low or minimal disease activity. Patients should be assessed regularly and, if the target is not attained, treatment should be escalated to the next phase of the algorithm. The 2017 task force arrived at a single set of recommendations for axSpA and peripheral

[a] Rheumatology Department, Saint-Joseph University, Alfred Naccache Boulevard, Achrafieh, PO Box 166830, Beirut, Lebanon; [b] Hotel-Dieu de France Hospital, Beirut, Lebanon; [c] Rheumatology Department, Ghent University Hospital, C. Heymanslaan 10, Gent 9000, Belgium; [d] Inflammation Research Center, VIB, Technologiepark-Zwijnaarde 71, 9052 Gent, Belgium
* Corresponding author. Rheumatology Department, Ghent University Hospital, C. Heymanslaan 10, Gent 9000, Belgium.
E-mail address: philippe.carron@ugent.be

Rheum Dis Clin N Am 46 (2020) 315–329
https://doi.org/10.1016/j.rdc.2020.01.006
0889-857X/20/© 2020 Elsevier Inc. All rights reserved.

SpA, including PsA.[1] Although no T2T study has been performed in axSpA, it is deemed that a predefined target algorithm with tight control of inflammation could also improve outcomes in axSpA, given the correlation between damage progression and disease activity.[2,3]

In clinical practice, validated clinical measurement of disease activity has been used to define the target for remission and adjust the treatment accordingly.[1,4] Increasingly, the importance of imaging modalities, especially MRI, has risen not only in diagnosing but also in monitoring of disease activity and prognostication of SpA.

The purpose of this article is to discuss current controversies regarding the use of imaging for monitoring disease activity and predicting treatment response and progression in axSpA with the emphasis on whether imaging remission should be the treatment target.

CLINICAL REMISSION AND IMAGING REMISSION

At present, there is evidence supporting that high disease activity is associated with radiographic progression and syndesmophyte formation in SpA, whereas remission or inactive disease is associated with inhibition of structural progression.[5] In fact, clinical remission or inactive disease is defined as "the absence of clinical and laboratory evidence of significant disease".[1] The Ankylosing Spondylitis Disease Activity Score (ASDAS) is the preferred outcome measure of disease activity in axSpA, recommended by the task force in the most recent T2T recommendations.[1] ASDAS has a better correlation with inflammatory biomarkers and MRI findings compared with the Bath Ankylosing Spondylitis Disease Activity Index (BASDAI). ASDAS remission or inactive disease is defined as an ASDAS less than 1.3 and ASDAS partial remission is defined as a value less than or equal to two units on a 0 to 10 scale in each of the four domains: patient global, function, pain, and inflammation. In PsA, Disease Activity Index for Psoriatic Arthritis (DAPSA) or minimal disease activity (MDA) are used to define clinical remission.[1]

Overall, the mainstay of T2T is to aim for clinical remission or inactive disease and, if unachievable, a state of low or minimal disease activity is an acceptable target.[1] Furthermore, the role of imaging in the assessment of disease activity has not yet been supported by evidence.[1] Nevertheless, recently conducted clinical trials have defined the concept of "imaging remission" with MRI scoring systems: Spondyloarthritis Research Consortium of Canada (SPARCC) sacroiliac joints (SIJ), spine 6-discovertebral unit, and the Berlin scoring system (modification of the Ankylosing Spondylitis Spine MRI Score for Activity [ASspiMRI-a]).

MRI, with its ability to detect active and structural lesions early after symptom onset, is considered as the optimal imaging modality in patients with clinically suspected SpA and is currently the main contributor for early diagnosis of SpA. This is also the reason why a positive MRI of the SIJ makes part of the 2009 Assessment of SpondyloArthritis International Society (ASAS) classification criteria for axSpA.[6] Furthermore, it has been well established that MRI findings are valuable in clinical trials and clinical practice because it can detect inflammation before structural damage develops. Notwithstanding, there is no consensus on a standardized definition of MRI remission. As a consequence, several trials have defined MRI remission in axSpA differently. In the EMBARK trial,[7] MRI remission of the SIJ and the spine was defined as SPARCC MRI SIJ score less than or equal to two and SPARCC MRI spinal 6-discovertebral unit score less than or equal to three, respectively. In the trial by Braun and colleagues,[8] remission thresholds were the validated SPARCC (SIJ) less than two and unvalidated Berlin (spine) less than or equal to two, whereas in the ABILITY-1 trial,[9] more stringent thresholds for MRI remission were used: a SPARCC score less than two for the SIJ, spine, or both.

Besides involvement of SIJ and spine, SpA can also manifest in peripheral joints and entheses that are visualized with MRI. Whole-body MRI (WBMRI) potentially allows assessment of the entire musculoskeletal system in one scan and seems like a promising tool for objective assessment and monitoring of axial and peripheral inflammatory activity in future clinical trials. However, further work on WBMRI indices as a sensitive objective outcome measure is justified to get them validated in independent cohorts and leading to a definition of WBMRI remission.

MONITORING OF DISEASE ACTIVITY DURING TREATMENT

Structural damage of the spine and SIJ is assessed on conventional radiographs (CR). Ankylosing spondylitis (AS) is characterized by the presence and development of syndesmophytes and sacroiliitis. With the modified Stoke Ankylosing Spondylitis Spine Score (mSASSS) spinal structural damage is measured most accurately, whereas the modified New York criteria are preferred to assess radiographic sacroiliitis.[10] To monitor structural changes in SpA, CR and MRI are mainly used (**Table 1**).[11] CR of the SIJ and/or spine may be performed on a 2-year follow-up basis to monitor structural changes over time. Computed tomography (CT) is also useful for the detection of structural changes in the SIJ because of its superior sensitivity and specificity in relation to CR. However, both methods are unable to visualize active inflammation and CT is associated with high radiation exposure mostly in young patients with axSpA. Nevertheless, this argument has been refuted with the entrance of low-dose CT imaging technique in the axSpA field. With low-dose CT the exposure to radiation is similar to that of CR with the advantage of properly displaying a three-dimensional structure, such as the SIJ. Still, it is understandable that MRI is given preference in clinical practice and for classification of axSpA, because it has led to a better understanding of the pathophysiology of the underlying structural progression in axSpA by identifying

Table 1 Use of imaging in axial spondyloarthritis		
	In Clinical Practice	**In Clinical Trials**
For diagnosis of SpA	CR MRI CR and MRI	CR MRI CR and MRI SPECT-CT[a]
For monitoring of disease activity	MRI[a]	MRI WBMRI[a] ^{18}F-fluoride PET-CT[a]
For monitoring of disease chronicity/ structural damage	CR MRI[a] CT[a]	CR MRI CT Low-dose CT[a]
For evaluating response to treatment	MRI[a]	MRI WBMRI[a]
For predicting progression (risk profiling)	MRI[a]	CR MRI WBMRI[a] ^{18}F-fluoride PET-CT[a]

Abbreviations: CT, computed tomography; SPECT, single-photon emission computed tomography.
  [a] Could be an option, more data needed regarding its use.

active inflammatory lesions (primarily bone marrow edema [BME]/osteitis) and more chronic structural lesions (bone erosions, fatty infiltration, sclerosis, backfill, and new bone formation/ankylosis).[12] Hence, MRI provides an objective measure and allows assessment of currently active inflammation in patients with SpA. It has gained a decisive role in follow-up and response to therapy in clinical trials and may possibly lead to treatment adjustment in clinical practice.

The question whether a repetition of MRI scans to monitor a patient in remission makes clinical sense has been overviewed in several studies. These trials have followed patients on biologic disease-modifying antirheumatic drugs (bDMARDs) and compared MRI inflammation at baseline and during and after treatment. In one study, 14 patients with axSpA on etanercept (ETN) with a control group were followed and repetitive MRI scans (at Weeks 0, 6, 24, and 102) were done showing a significant reduction of active inflammatory lesions of the spine in the ETN arm (mean ASspiMRI-a decreased from 23.7 ± 13.3 at Weeks 0–5 ± 5.4 at Week 102).[13] However, some patients still presented with spinal inflammation after 2 years of ETN therapy and no correlation was found between MRI changes and clinical measures of disease activity. Another study with 12 patients treated with ETN showed a significant and rapid regression of active inflammatory spinal lesions on MRI after only 6 weeks of treatment and reduction of inflammation by 69% ($P = .012$) after 24 weeks.[14] Moreover, no progression of chronic lesions of the spine occurred in the ETN group. Another trial obtained repetitive MRI scans (at Weeks 0, 12, and 52) in 38 patients with active AS treated with adalimumab and, at Week 12, 53.6% and 52.9% reduction in the mean SPARCC score of the spine and SIJ, respectively, was observed.[15] In contrast, a 9.4% increase in spine score was noted in the placebo arm at Week 12. A reduction of MRI spinal inflammation was found in ASAS responders but also in ASAS nonresponders.[15] Another observational study assessed spinal MRI results in 13 patients with AS treated with secukinumab.[16] At Week 94, a regression of 75% and 83% in the Berlin score was achieved in ASAS20 and ASAS40 responders, respectively, with a good correspondence in the same subjects between inflammation reduction of the spine and clinical response at Week 94.[16] A larger study, the EMBARK,[7,17,18] assessed treatment response with clinical outcomes and also repetitive MRI scans showing reduction of inflammatory MRI lesions at Week 12 that was sustained at Week 104 in patients with ETN-treated axSpA. The RAPID-axSpA phase III trial[19] included 315 certolizumab pegol (CZP)-treated axSpA patients and also demonstrated early reduction in MRI inflammation at Week 12, which sustained up to Year 4. Additionally, the largest reduction in MRI inflammation of the spine and SIJ happened during the first year after initiation of tumor necrosis factor inhibitors (TNFi) in a 5-year follow-up study of axSpA/AS.[20]

Overall, considerable reduction of inflammation on MRI was observed after a treatment period with TNFi and interleukin-17 inhibitors in patients who experienced a clear clinical response. An illustrative example is shown in **Fig. 1**. However, do all patients with a clinical response show inflammation reduction on MRI? Is this also true the other way around: does MRI remission in the spine and SIJ occur in all patients with clinical remission? To discuss this issue, an important clinical question emerges whether MRI findings are correlated to clinical and patient-reported outcomes.

CORRELATION AMONG IMAGING, CLINICAL OUTCOMES, AND PATIENT-REPORTED OUTCOMES

Currently, only clinical remission is suggested as a treatment target in the 2017 updated EULAR recommendations for axSpA.[1] The rationale behind this is the need

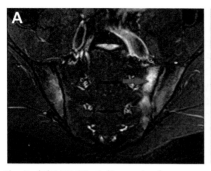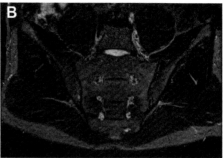

Fig. 1. (A) MRI-SIJ at diagnosis of a young male patient with nonradiographic axial spondyloarthritis, showing extensive bilateral bone marrow edema with a deep and intense lesion in the upper left sacral quadrant (arrow) on the baseline STIR image. ASDAS-CRP = 3.4 = high disease activity. (B) MRI-SIJ (STIR sequence) of the same patient after 6 months treatment with a TNFi, showing almost complete disappearance of bone marrow edema. ASDAS-CRP = 0.6 = inactive disease. CRP, C-reactive protein; STIR, short TI inversion recovery.

to better understand the correlation between objective parameters of disease activity (eg, MRI and C-reactive protein [CRP]), clinical and patient-reported measures of disease activity, and their relationship and impact on spinal mobility in SpA.

First, concerning the correlation with disease activity, there are conflicting data in the literature. A small study that included 46 patients with active AS found no correlation between Berlin MRI score of the spine and BASDAI, patient global, CRP, and erythrocyte sedimentation rate.[21] In the GO-RAISE study, ASspiMRI-a scores have shown to correlate well with ASDAS ($r = 0.35$; $P = .004$) but weakly with BASDAI ($r = 0.11$).[22] Similarly, in a study with 221 AS patients, the Berlin MRI activity correlated (weakly to moderately) with ASDAS ($r = 0.23$ at Week 102) and CRP ($r = 0.32$ at Week 102) but not with BASDAI ($r = 0.14$; $P = .063$ at Week 102).[23] Another study found no correlation between ASDAS, BASDAI, the extent of inflammatory lesions on MRI, and CRP ($r = 0.08$ and 0.06) in 100 patients with axSpA.[24] Moreover, 2-year follow-up data from the DESIR cohort found a significant correlation (in men but not in women) between ASDAS and SIJ inflammation on MRI ($\beta = 2.4$; 95% confidence interval, 1.13–3.69). Consequently, an increase of 1 U in ASDAS coincides with a 2.4-U increase in SIJ SPARCC score. However, this association was not found with BASDAI, which is a fully patient reported outcome, thus not reflecting very well inflammation compared with ASDAS.[25] Additionally, 12-year data from the OASIS cohort found that disease activity was correlated to radiographic progression (using the mSASSS): per 1 U in ASDAS increase, a progression of 0.7 mSASSS units could be estimated.[2]

Second, concerning the correlation to physical functioning, a nonstatistically significant association was found between MRI spine scores and the Bath Ankylosing Spondylitis Metrology Index (BASMI).[21] Another study on 214 patients with AS showed a weak correlation between MRI inflammation and spinal mobility assessed by BASMI (Spearman $\rho = 0.3$; $P<.001$) and a moderate correlation between radiographic damage and BASMI ($\rho = 0.6$; $P<.001$).[26] Therefore, it seems that spinal mobility impairment at the start of the disease mostly is determined by spinal inflammation and in contrast by irreversible structural damage of the spine later on.

More recent trials had a particular interest in defining the relationship between improvement of clinical disease activity and decrease of MRI inflammation over time. The RAPID-axSpA trial evaluated MRI remission in 163 patients with axSpA on

CZP after 96 weeks of follow-up. Intriguingly, a high proportion (65.9%) of patients not achieving clinical remission had MRI remission and 57.5% achieving clinical remission had no MRI inflammation at Week 96, demonstrating the absence of concordance between clinical remission and MRI remission.[8] Another trial, the EMBARK, that included 215 nonradiographic axSpA patients on ETN, showed that achievement of MRI remission of spine or SIJ inflammation (assessed by SPARCC score) at baseline, Week 12, and Week 104 were not significantly correlated with ASDAS remission.[7] An interesting observation is that patients with MRI remission of the spine achieved more ASDAS-low disease activity than patients with MRI remission of the SIJ ($P = .02$).[7] On the contrary, in the ABILITY-1 trial,[9] including 185 nonradiographic axSpA patients on adalimumab, a better numerical agreement was seen between clinical and MRI remission in the SIJ than in the spine, probably related to the presence of nonspecific lesions in the spine and the use of more stringent MRI thresholds than the EMBARK. Furthermore, among patients who attained ASDAS remission, only 40% achieved overall MRI remission in SIJ and spine at Year 1 and 44% at Year 2.[9] Additionally, in the ABILITY-1 trial, a subgroup analysis was performed in patients with objective evidence of inflammation on MRI and an elevated CRP (MRI/CRP-positive subpopulation). It showed that the clinical improvement on adalimumab was higher in the MRI/CRP-positive subpopulation compared with the MRI- and CRP-negative subpopulation.[9]

In the CRESPA trial, a placebo-controlled trial in very early, treatment-naive, peripheral SpA, all patient were evaluated by extensive ultrasound (US) studies and modified WBMRI confirming the general understanding that peripheral SpA mainly affects joints and entheses of the lower limbs.[27,28] A good concordance (>80%) between swollen joints and WBMRI and US was found, which was not the case for tender joints and enthesitis. Both US and WBMRI were also able to detect subclinical synovitis; whereas this was comparable for US and WBMRI at the level of the knee joints, WBMRI demonstrated far more subclinical ankle synovitis compared with US (**Fig. 2**). Still, the significance of this subclinical imaging finding is unclear.

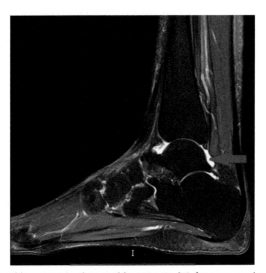

Fig. 2. Subclinical ankle synovitis, detected by WBMRI (T2 fat-saturated sequence), in a patient with early peripheral spondyloarthritis in clinical remission. The *red arrow* points at significant tibiotalar joint effusion.

Overall, there is an association between structural lesions on imaging and spinal mobility but a more doubtful association between inflammatory lesions on MRI and clinical disease activity, suggesting that imaging is an important surrogate marker but is only one of the many parameters to guide treatment decisions. Nevertheless, it is striking that better treatment responses with TNFi are associated with patients having more objective signs of inflammation, such as elevated baseline CRP or higher SPARCC MRI SIJ scores.[8,29] More data are needed to better clarify the role of MRI in clinical practice for monitoring patients in remission. Yet, reassessment by MRI may still be helpful in secondary failure of TNFi or to rule out other causes of back pain mimicking axSpA.[30]

IMAGING TO PREDICT CLINICAL RESPONSE

Another important clinical question is whether imaging can predict relapse in patients with sustained clinical remission and give guidance to clinicians to decide when to taper bDMARDs.

It is generally believed that new bone formation occurs more frequently at the areas of inflammatory spinal lesions on MRI.[5,31] Some data have shown that inflammatory corner lesions and the combination of inflammatory and fatty lesions on MRI strongly predict the development of new syndesmophytes.[5,12,32] There is increasing evidence supporting MRI as a prognostic tool in the prediction of radiographic progression in SpA.[31] Consequently, knowing that inflammatory lesions could progress to structural damage, one can think that in a patient in remission, the detection of subclinical inflammation could have a prognostic impact and influence treatment decisions by alerting the clinician to monitor closely and possibly wait to taper bDMARDs. Yet, there is limited evidence whether MRI can be used in this indication and because the data on correlation between inflammatory lesions on MRI and clinical disease activity are conflicting, it is still unclear whether the presence of subclinical inflammation is associated with a nonresponse or relapse.

For comparison with peripheral SpA, patients included in the CRESPA trial underwent a second modified WBMRI once they reached a status of sustained clinical remission.[27,28] No prediction of clinical remission or relapse based on baseline WBMRI was found. Similarly, when comparing patients relapsing after treatment discontinuation and those in sustained remission, no statistical difference was observed in baseline and remission WBMRI inflammatory indices.[33]

Overall, it would be interesting to investigate individual classification of axSpA patients based on their risk profile for progression by taking into consideration not only their MRI findings but also other factors of progression (eg, male gender, erythrocyte sedimentation rate, CRP, ASDAS, BASDAI, baseline syndesmophytes) to have a better prediction of outcomes and progression of the disease.

IMAGING-DRIVEN TREAT-TO-TARGET STRATEGY IN SPONDYLOARTHRITIS

A new concept of T2T has emerged in the management of SpA similarly to rheumatoid arthritis, where this strategy was proven to be effective in reducing structural damage.[34,35] The T2T strategy is established on predefining a treatment target and escalating therapy in case such target is not achieved. In PsA the T2T approach with minimal disease activity (defined as the treatment target for clinical remission) in the Tight Control in Psoriatic Arthritis (TICOPA) trial has shown better joint outcomes without increased number of serious adverse events.[36] In axSpA, three studies are currently being conducted on the T2T strategy: the Tight Control in Spondyloarthritis study (TICOSPA, NCT03043846), the STRIKE study (NCT02897115, terminated because of slow recruitment), and the TReat-to-tArget with seCukinumab in Axial Spondyloarthritis study (TRACE, NCT03639740).

Recently, the treatment targets to use for clinical remission in SpA were recommended by international experts[1]; however, the question whether imaging, mainly MRI remission, could guide treatment decisions remains unanswered. In rheumatoid arthritis, studies have evaluated the use of US or MRI for guiding treatment decisions compared with routine clinical practice, but they failed to demonstrate improved disease activity or reduced structural progression and have led to more intensified treatment.[37,38]

Although no results are yet available of trials of this T2T strategy in axSpA, it is deemed that such an approach could improve outcomes in axSpA, given the correlation of structural damage progression with disease activity.

NEW EMERGING IMAGING MODALITIES
Positron Emission Tomography

PET is a sensitive nuclear imaging technique that allows for visualization and quantification of metabolic activity at different target sites (bone marrow, synovium, entheses) within the whole body. Images are often converged with CT or MRI for anatomic references. The performance of these hybrid techniques, especially the specificity, depends on the radionuclide tracer used. Isotopes such as ^{18}F-fluoro-deoxy-glucose (^{18}F-FDG), captured by inflamed synovium, and the macrophage tracer ^{11}C-PK11195 showed to be of little use for detection of inflammatory processes in the spine or SIJ of AS patients with high disease activity.[39] One study performed sequential ^{18}F-FDG PET-CT before and 3 months after initiation of a TNFi in active axSpA patients but found no decrease in ^{18}F-FDG uptake in the SIJ despite a significant decrease in disease activity.[40] No studies have been performed to assess (change in) ^{18}F-FDG or ^{11}C-PK11195 tracer uptake in the spine or SIJ of axSpA patients achieving clinical remission.

In contrast, targeting osteoblastic activity with the bone tracer ^{18}F-fluoride proved to be more useful to assess disease activity because new bone formation is a hallmark of AS.[39] After injection ^{18}F-fluoride is rapidly incorporated in hydroxyapatite crystals, which form the mineral fluoroapatite of the bone, especially at sites of high bone turnover. The concentration of the ^{18}F-fluoride tracer reflects metabolic activity in terms of local blood perfusion and *in vivo* bone remodeling. Recent *in vivo* evidence confirmed that the histopathologic substrate of ^{18}F-fluoride PET-positive lesions in the spine of active AS patients consists of osteoid and calcium depositions.[41]

The correlation between osteoblastic activity (= high ^{18}F-fluoride uptake) and BME in the spine or SIJ of active AS patients is controversial. Studies comparing ^{18}F-fluoride-avid lesions on PET-CT with concomitant BME on MRI of the spine or the SIJ, reporting conflicting results especially regarding the spine, warrant careful interpretation because these lesions do not always show a complete overlap within the same quadrant.[42,43] In contrast, a study using hybrid ^{18}F-fluoride PET-MRI depicted an association between ^{18}F-fluoride uptake and BME rather than structural alterations in the SIJ of active AS patients.[44]

Regarding structural lesions, ^{18}F-fluoride tracer uptake on PET-CT is not correlated with the number of erosions or ankylosis on CT of the SIJ[42] nor the number of quadrants affected by fatty degeneration on MRI of the spine and SIJ in active AS patients.[44] This evidence seems in contrast with the current pathophysiologic paradigm of AS, which postulates that axial inflammation needs to disappear before fatty degeneration can occur, followed by chondral metaplasia and osteoproliferation. Yet, ^{18}F-fluoride PET can possibly detect early bone remodeling (osteoid tissue that is not yet mineralized) before structural lesions become apparent on CT or MRI and so might be useful in monitoring disease activity of AS patients.

Additionally, Idolazzi and colleagues[45] reported a good correlation between the number of ^{18}F-fluoride PET-positive lesions and disease activity parameters, such as BASDAI, ASDAS, and BASFI. However, although limited evidence also suggests that ^{18}F-fluoride uptake in the SIJ of active AS patients significantly declines in TNFi responders compared with nonresponders,[41] patients in clinical remission often show persistent ^{18}F-fluoride PET-positive lesions suggestive for disease progression, even when treated with TNFi.[45]

In summary, the prognostic role of hybrid PET techniques in SpA patients in clinical remission remains to be elucidated. Also, considering its high radiation dose ($\pm$ 5 mSv), currently available evidence does not support the routine clinical use of ^{18}F-fluoride PET-CT for monitoring of bone remodeling in axSpA patients.

Scintigraphy

Conventional planar bone scintigraphy, using 99m-technetium-labeled methylene diphosphate as a radionuclide tracer for increased bone turnover, plays no significant role in the diagnosis of sacroiliitis given its poor sensitivity and bad correlation with MRI findings in AS.[12,46] Low sensitivity, which may be caused by the complex anatomy of the SIJ and the lack of anatomic precision of planar bone scintigraphy, could be overcome by single-photon emission CT (SPECT). This hybrid technique, combining three-dimensional functional and anatomic information, allows for a more accurate quantification of radionuclide tracer uptake in the SIJ compared with an adjacent background reference (usually the sacrum). SPECT-CT shows better diagnostic performance in axSpA (early disease stages and established AS[47,48]) compared with planar bone scintigraphy and proved to have a good agreement with sacroiliitis on MRI using a qualitative[49] or semiquantitative approach.[50] One study examined a group of inactive axSpA with planar bone scintigraphy and found significant subclinical radionuclide tracer uptake in the SIJ and peripheral joints.[51] However, more studies are required to determine the prognostic significance of subclinical radionuclide bone tracer uptake assessed by planar scintigraphy and/or SPECT in axSpA patients in clinical remission.

Of note, a pilot study investigating the role of 99m-Tc labeled CZP (= immunoscintigraphy) in a small group of axSpA patients showed an excellent agreement between radionuclide tracer uptake assessed by SPECT and BME assessed by MRI within the corresponding quadrant of the SIJ (**Fig. 3**).[52]

Whole-Body MRI

WBMRI is an emerging technique enabling a comprehensive and simultaneous assessment of axial and peripheral joints and entheses. It captures inflammatory and structural lesions, such as BME, soft tissue inflammation, and bone erosions at multiple sites in a single radiologic examination. Consensus-based and semiquantitative scoring methods with a primary focus on peripheral arthritis and enthesitis have recently been developed and validated to objectively assess SpA patients' overall inflammatory burden.[53] WBMRI inflammatory indices generally show poor correlation with clinical evaluation, that is, tenderness at peripheral joints and entheses in axSpA[54] and peripheral SpA.[55] TNFi proved to induce a significant reduction of WBMRI inflammatory indices rapidly after treatment initiation[56,57] and in parallel with a significant decline in clinical disease activity outcome measures reflecting remission induction in axSpA[58] and early peripheral SpA patients (manuscript under preparation, 2019, P. Carron). However, studies in axial and early peripheral SpA

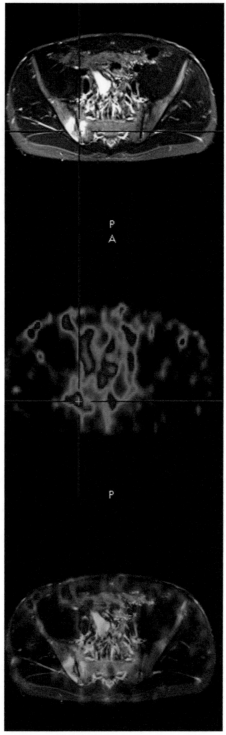

Fig. 3. Fusion of MRI image (STIR sequence) and SPECT image (4–6 hours after 99m-Tc-CZP intravenous injection) of the sacroiliac joints of a patient with active axial spondyloarthritis. STIR, short TI inversion recovery.

report residual inflammatory activity despite achievement of a significant clinical response, which is at least partially age-related and involves sites prone to mechanical load and osteoarthritis.[33,57] The prognostic value of residual subclinical inflammation is questionable, because WBMRI inflammatory indices assessed at time of clinical remission were not predictive for relapse in early peripheral SpA.[33] This could possibly be attributed to the former findings, because most subclinically affected joints and entheses at remission WBMRI were not clinically involved at disease onset in these patients (manuscript under preparation, 2019, P. Carron).

In conclusion, WBMRI seems to be a promising tool for objective assessment and monitoring of the global inflammatory load in SpA patients. However, WBMRI remission cannot be used as a treatment target yet given the lack of a validated definition and uncertainty about the prognostic meaning of subclinical inflammatory lesions.

SUMMARY

T2T based on imaging remission has not yet proven its efficacy in axSpA. Imaging plays an essential role in diagnosis and classification of axSpA. Regarding the ability to predict treatment response and guidance for tapering medication when patients experience a clinical remission state, more research is needed. Nevertheless, imaging is currently one of the many parameters to take into consideration in therapeutic decision making. In fact, because of the lack of strong evidence correlating clinical disease activity and MRI findings, routine MRI assessment is still not recommended in patients with axSpA in clinical remission, although it may be helpful in some circumstances to rule-out other causes of back pain. However, it is striking that better treatment responses with biologic treatment are observed in patients having more objective signs of inflammation, such as elevated baseline CRP or higher SPARCC MRI SIJ scores.

Emerging imaging tools, such as WBMRI and ^{18}F-fluoride PET-CT, have shown some evidence in monitoring of disease activity in AS, but their clinical application in patients achieving clinical remission is premature.

Overall, to optimize the use of imaging in daily clinical practice, research and technical advances in imaging are awaited to better define its practical role in monitoring and prognosticating SpA patients in clinical remission.

DISCLOSURE

Dr. A.S. De Craemer is supported by the Special Research Fund of the Ghent University (BOF, 01D01718). Drs. K. Aouad and P. Carron have nothing to disclose.

REFERENCES

1. Smolen JS, Schöls M, Braun J, et al. Treating axial spondyloarthritis and peripheral spondyloarthritis, especially psoriatic arthritis, to target: 2017 update of recommendations by an international task force. Ann Rheum Dis 2018;77(1):3–17.

2. Ramiro S, van der Heijde D, van Tubergen A, et al. Higher disease activity leads to more structural damage in the spine in ankylosing spondylitis: 12-year longitudinal data from the OASIS cohort. Ann Rheum Dis 2014;73(8):1455–61.

3. Poddubnyy D, Protopopov M, Haibel H, et al. High disease activity according to the Ankylosing Spondylitis Disease Activity Score is associated with accelerated radiographic spinal progression in patients with early axial spondyloarthritis: results from the GErman SPondyloarthritis Inception Cohort. Ann Rheum Dis 2016;75(12):2114–8.

4. van der Heijde D, Ramiro S, Landewé R, et al. 2016 update of the ASAS-EULAR management recommendations for axial spondyloarthritis. Ann Rheum Dis 2017; 76(6):978–91.

5. Aouad K, Ziade N, Baraliakos X. Structural progression in axial spondyloarthritis. Joint Bone Spine 2019. https://doi.org/10.1016/j.jbspin.2019.04.006.

6. Rudwaleit M, van der Heijde D, Landewé R, et al. The development of Assessment of SpondyloArthritis International Society classification criteria for axial spondyloarthritis (part II): validation and final selection. Ann Rheum Dis 2009; 68(6):777–83.

7. Dougados M, van der Heijde D, Sieper J, et al. Effects of long-term etanercept treatment on clinical outcomes and objective signs of inflammation in early non-radiographic axial spondyloarthritis: 104-week results from a randomized, placebo-controlled study. Arthritis Care Res (Hoboken) 2017;69(10):1590–8.

8. Braun J, Baraliakos X, Hermann K-G, et al. Effect of certolizumab pegol over 96 weeks of treatment on inflammation of the spine and sacroiliac joints, as measured by MRI, and the association between clinical and MRI outcomes in patients with axial spondyloarthritis. RMD Open 2017;3(1):e000430.

9. van der Heijde D, Sieper J, Maksymowych WP, et al. Clinical and MRI remission in patients with nonradiographic axial spondyloarthritis who received long-term open-label adalimumab treatment: 3-year results of the ABILITY-1 trial. Arthritis Res Ther 2018;20(1):61.

10. van der Heijde D, Landewé R. Selection of a method for scoring radiographs for ankylosing spondylitis clinical trials, by the Assessment in Ankylosing Spondylitis Working Group and OMERACT. J Rheumatol 2005;32(10):2048–9.

11. Østergaard M, Lambert RGW. Imaging in ankylosing spondylitis. Ther Adv Musculoskelet Dis 2012;4(4):301–11.

12. Mandl P, Navarro-Compán V, Terslev L, et al. EULAR recommendations for the use of imaging in the diagnosis and management of spondyloarthritis in clinical practice. Ann Rheum Dis 2015;74(7):1327–39.

13. Baraliakos X, Brandt J, Listing J, et al. Outcome of patients with active ankylosing spondylitis after two years of therapy with etanercept: clinical and magnetic resonance imaging data. Arthritis Rheum 2005;53(6):856–63.

14. Rudwaleit M, Baraliakos X, Listing J, et al. Magnetic resonance imaging of the spine and the sacroiliac joints in ankylosing spondylitis and undifferentiated spondyloarthritis during treatment with etanercept. Ann Rheum Dis 2005;64(9): 1305–10.

15. Lambert RGW, Salonen D, Rahman P, et al. Adalimumab significantly reduces both spinal and sacroiliac joint inflammation in patients with ankylosing spondylitis: a multicenter, randomized, double-blind, placebo-controlled study. Arthritis Rheum 2007;56(12):4005–14.

16. Baraliakos X, Borah B, Braun J, et al. Long-term effects of secukinumab on MRI findings in relation to clinical efficacy in subjects with active ankylosing spondylitis: an observational study. Ann Rheum Dis 2016;75(2):408–12.

17. Maksymowych WP, Wichuk S, Dougados M, et al. Modification of structural lesions on MRI of the sacroiliac joints by etanercept in the EMBARK trial: a 12-week randomised placebo-controlled trial in patients with non-radiographic axial spondyloarthritis. Ann Rheum Dis 2018;77(1):78–84.

18. Maksymowych WP, Dougados M, van der Heijde D, et al. Clinical and MRI responses to etanercept in early non-radiographic axial spondyloarthritis: 48-week results from the EMBARK study. Ann Rheum Dis 2016;75(7):1328–35.

19. van der Heijde D, Baraliakos X, Hermann K-GA, et al. Limited radiographic progression and sustained reductions in MRI inflammation in patients with axial spondyloarthritis: 4-year imaging outcomes from the RAPID-axSpA phase III randomised trial. Ann Rheum Dis 2018;77(5):699–705.

20. Pedersen SJ, Weber U, Said-Nahal R, et al. Structural progression rate decreases over time on serial radiography and magnetic resonance imaging of sacroiliac joints and spine in a five-year follow-up study of patients with ankylosing spondylitis treated with tumour necrosis factor inhibitor. Scand J Rheumatol 2019;48(3):185–97.

21. Rudwaleit M, Schwarzlose S, Hilgert ES, et al. MRI in predicting a major clinical response to anti-tumour necrosis factor treatment in ankylosing spondylitis. Ann Rheum Dis 2008;67(9):1276–81.

22. Braun J, Baraliakos X, Hermann K-GA, et al. Golimumab reduces spinal inflammation in ankylosing spondylitis: MRI results of the randomised, placebo-controlled GO-RAISE study. Ann Rheum Dis 2012;71(6):878–84.

23. Machado P, Landewé RBM, Braun J, et al. MRI inflammation and its relation with measures of clinical disease activity and different treatment responses in patients with ankylosing spondylitis treated with a tumour necrosis factor inhibitor. Ann Rheum Dis 2012;71(12):2002–5.

24. Kiltz U, Baraliakos X, Karakostas P, et al. The degree of spinal inflammation is similar in patients with axial spondyloarthritis who report high or low levels of disease activity: a cohort study. Ann Rheum Dis 2012;71(7):1207–11.

25. Navarro-Compán V, Ramiro S, Landewé R, et al. Disease activity is longitudinally related to sacroiliac inflammation on MRI in male patients with axial spondyloarthritis: 2-years of the DESIR cohort. Ann Rheum Dis 2016;75(5):874–8.

26. Machado P, Landewé R, Braun J, et al. Both structural damage and inflammation of the spine contribute to impairment of spinal mobility in patients with ankylosing spondylitis. Ann Rheum Dis 2010;69(8):1465–70.

27. Carron P, Varkas G, Cypers H, et al. Anti-TNF-induced remission in very early peripheral spondyloarthritis: the CRESPA study. Ann Rheum Dis 2017;76(8):1389–95.

28. Carron P, Varkas G, Renson T, et al. High rate of drug-free remission after induction therapy with golimumab in early peripheral spondyloarthritis. Arthritis Rheumatol 2018;70(11):1769–77.

29. Sieper J, van der Heijde D, Dougados M, et al. Efficacy and safety of adalimumab in patients with non-radiographic axial spondyloarthritis: results of a randomised placebo-controlled trial (ABILITY-1). Ann Rheum Dis 2013;72(6):815–22.

30. Maksymowych WP. The role of MRI in the evaluation of spondyloarthritis: a clinician's guide. Clin Rheumatol 2016;35(6):1447–55.

31. Schwartzman M, Maksymowych WP. Is there a role for MRI to establish treatment indications and effectively monitor response in patients with axial spondyloarthritis? Rheum Dis Clin North Am 2019;45(3):341–58.

32. Baraliakos X, Heldmann F, Callhoff J, et al. Which spinal lesions are associated with new bone formation in patients with ankylosing spondylitis treated with anti-TNF agents? A long-term observational study using MRI and conventional radiography. Ann Rheum Dis 2014;73(10):1819–25.

33. Renson T, Carron P, Krabbe S, et al. FRI0177 assessing the value of whole body magnetic resonance imaging as to clinical examination to predict remission and relapse in early peripheral spondyloarthritis. Ann Rheum Dis 2018;77(Suppl 2):630–1.

34. Machado PM, Deodhar A. Treat-to-target in axial spondyloarthritis: gold standard or fools' gold? Curr Opin Rheumatol 2019;31(4):344–8.
35. Grigor C, Capell H, Stirling A, et al. Effect of a treatment strategy of tight control for rheumatoid arthritis (the TICORA study): a single-blind randomised controlled trial. Lancet 2004;364(9430):263–9.
36. Coates LC, Moverley AR, McParland L, et al. Effect of tight control of inflammation in early psoriatic arthritis (TICOPA): a UK multicentre, open-label, randomised controlled trial. Lancet 2015;386(10012):2489–98.
37. Møller-Bisgaard S, Hørslev-Petersen K, Ejbjerg B, et al. Effect of magnetic resonance imaging vs conventional treat-to-target strategies on disease activity remission and radiographic progression in rheumatoid arthritis: the IMAGINE-RA randomized clinical trial. JAMA 2019;321(5):461–72.
38. Dale J, Stirling A, Zhang R, et al. Targeting ultrasound remission in early rheumatoid arthritis: the results of the TaSER study, a randomised clinical trial. Ann Rheum Dis 2016;75(6):1043–50.
39. Bruijnen STG, van der Weijden MAC, Klein JP, et al. Bone formation rather than inflammation reflects ankylosing spondylitis activity on PET-CT: a pilot study. Arthritis Res Ther 2012;14(2):R71.
40. Kaijasilta J-P, Kerola A, Tuompo R, et al. AB0838 the efficacy of adalimumab and sulfasalazine in alleviating axial and aortic inflammation detected in PET/CT in patients with axial spondyloarthritis. Ann Rheum Dis 2018;77(Suppl 2):1547.
41. Bruijnen STG, Verweij NJF, van Duivenvoorde LM, et al. Bone formation in ankylosing spondylitis during anti-tumour necrosis factor therapy imaged by 18F-fluoride positron emission tomography. Rheumatology (Oxford) 2018;57(4):631–8.
42. Raynal M, Bouderraoui F, Ouichka R, et al. Performance of 18F-sodium fluoride positron emission tomography with computed tomography to assess inflammatory and structural sacroiliitis on magnetic resonance imaging and computed tomography, respectively, in axial spondyloarthritis. Arthritis Res Ther 2019;21:119.
43. Fischer DR, Pfirrmann CWA, Zubler V, et al. High bone turnover assessed by 18F-fluoride PET/CT in the spine and sacroiliac joints of patients with ankylosing spondylitis: comparison with inflammatory lesions detected by whole body MRI. EJNMMI Res 2012;2(1):38.
44. Buchbender C, Ostendorf B, Ruhlmann V, et al. Hybrid 18F-labeled fluoride positron emission tomography/magnetic resonance (MR) imaging of the sacroiliac joints and the spine in patients with axial spondyloarthritis: a pilot study exploring the link of MR bone pathologies and increased osteoblastic activity. J Rheumatol 2015;42(9):1631–7.
45. Idolazzi L, Salgarello M, Gatti D, et al. 18F-fluoride PET/CT for detection of axial involvement in ankylosing spondylitis: correlation with disease activity. Ann Nucl Med 2016;30(6):430–4.
46. Song IH, Carrasco-Fernández J, Rudwaleit M, et al. The diagnostic value of scintigraphy in assessing sacroiliitis in ankylosing spondylitis: a systematic literature research. Ann Rheum Dis 2008;67(11):1535–40.
47. Kim Y, Suh M, Kim YK, et al. The usefulness of bone SPECT/CT imaging with volume of interest analysis in early axial spondyloarthritis. BMC Musculoskelet Disord 2015;16:9.
48. Zilber K, Gorenberg M, Rimar D, et al. Radionuclide methods in the diagnosis of sacroiliitis in patients with spondyloarthritis: an update. Rambam Maimonides Med J 2016;7(4).
49. Pipikos T, Koutsikos J, Bakalis S, et al. OP668 radiographic suspicious changes in the sacroiliac joints: the role of bone single photon emission computed

tomography (SPECT) scintigraphy. Eur J Nucl Med Mol Imaging 2013;40(Suppl 2):S1–477.

50. Parghane RV, Singh B, Sharma A, et al. Role of 99mTc-methylene diphosphonate SPECT/CT in the detection of sacroiliitis in patients with spondyloarthropathy: comparison with clinical markers and MRI. J Nucl Med Technol 2017;45(4):280–4.

51. Gheita TA, Azkalany GS, Kenawy SA, et al. Bone scintigraphy in axial seronegative spondyloarthritis patients: role in detection of subclinical peripheral arthritis and disease activity. Int J Rheum Dis 2015;18(5):553–9.

52. Carron P, de Hooge M, Renson T, et al. Sat0525 immunoscintigraphy of sacroiliac joints shows very good agreement with inflammation on MRI in axial spondyloarthritis patients. Ann Rheum Dis 2019;78(Suppl 2):1354.

53. Krabbe S, Eshed I, Gandjbakhch F, et al. Development and validation of an OMERACT MRI whole-body score for inflammation in peripheral joints and entheses in inflammatory arthritis (MRI-WIPE). J Rheumatol 2019;46(9):1215–21.

54. Krabbe S, Eshed I, Juul Sørensen I, et al. Whole-body magnetic resonance imaging inflammation in peripheral joints and entheses in axial spondyloarthritis: distribution and changes during adalimumab treatment. J Rheumatol 2019; 47(1):50–8.

55. Renson T, Carron P, Krabbe S, et al. FRI0214 clinical evaluation correlates poorly with ultrasound and magnetic resonance imaging of joints and entheses in early peripheral spondyloarthritis. Ann Rheum Dis 2018;77(Suppl 2):648.

56. Krabbe S, Østergaard M, Eshed I, et al. Whole-body magnetic resonance imaging in axial spondyloarthritis: reduction of sacroiliac, spinal, and entheseal inflammation in a placebo-controlled trial of adalimumab. J Rheumatol 2018;45(5): 621–9.

57. Krabbe S, Østergaard M, Eshed I, et al. FRI0591 Whole-body MRI demonstrates reduction of inflammation in peripheral joints and entheses during tnf-inhibitor treatment in patients with axial spondyloarthritis, but also age-dependent persistent inflammation in joints prone to osteoarthritis. Ann Rheum Dis 2018;77(Suppl 2):819.

58. Karpitschka M, Godau-Kellner P, Kellner H, et al. Assessment of therapeutic response in ankylosing spondylitis patients undergoing anti-tumour necrosis factor therapy by whole-body magnetic resonance imaging. Eur Radiol 2013;23(7): 1773–84.

Treatment and Outcomes

Axial Psoriatic Arthritis
A Distinct Clinical Entity in Search of a Definition

Xabier Michelena, MD[a,b,c], Denis Poddubnyy, MD, MSc (Epi)[d,e],
Helena Marzo-Ortega, MD, PhD[a,b],*

KEYWORDS

- Axial involvement • Axial spondyloarthritis • Axial psoriatic arthritis
- Psoriatic arthritis • Psoriatic spondylitis

KEY POINTS

- Axial involvement in psoriatic arthritis is a prevalent entity and must be taken into account in disease management.
- Axial psoriatic arthritis can be asymptomatic, tends to present with asymmetric sacroiliitis, more cervical involvement, and nonmarginal "chunky" syndesmophytes.
- HLA-B27 drives a more severe phenotype (similar to axial spondyloarthritis) with significant radiographic changes.
- A consensus on a definition is needed to unify research efforts and help with the clinical management of axial psoriatic arthritis.

INTRODUCTION

Psoriatic arthritis (PsA) is a chronic inflammatory condition affecting multiple tissues including skin and joints. PsA has traditionally been considered part of the spondyloarthritis (SpA) group. This stems from the observations made by Moll and Wright in 1974,[1] who justified the inclusion of PsA as part of the SpA group due to the high prevalence of sacroiliac and spine involvement seen in PsA. Since then, substantial efforts have been made to describe axial involvement in PsA and whether this may indeed represent a distinct entity or the consequence of the coexistence of psoriasis and axial spondyloarthritis (axSpA). Furthermore, there is no consensus on the definition of axial PsA hindering the extrapolation of results from the limited pool of available studies.

[a] NIHR Leeds Biomedical Research Centre, Leeds Teaching Hospitals NHS Trust, Leeds, UK; [b] Leeds Institute of Rheumatic and Musculoskeletal Medicine, University of Leeds, Chapel Allerton Hospital, Second Floor, Chapeltown Road, Leeds LS7 4SA, UK; [c] Hospital Universitari de Bellvitge-IDIBELL, Hospitalet de Llobregat, Barcelona, Spain; [d] Department of Gastroenterology, Infectious Diseases and Rheumatology, Charité—Universitätsmedizin Berlin, Campus Benjamin Franklin, Hindenburgdamm 30, Berlin 12203, Germany; [e] German Rheumatism Research Centre, Berlin, Germany
* Corresponding author. Leeds Institute of Rheumatic and Musculoskeletal Medicine, University of Leeds, Chapel Allerton Hospital, Second Floor, Chapeltown Road, Leeds LS7 4SA, UK.
E-mail address: H.Marzo-Ortega@leeds.ac.uk

Rheum Dis Clin N Am 46 (2020) 331–345
https://doi.org/10.1016/j.rdc.2020.01.009
rheumatic.theclinics.com
0889-857X/20/© 2020 Elsevier Inc. All rights reserved.

The purpose of this review is to summarize the current understanding of axial involvement in PsA and highlight the need for a definition to facilitate further characterization of this clinical entity.

CLASSIFICATION OF PSORIATIC ARTHRITIS AND PHENOTYPES

In 1973, Moll and Wright[2] described PsA as a distinct clinical entity from rheumatoid arthritis and published the first classification criteria for PsA. These criteria incorporated a description of 5 clinical subtypes: predominant distal interphalangeal joint disease, asymmetrical oligoarthritis, polyarthritis, spondylitis, and arthritis mutilans. Subsequently, modifications to the original criteria were proposed by several authors,[3–8] but it was not until 2006 when a large prospective international study outlined the CASPAR (Classification Criteria for Psoriatic Arthritis) criteria.[9] Whereas CASPAR criteria showed good sensitivity and specificity, the mandatory entry criteria referring to inflammatory articular disease (joint, spine, or enthesis) is quite loose. This is of particular relevance in the context of spinal inflammatory disease, where there is considerable heterogeneity on what physicians consider axial involvement.

More recently, there has been controversy on whether the clinical subtypes should be abandoned[10,11] as the "new" criteria enclosed all, and available treatments at the time (tumor necrosis factor [TNF] inhibitors) appeared efficacious on all subtypes in real life. With the introduction of novel drug therapies targeting different pathogenic pathways (IL-12/23, PDE4, IL-17), the recognition of these domains is essential to direct management[12] despite the disparity in the available amount of data relating to each of the domains. Added to that, extra-articular manifestations and comorbidities[13] are crucial to the management strategy adopted.

In addition to CASPAR, some patients with PsA and spinal involvement may be classified according to the ASAS (Assessment of Spondyloarthritis International Society) classification criteria adding to the controversy of whether axial PsA constitutes a distinct clinical entity or simply represents axSpA with concurrent skin psoriasis. This can be achieved by either the imaging or the so-called clinical arm. There are, however, 2 important caveats of these criteria in the context of PsA with axial involvement, namely that the imaging arm relies on the presence of sacroiliitis (either on plain radiograph or MRI), a feature that is not universal in PsA, in which an estimated 35% may have isolated spondylitis without sacroiliitis[14–16]; and that the clinical arm requires the presence of HLA-B27 (plus 2 additional SpA features, to include skin psoriasis), which may only be present in 23% to 43% of axial PsA.[14,17–20] Furthermore, the ASAS classification criteria require the presence of chronic back pain with onset before 45 years of age that might not be the case in a considerable number of patients with PsA.

NOMENCLATURE

The current understanding of what constitutes axial psoriatic arthritis has been hampered by the lack of a definition to facilitate the conduct of research into this area. Indeed, there are many different terms used to refer to spinal affection in the context of PsA, such as "psoriatic spondyloarthropathy",[21] "axial psoriatic arthritis",[22] and "psoriatic spondylitis",[23] that have been used interchangeably in the medical literature. Axial psoriatic arthritis might be the preferred term as psoriatic spondylitis may imply that only the spine is affected (without sacroiliac joint [SIJ] involvement) and psoriatic spondyloarthropathy includes an outdated term ("spondyloarthropathy") that is currently substituted by the term spondyloarthritis. For the purpose of this review and to harmonize with the current nomenclature relating to spondyloarthritis, we will be using the terminology axial psoriatic arthritis abbreviated as axial PsA (axPsA) throughout.

GENETICS

Several genes have been associated with psoriasis, PsA in general and axPsA in particular. Although the studied cohorts are very heterogeneous with different defini- tions of axial disease, some studies have shown that HLA-B27 has the strongest association with sacroiliitis in patients with PsA.[24–30] Others, however, argue that HLA-B27 is not a true marker of axial PsA as no association to a specific HLA could be made in their cohorts.[31] In the same line, a recent study showed that HLA-B0801 had the strongest association with radiographic sacroiliitis; however, when dividing the cohort HLA-B0801 was associated with unilateral sacroiliitis, whereas HLA-B27 was associated with bilateral sacroiliitis,[19] corroborating the possible distinct clinical phenotypes of axial PsA and radiographic axial SpA, traditionally known as ankylosing spondylitis (AS).

These data are consistent with results from clinical observational studies where a variable prevalence of HLA-B27 was reported in subjects with axPsA.[14,17–20] Data from these cohorts also suggest that the smaller subset of axPsA in which the diag- nosis has been substantiated by imaging, and which is HLA-B27-positive, seems to be the subset with more radiographic, bilateral SIJ damage,[18] and/or MRI findings of acute inflammatory lesions[32] similar to those seen in HLA-B27-positive axSpA.[33] Here, these data suggest 2 distinct subtypes of the axial phenotype within the already heterogeneous PsA population underpinned, at least in part, by HLA-B27 (**Table 1**).

Polymorphisms in the IL-23 receptor provide further evidence that AS and axPsA might have a different genetic background becasue rs12401432 GG homozygosity was related to axial involvement in PsA[34] and rs11209032 was previously found to be associated with AS.[35,36] Further HLA associations have been reported, such as HLA-Bw38,[25] HLA-Cw*0802,[37] HLA Cw2 and DRw52,[26] HLA-B39,[38] and HLA-B17/ Cw6.[39] Singularly, HLA-B46 was found to be associated with radiographic sacroiliitis in a Japanese cohort[40]; a finding that has not been investigated in the white population.

PREVALENCE

The prevalence of axial involvement in PsA varies between 12.5% and 78%. This considerable heterogeneity is largely because of the varied definitions and inclusion criteria used by the different authors. Most of the studies performed required radio- graphic evidence of SIJ disease fulfilling the modified New York radiographic criteria[14,41,42] as entry criterion. Inflammatory back pain (IBP)[43] was an added criterion by some authors, whereas others required solely the presence of IBP to classify them as axial PsA.[17,44,45] These varied scenarios allowed for different values of the preva- lence of asymptomatic sacroiliitis in PsA being reported and spanning from 15.7% to 55% in some cohorts.[20,42,46,47]

CLINICAL MANIFESTATIONS

IBP is the pivotal symptom of inflammatory affection of the axial skeleton. Symptoms of IBP have been shown to work well as a screening tool for primary care referral to rheumatology; although in itself IBP has a low specificity for the diagnosis of axSpA in a rheumatology setting.[48]

Table 1
Clinical and imaging characteristics of axial psoriatic arthritis and axial spondyloarthritis according to HLA-B27 status

	axPsA		axSpA	
	HLA-B27+	HLA-B27−	HLA-B27+	HLA-B27−
Estimated prevalence	23%–43% of axPsA[14,17–20]	57%–77% of axPsA	≈ 90%[85,86] of axSpA	10% axSpA
Age of presentation	Younger (<40 y)[18,53]	Older (>40 y)	Younger (≈30 y)[87]	Older (≈35 y)
Male:female ratio/ %	1:7[18]	1:1	51%–96%[88]	37%–95%
Radiographic features	Bilateral symmetric sacroiliitis[18]	Asymmetrical sacroiliitis	More radiographic sacroiliitis[89]	Less radiographic sacroiliitis
Concomitant spondylitis	Sacroiliitis with spondylitis[14]	Isolated spondylitis	Sacroiliitis with spondylitis	Sacroiliitis with spondylitis
Pattern of spinal involvement	Lumbar spine, SIJ less cervical involvement	More cervical involvement[51]	Lumbar spine, SIJ, rare isolated cervical involvement[90] No HLA-B27 subset data available	Lumbar spine, SIJ, rare isolated cervical involvement
Radiographic progression	More radiographic progression[20]	Less radiographic progression	Heterogeneity in results[88]: HLA-B27+ men progress more[91]	Heterogeneity in results: HLA-B27- men progress less
MRI features	More BMO[32]	Less BMO	More BMO[69,92]	Less BMO
Extra-articular manifestations	More uveitis.[18] IBD data not available	Less uveitis	More uveitis,[93] less Pso.[89] No evidence in IBD[94]	Less uveitis, more Pso. No evidence in IBD

Abbreviations: BMO, bone marrow edema; IBD, inflammatory bowel disease; Pso, psoriasis.
Data from Refs.[14,17–20,32,51,53,69,85–94]

Different criteria have been developed to increase the sensitivity and specificity of the definition of IBP. In a recent study, Yap and colleagues[47] evaluated the performance of the existing IBP criteria: Calin, Berlin, and ASAS in the detection of axPsA. Sensitivity of all 3 criteria was found to be low, with 33 of the patients displaying axial disease on imaging despite not complaining of back pain. In a similar study from Turkey, poor sensitivity was noted, especially in women.[49] More recently, Haroon and colleagues[50] found that the sensitivity of the ASAS criteria was low in established disease but performed better in the context of active disease. Furthermore, a comparison between AS and axPsA patients showed that IBP reporting was higher in the AS group, who had more symptoms of thoracic and buttock pain when compared with the axPsA[14] group. Here, these data suggest that IBP might not be a good tool for identifying axPsA and this might be supported by the considerable amount of patients with asymptomatic axPsA. Furthermore, the high frequency of cervical spine involvement in axPsA[51] is also an important consideration as patients may only present with neck pain as opposed to low back pain.

The importance of diagnosing axial disease in PsA underlies its association with disease severity and more peripheral involvement,[17,19,27,28,52] with some cohorts also showing a higher prevalence of peripheral joint erosions.[19,28,52] With regard to the dermatologic domain, patients with axPsA tend to have more severe skin psoriasis[17,19] in addition to nail involvement[14,17] than patients with PsA with peripheral involvement without axial disease.

Looking at the demographics of the reported populations, patients with axPsA are younger[14,17,19] than those with only peripheral PsA, and early onset PsA tends to have more axial symptoms and sacroiliitis.[30,53] However, when compared with AS populations, patients with axPsA are older.[14,54–56]

With regard to gender, no differences were reported between axPsA and only peripheral PsA in the Bath cohort,[14] whereas a higher prevalence of men in the axPsA group was found in the Turkey cohort.[57] Male sex may also be a risk factor for development[43] of axPsA and, interestingly, may also determine less peripheral involvement, as shown in the Iberoamerican spondyloarthritis cohort.[58] When dividing axPsA into HLA-B27-positive and HLA-B27-negative, a male prevalence was noted in HLA-B27-positive subjects.[18]

There is also a paucity of data regarding extra-articular manifestations in axPsA. Cases with axial involvement were significantly more likely to have a history of inflammatory bowel disease in the Jadon and colleagues[14] study and a trend was noticed in history of uveitis, the latter was also confirmed in the Dublin cohort reaching statistical significance.[19] Considering HLA-B27 status, uveitis was more prevalent in patients with HLA-B27-positive axPsA.[18]

Cardiovascular comorbidities are an important consideration in psoriatic disease. Few data on cardiovascular disease are available in axPsA, with no differences in prevalence when comparing it with non-axPsA in the Corrona registry.[17] Interestingly, the Turkish group reported more smokers in the axial subset,[57] and a recent study by Queiro and colleagues[59] described axial involvement during evolution of PsA as an independent factor associated with obesity.

Finally, prospective data are scarce on clinical symptoms in patients with axPsA. The Toronto group described, in data from a follow-up of up to 10-years, a decline in the number of patients with neck pain, back pain, neck stiffness and back stiffness, suggesting that clinical symptoms may ease or even disappear over time.

IMAGING

Sacroiliitis is the defining radiographic feature of axSpA and a central criterion in its diagnosis. Yet, up to 35% of patients with axPsA will only present with spondylitis without radiographic changes in the SIJs[14–16] (**Fig. 1**). When SIJ involvement is present, it tends to be asymmetrical and more unilateral as compared with AS described by McEwen and colleagues[60] in 1971 and confirmed in subsequent cohorts. Furthermore, complete ankylosis of the SIJs is infrequent in axPsA.[14]

When it comes to the spine, differential characteristics have also been outlined. AS presents more severe changes, particularly in the lumbar spine,[55] whereas axPsA has a predilection for involving the cervical spine. A study focusing on this segment confirmed a frequency of 70% of cervical radiological involvement in patients with PsA together with a high frequency of posterior elements fusion (zygo-apophyseal or facet joints) in an established cohort with a mean duration of 10 years.[51] The morphology of syndesmophytes also differs between both diseases with nonmarginal, asymmetrical, and "chunky" syndesmophytes in axPsA versus marginal, symmetric, well-delimited syndesmophytes described in established axSpA or AS.

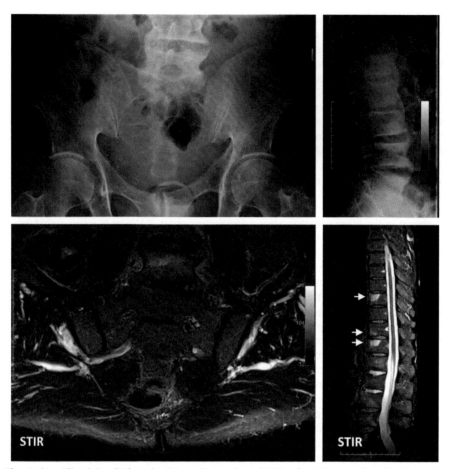

Fig. 1. Sacroiliac joint (SIJ) and spine radiograph and MRI of axial psoriatic arthritis. A 65-year-old male patient with known psoriasis for more than 30 years and intermittent inflammatory back pain for 20 years; HLA-B27 is negative and normal CRP. The radiograph of the SIJ is normal with no bone marrow edema (BMO) in the MRI. The radiograph of the spine shows chunky nonmarginal syndesmophytes with typical vertebral corner BMO (arrows) in the MRI.

One of the main clinical challenges in the diagnosis of axPsA is the differential with another common condition that may present with similar syndesmophyte appearance: diffuse idiopathic skeletal hyperostosis (DISH). A study conducted by Haddad and colleagues[61] found that both diseases can coexist with a 8.3% prevalence of DISH in patients with PsA similar to the general population. The physiopathology underlying DISH remains ill understood and possible common underlying mechanisms of aberrant new bone formation underpinning both diseases have not yet been identified.[62–64]

The Bath Ankylosing Spondylitis Radiology Index (BASRI) and the Modified Stokes Ankylosing Spondylitis Spinal Score (mSASSS) are available tools to score radiographic damage in the spine in axSpA. Both BASRI and mSASSS were tested in a study[15] with PsA patients and good correlation with metrology and clinical measures was found. To encompass characteristic features of axPsA, mainly the cervical zygo-apophyseal involvement, the same authors designed the Psoriatic Arthritis Spondylitis Radiology Index,[65] which correlated well with both metrology and patient-reported outcomes.

Sensitivity to change of these indexes in axPsA was confirmed by 1 study showing a 24% radiographic progression over 3.5 years that was detected equally by all indexes.[66]

There are few prospective studies in axPsA addressing radiographic progression. The Toronto group reported 10-year follow-up data of their axPsA cohort (considering clinical and radiographic criteria),[20] finding that 51.7% of the patients with no evidence of sacroiliitis at baseline developed grade 2 or 3 sacroiliitis; and 52% with grade 2 progressed to grade 3 or 4 sacroiliitis. Regarding the spine, approximately 15% to 20% patients without syndesmophytes at study entry had developed syndesmophytes after 10 years. HLA-B27-positive patients developed more lumbar syndesmophytes in comparison with HLA-B27-negative axPsA patients. More prospective data are needed to assess radiographic progression in axPsA and allow for meaningful comparisons with axSpA.

MRI data in axPsA are scarce. A study with 125 patients of the Toronto cohort described that spinal MRI in PsA patients were mainly requested because of suspicion of inflammatory disease (51.1%).[67] The most common features reported were erosions (15.6%) and bone marrow edema (18.5%). Considering those cases with IBP, only 44.6% of the scans presented changes compatible with spondyloarthritis. Two other studies have addressed the role of MRI in axial PsA with discordant results. Williamson and colleagues[68] performed MRI of the SIJs in 103 patients with PsA finding abnormalities in 38% of the cases but no correlation of these with clinical signs or HLA-B27 status. By contrast, Castillo-Gallego and colleagues[32] reported a significant correlation between HLA-B27 and the extent of bone marrow edema in axial PsA patients, suggesting that HLA-B27 is a marker of disease severity and progression much as shown in axSpA.[69] This disparity in the findings from both studies might be related to the different methodologies used as the first study only considered abnormal/normal scan, whereas the latter used a semi-quantitative scoring of the lesions.

ASSESSMENT

A question that remains in the research agenda is what tools are best placed to assess axial involvement in PsA. The lack of objective biomarkers in the assessment of spinal disease has led to the reliance on subjective or patient-reported measures of disease activity such as the Bath AS Disease Activity Index (BASDAI), Bath AS Functional Index (BASFI), or visual analog scale spinal measurements of pain or global disease activity. BASDAI has been shown to correlate well with patient perception of arthritis, although it did not discriminate between high and low disease activity in 2 studies.[70,71] Nevertheless, BASDAI showed good to moderate discriminative power in disease activity in another study,[72] with more recent data[73] confirming that the AS Disease Activity Score (ASDAS) and BASDAI have similar discriminative power and can be used interchangeably.

Regarding spinal mobility assessment, measures included in the Bath AS Metrology Index are reproducible in axPsA as well as in AS.[74,75] They also correlated adequately with radiographic damage assessed by mSASSS with an enhanced correlation in axPsA between cervical mobility and cervical mSASSS.[76]

In relation to functional disability, a study evaluated HAQ, BASFI, Dougados-FI, and SF-36-PF questionnaires that performed accurately in axPsA.[77]

TREATMENT

Data exploring treatment response in axPsA are very limited, with only a handful of studies that have specifically addressed different treatment strategies (**Table 2**). The most recent Group for Research and Assessment of Psoriasis and Psoriatic Arthritis

Table 2
Studies evaluating treatment response in axial psoriatic arthritis

	Lubrano et al,[78] 2011	Lubrano et al,[79] 2016	Haroon et al,[80] 2018	MAXIMISE Trial (NCT02721966) Primary Results
Design	Multicenter observational study	Single-center observational study	Single-center open-label controlled trial	Muticenter RDBCT phase 3 trial
Inclusion criteria	CASPAR criteria IBP AND/or radiological axial involvement Eligible for TNFi according to local guidelines	CASPAR criteria IBP AND/or radiological axial involvement Eligible for TNFi according to local guidelines	CASPAR criteria OR mNY criteria IBP with spinal VAS score $\geq$4 and BASDAI $\geq$4 MRI-proven SIJ BMO Naive to biologics	CASPAR criteria IBP with spinal VAS score $\geq$4 and BASDAI $\geq$4 Inadequate response to 2 NSAIDs Naive to biologics
Sample size	32	58	15 axPsA, 15 AS, 10 controls (chronic LBP)	503
Primary outcome	BASDAI 50 response at week 52	BASDAI 50 response at week 52	Mean change in ASDAS at week 2	ASAS20 response with SEC 300 mg at week 12
Intervention	Etanercept 50 mg s.c. w	Adalimumab 40 mg eow OR Etanercept 50 mg w OR Golimumab 50 mg mo	Triamcinolone acetonide 80 mg i.m depot	Arm 1: SEC 300 mg Arm 2: SEC 150 mg Arm 3: placebo
Results	72% patients achieved BASDAI 50	Percentages of patients achieving: BASDAI 50 31.2% CPDAI <4 35.4% DAPSA $\leq$3.3 22.9% PR 22.9% MDA 50%	Mean change in ASDAS: axPsA: 1.43 $\pm$ 0.39 AS: 1.03 $\pm$ 0.30 Controls: 0.81 $\pm$ 0.26	63.1% responders with SEC 300 mg vs 31.3% with placebo with an OR 3.81 (P<.0001)

Abbreviations: ASDAS, ankylosing spondylitis disease activity score; BASDAI, bath ankylosing spondylitis disease activity index; BMO, bone marrow edema; CPDAI, composite psoriatic disease activity index; DAPSA, disease activity index for psoriatic arthritis; IBP, inflammatory back pain; LBP, low back pain; MDA, minimal disease activity; mNY, modified New York; NSAID, nonsteroidal anti-inflammatory drug; PR, partial remission; RDBCT, randomized double-blind clinical trial; SEC, Secukinumab; TNFi, TNF inhibitors; VAS, visual analog scale.
Data from Refs.[78–81]

(GRAPPA) recommendations outlined treatment advice on axial involvement based on studies performed in axSpA.[12] Trial design in axPsA has been hampered by the lack of a consensus or validated definition; and assessment of axial involvement in most phase III trials looking at the efficacy of biologic drugs in PsA has been poorly reported or not performed at all. Some smaller studies[78–80] limited the studied population to cases with radiographic evidence of axial PsA.

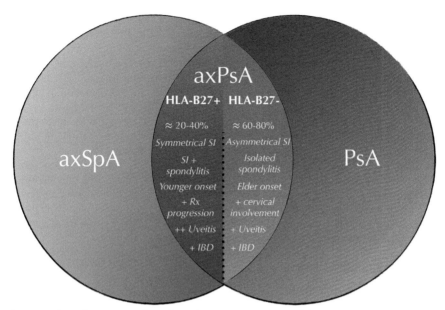

Fig. 2. Distinct phenotypes of axial involvement in axial spondyloarthritis and axial psoriatic arthritis. IBD, inflammatory bowel disease; Rx, radiographic; SI, sacroiliitis.

The limited available data to date coming largely from observational studies suggest that TNF inhibitors are efficacious in axial PsA. The only randomized controlled study available to date is the MAXIMISE (EudraCT number 2016–000814–31) trial, which tests the efficacy of an IL-17 inhibitor in axPsA with promising preliminary results.[81] With regard to IL-12/23 inhibition, although an initial post-hoc analysis of its pivotal studies showed significant improvement in BASDAI and ASDAS in patients with PsA with physician reported spondylitis,[82] subsequent placebo-controlled trials failed to demonstrate efficacy in axSpA (radiographic and nonradiographic).[83] This was somehow surprising in view of the proven efficacy of these drugs in psoriasis and PsA with peripheral involvement. These dichotomous responses in spine and peripheral joints suggest tissue-specific pathogenic variations, with recent data pointing toward specific IL-17A production independently of IL-23R expression at the spinal entheses.[84] Nonetheless, it cannot be excluded that the response to therapy might be different in primary axial SpA and axial PsA, which warrants clinical studies in this patient population.

SUMMARY

The current understanding from the literature and clinical experience is that axPsA is indeed a distinct entity from axSpA. Although the genetic endotype remains elusive, there is clear evidence that the major histocompatibility complex (MHC) class I HLA-B27 has a strong association with axPsA, and also determines a phenotype more similar to axSpA with more severe radiographic changes, as evaluated by plain radiographs and MRI. Hence, it seems that, although HLA-B27 might not determine axial involvement in most of the PsA population affected by spinal or axial symptoms, it acts as a marker of its severity and expression supporting the concept of PsA being an "MHC-I-opathy" as a result of the interaction between the MHC-I alleles and tissue-specific factors driving the clinical presentation. Characteristic clinical aspects and different treatment responses also endorse its distinct nature identifying 2 distinct phenotypes within the axial PsA subtype as shown in **Table 1** and **Fig. 2.**

From an imaging standpoint, the occurrence of isolated spondylitis sparing the SIJ and the high prevalence of asymptomatic sacroiliitis complicates the assembly of universal axial PsA criteria. The only randomized trial on this entity (MAXIMISE) favored a purely clinical entry criterion, with back pain without objective confirmation of inflammatory affection of the axial skeleton being the only requisite in patients with PsA, in stark contrast with other studies that demanded definite radiographic SIJ changes or MRI-proven inflammation to define their population. The imaging data of the MAXIMISE trial could shed some light on our insight into this condition.

In summary, prospective, longitudinal cohorts are needed to allow for the characterization of axial involvement in PsA. A joint initiative between the ASAS and GRAPPA specialist groups is currently underway aimed to develop a data-driven consensus definition of axial involvement in PsA that will allow for homogeneity in clinical trial design. Once a definition is formulated, efforts should be placed in the development of enhanced assessment tools and management strategies of axPsA.

ACKNOWLEDGMENTS

H. Marzo-Ortega and X. Michelena are supported by the NIHR Leeds Biomedical Research Centre. The views expressed are those of the authors and not necessarily those of the (UK) National Health Service (NHS), the NIHR, or the (UK) Department of Health. X. Michelena's work is supported by the Catalan Society of Rheumatology.

DISCLOSURE

X. Michelena has received speaking fees from UCB, Novartis, and Sanofi-Genzyme. D. Poddubnyy: research grants from AbbVie, Lilly, MSD, Novartis, and Pfizer. Consultancy/speaker fees from AbbVie, BMS, Celgene, Janssen, Lilly, MSD, Novartis, Pfizer, Roche, and UCB; H. Marzo-Ortega: research grants from Janssen and Novartis. Consultancy/Speaker from AbbVie, Celgene, Eli-Lilly, Janssen, Novartis, Takeda, UCB.

REFERENCES

1. Moll JM, Haslock I, Macrae IF, et al. Associations between ankylosing spondylitis, psoriatic arthritis, Reiter's disease, the intestinal arthropathies, and Behcet's syndrome. Medicine (Baltimore) 1974;53:343–64.
2. Moll JM, Wright V. Psoriatic arthritis. Semin Arthritis Rheum 1973;3:55–78.
3. Gladman DD, Shuckett R, Russell ML, et al. Psoriatic arthritis (PSA)—an analysis of 220 patients. Q J Med 1987;62:127–41.
4. McGonagle D, Conaghan PG, Emery P. Psoriatic arthritis: a unified concept twenty years on. Arthritis Rheum 1999;42:1080–6.
5. Fournié B, Crognier L, Arnaud C, et al. Proposed classification criteria of psoriatic arthritis. A preliminary study in 260 patients. Rev Rhum Engl Ed 1999;66:446–56.
6. Bennet R. Psoriatic arthritis. In: Mc Carty D, editor. Arthritis and allied conditions. 9th edition. Philadelphia: Lea & Febiger; 1979. p. 645.
7. Vasey F, Espinoza L. Psoriatic arthropathy. In: Calin A, editor. Spondyloarthropaties. Orlando (FL): Grune & Stratton; 1984. p. 151–85.
8. Dougados M, van der Linden S, Juhlin R, et al. The European Spondylarthropathy Study Group preliminary criteria for the classification of spondylarthropathy. Arthritis Rheum 1991;34:1218–27.

9. Taylor W, Gladman D, Helliwell P, et al. Classification criteria for psoriatic arthritis: development of new criteria from a large international study. Arthritis Rheum 2006;54:2665–73.

10. Taylor WJ, Zmierczak H-G, Helliwell PS. Problems with the definition of axial and peripheral disease patterns in psoriatic arthritis. J Rheumatol 2005;32:974–7.

11. Coates LC, Helliwell PS. Classification and categorisation of psoriatic arthritis. Clin Rheumatol 2008;27:1211–6.

12. Coates LC, Murphy R, Helliwell PS. New GRAPPA recommendations for the management of psoriasis and psoriatic arthritis: process, challenges and implementation. Br J Dermatol 2016;174:1174–8.

13. Moltó A, Dougados M. Comorbidities in spondyloarthritis including psoriatic arthritis. Best Pract Res Clin Rheumatol 2018;32:390–400.

14. Jadon DR, Sengupta R, Nightingale A, et al. Axial Disease in Psoriatic Arthritis study: defining the clinical and radiographic phenotype of psoriatic spondyloarthritis. Ann Rheum Dis 2017;76:701–7.

15. Lubrano E, Marchesoni A, Olivieri I, et al. The radiological assessment of axial involvement in psoriatic arthritis: a validation study of the BASRI total and the modified SASSS scoring methods. Clin Exp Rheumatol 2009;27:977–80.

16. Wakhlu A, Chandran V, Phumethum V, et al. Comparison between INSPIRE and Domjan method for measuring lumbar lateral flexion in patients of psoriatic arthritis (PsA) and correlation with radiographic damage. Clin Rheumatol 2019; 38:1063–6.

17. Mease PJ, Palmer JB, Liu M, et al. Influence of axial involvement on clinical characteristics of psoriatic arthritis: analysis from the corrona psoriatic arthritis/spondyloarthritis registry. J Rheumatol 2018;45:1389–96.

18. Queiro R, Sarasqueta C, Belzunegui J, et al. Psoriatic spondyloarthropathy: a comparative study between HLA-B27 positive and HLA-B27 negative disease. Semin Arthritis Rheum 2002;31:413–8.

19. Haroon M, Winchester R, Giles JT, et al. Clinical and genetic associations of radiographic sacroiliitis and its different patterns in psoriatic arthritis. Clin Exp Rheumatol 2017;35:270–6.

20. Chandran V, Barrett J, Schentag CT, et al. Axial psoriatic arthritis: update on a longterm prospective study. J Rheumatol 2009;36:2744–50.

21. Hanly JG, Russell ML, Gladman DD. Psoriatic spondyloarthropathy: a long term prospective study. Ann Rheum Dis 1988;47:386–93.

22. Feld J, Chandran V, Haroon N, et al. Axial disease in psoriatic arthritis and ankylosing spondylitis: a critical comparison. Nat Rev Rheumatol 2018;14:363–71.

23. Lambert JR, Wright V. Psoriatic spondylitis: a clinical and radiological description of the spine in psoriatic arthritis. Q J Med 1977;46:411–25.

24. Eastmond CJ, Woodrow JC. The HLA system and the arthropathies associated with psoriasis. Ann Rheum Dis 1977;36:112–20.

25. Kantor SM, Hsu SH, Bias WB, et al. Clinical and immunogenetic subsets of psoriatic arthritis. Clin Exp Rheumatol 1984;2:105–9.

26. Gladman DD, Anhorn KA, Schachter RK, et al. HLA antigens in psoriatic arthritis. J Rheumatol 1986;13:586–92.

27. Suarez-Almazor ME, Russell AS. Sacroiliitis in psoriasis: relationship to peripheral arthritis and HLA-B27. J Rheumatol 1990;17:804–8.

28. Marsal S, Armadans-Gil L, Martínez M, et al. Clinical, radiographic and HLA associations as markers for different patterns of psoriatic arthritis. Rheumatology 1999;38:332–7.

29. Liao H-T, Lin K-C, Chang Y-T, et al. Human leukocyte antigen and clinical and demographic characteristics in psoriatic arthritis and psoriasis in Chinese patients. J Rheumatol 2008;35:891–5.

30. Queiro R, Alperi M, Lopez A, et al. Clinical expression, but not disease outcome, may vary according to age at disease onset in psoriatic spondylitis. Joint Bone Spine 2008;75:544–7.

31. Trabace S, Cappellacci S, Ciccarone P, et al. Psoriatic arthritis: a clinical, radiological and genetic study of 58 Italian patients. Acta Derm Venereol Suppl (Stockh) 1994;186:69–70.

32. Castillo-Gallego C, Aydin SZ, Emery P, et al. Brief report: magnetic resonance imaging assessment of axial psoriatic arthritis: extent of disease relates to HLA-B27. Arthritis Rheum 2013;65:2274–8.

33. van Onna M, Jurik AG, van der Heijde D, et al. HLA-B27 and gender independently determine the likelihood of a positive MRI of the sacroiliac joints in patients with early inflammatory back pain: a 2-year MRI follow-up study. Ann Rheum Dis 2011;70(11):1981–5.

34. Catanoso MG, Boiardi L, Macchioni P, et al. IL-23A, IL-23R, IL-17A and IL-17R polymorphisms in different psoriatic arthritis clinical manifestations in the northern Italian population. Rheumatol Int 2013;33:1165–76.

35. Rahman P, Inman RD, Gladman DD, et al. Association of interleukin-23 receptor variants with ankylosing spondylitis. Arthritis Rheum 2008;58:1020–5.

36. Rueda B, Orozco G, Raya E, et al. The IL23R Arg381Gln non-synonymous polymorphism confers susceptibility to ankylosing spondylitis. Ann Rheum Dis 2008; 67:1451–4.

37. Queiro R, Gonzalez S, Lopez-Larrea C, et al. HLA-C locus alleles may modulate the clinical expression of psoriatic arthritis. Arthritis Res Ther 2006;8(6):R185.

38. Crivellato E, Zacchi T. HLA-B39 and the axial type of psoriatic arthritis. Acta Derm Venereol 1987;67:249–50.

39. Torre Alonso JC, Rodriguez Perez A, Arribas Castrillo JM, et al. Psoriatic arthritis (PA): a clinical, immunological and radiological study of 180 patients. Br J Rheumatol 1991;30:245–50.

40. Ikumi K, Kobayashi S, Tamura N, et al. HLA-B46 is associated with severe sacroiliitis in Japanese patients with psoriatic arthritis. Mod Rheumatol 2019;29(6): 1017–22.

41. Battistone MJ, Manaster BJ, Reda DJ, et al. The prevalence of sacroiliitis in psoriatic arthritis: new perspectives from a large, multicenter cohort. A Department of Veterans Affairs Cooperative Study. Skeletal Radiol 1999;28:196–201.

42. Carvalho PD, Savy F, Moragues C, et al. Axial involvement according to ASAS criteria in an observational psoriatic arthritis cohort. Acta Reumatol Port 2017; 42:176–82.

43. Chandran V, Tolusso DC, Cook RJ, et al. Risk factors for axial inflammatory arthritis in patients with psoriatic arthritis. J Rheumatol 2010;37:809–15.

44. Kalyoncu U, Bayindir Ö, Ferhat Öksüz M, et al. The Psoriatic Arthritis Registry of Turkey: results of a multicentre registry on 1081 patients. Rheumatology (Oxford) 2017;56:279–86.

45. Lindström U, Bremander A, Haglund E, et al. Back pain and health status in patients with clinically diagnosed ankylosing spondylitis, psoriatic arthritis and other spondyloarthritis: a cross-sectional population-based study. BMC Musculoskelet Disord 2016;17:106.

46. Queiro R, Belzunegui J, González C, et al. Clinically asymptomatic axial disease in psoriatic spondyloarthropathy. A retrospective study. Clin Rheumatol 2002; 21:10–3.
47. Yap KS, Ye JY, Li S, et al. Back pain in psoriatic arthritis: defining prevalence, characteristics and performance of inflammatory back pain criteria in psoriatic arthritis. Ann Rheum Dis 2018;77(11):1573–7.
48. Poddubnyy D, Callhoff J, Spiller I, et al. Diagnostic accuracy of inflammatory back pain for axial spondyloarthritis in rheumatological care. RMD open 2018; 4:e000825.
49. Aydin SZ, Kilic L, Kucuksahin O, et al. Performances of inflammatory back pain criteria in axial psoriatic arthritis. Rheumatology (Oxford) 2017;56:2031–2.
50. Haroon M, Gallagher P, FitzGerald O. Inflammatory back pain criteria perform well in subset of patients with active axial psoriatic arthritis but not among patients with established axial disease. Ann Rheum Dis 2019;78(7):1003–4.
51. Salvarani C, Macchioni P, Cremonesi T, et al. The cervical spine in patients with psoriatic arthritis: a clinical, radiological and immunogenetic study. Ann Rheum Dis 1992;51(1):73–7.
52. Taccari E, Spadaro A, Riccieri V. Correlations between peripheral and axial radiological changes in patients with psoriatic polyarthritis. Rev Rhum Engl Ed 1996; 63:17–23.
53. Alonso S, Tejón P, Sarasqueta C, et al. Age at disease onset may help to further characterize the disease phenotype in psoriatic arthritis. Joint Bone Spine 2016; 83:533–7.
54. Gladman DD, Brubacher B, Buskila D, et al. Differences in the expression of spondyloarthropathy: a comparison between ankylosing spondylitis and psoriatic arthritis. Clin Invest Med 1993;16(1):1–7.
55. Helliwell PS, Hickling P, Wright V. Do the radiological changes of classic ankylosing spondylitis differ from the changes found in the spondylitis associated with inflammatory bowel disease, psoriasis, and reactive arthritis? Ann Rheum Dis 1998;57(3):135–40.
56. Perez Alamino R, Maldonado Cocco JA, Citera G, et al. Differential features between primary ankylosing spondylitis and spondylitis associated with psoriasis and inflammatory bowel disease. J Rheumatol 2011;38(8):1656–60.
57. Aydin SZ, Kucuksahin O, Kilic L, et al. Axial psoriatic arthritis: the impact of underdiagnosed disease on outcomes in real life. Clin Rheumatol 2018;37:3443–8.
58. Landi M, Maldonado-Ficco H, Perez-Alamino R, et al. Gender differences among patients with primary ankylosing spondylitis and spondylitis associated with psoriasis and inflammatory bowel disease in an iberoamerican spondyloarthritis cohort. Medicine (Baltimore) 2016;95(51):e5652.
59. Queiro R, Lorenzo A, Tejon P, et al. Obesity in psoriatic arthritis: comparative prevalence and associated factors. Medicine (Baltimore) 2019;98(28):e16400.
60. McEwen C, DiTata D, Lingg C, et al. Ankylosing spondylitis and spondylitis accompanying ulcerative colitis, regional enteritis, psoriasis and Reiter's disease. A comparative study. Arthritis Rheum 1971;14(3):291–318.
61. Haddad A, Thavaneswaran A, Toloza S, et al. Diffuse idiopathic skeletal hyperostosis in psoriatic arthritis. J Rheumatol 2013;40:1367–73.
62. Mader R, Verlaan JJ, Eshed I, et al. Diffuse idiopathic skeletal hyperostosis (DISH): where we are now and where to go next. RMD open 2017;3(1):e000472.
63. Mader R, Novofastovski I, Iervolino S, et al. Ultrasonography of peripheral entheses in the diagnosis and understanding of diffuse idiopathic skeletal hyperostosis (DISH). Rheumatol Int 2015;35(3):493–7.

64. Arad U, Elkayam O, Eshed I. Magnetic resonance imaging in diffuse idiopathic skeletal hyperostosis: similarities to axial spondyloarthritis. Clin Rheumatol 2017;36(7):1545–9.

65. Lubrano E, Marchesoni A, Olivieri I, et al. Psoriatic arthritis spondylitis radiology index: a modified index for radiologic assessment of axial involvement in psoriatic arthritis. J Rheumatol 2009;36:1006–11.

66. Ibrahim A, Gladman DD, Thavaneswaran A, et al. Sensitivity and specificity of radiographic scoring instruments for detecting change in axial psoriatic arthritis. Arthritis Care Res (Hoboken) 2017;69:1700–5.

67. Maldonado-Ficco H, Sheane BJ, Thavaneswaran A, et al. Magnetic resonance imaging in psoriatic arthritis. J Clin Rheumatol 2017;23:243–5.

68. Williamson L, Dockerty JL, Dalbeth N, et al. Clinical assessment of sacroiliitis and HLA-B27 are poor predictors of sacroiliitis diagnosed by magnetic resonance imaging in psoriatic arthritis. Rheumatology (Oxford) 2004;43:85–8.

69. Marzo-Ortega H, McGonagle D, O'Connor P, et al. Baseline and 1-year magnetic resonance imaging of the sacroiliac joint and lumbar spine in very early inflammatory back pain. Relationship between symptoms, HLA-B27 and disease extent and persistence. Ann Rheum Dis 2009;68(11):1721–7.

70. Taylor WJ, Harrison AA. Could the Bath Ankylosing Spondylitis Disease Activity Index (BASDAI) be a valid measure of disease activity in patients with psoriatic arthritis? Arthritis Rheum 2004;51(3):311–5.

71. Fernández-Sueiro JL, Willisch A, Pértega-Díaz S, et al. Validity of the Bath Ankylosing Spondylitis Disease Activity Index for the evaluation of disease activity in axial psoriatic arthritis. Arthritis Care Res (Hoboken) 2010;62:78–85.

72. Eder L, Chandran V, Shen H, et al. Is ASDAS better than BASDAI as a measure of disease activity in axial psoriatic arthritis? Ann Rheum Dis 2010;69(12):2160–4.

73. Kılıç G, Kılıç E, Nas K, et al. Comparison of ASDAS and BASDAI as a measure of disease activity in axial psoriatic arthritis. Clin Rheumatol 2015;34:515–21.

74. Gladman DD, Inman RD, Cook RJ, et al. International spondyloarthritis interobserver reliability exercise—the INSPIRE study: I. Assessment of spinal measures. J Rheumatol 2007;34(8):1733–9.

75. Fernández-Sueiro JL, Willisch A, Pértega-Díaz S, et al. Evaluation of ankylosing spondylitis spinal mobility measurements in the assessment of spinal involvement in psoriatic arthritis. Arthritis Rheum 2009;61:386–92.

76. Chandran V, O'Shea FD, Schentag CT, et al. Relationship between spinal mobility and radiographic damage in ankylosing spondylitis and psoriatic spondylitis: a comparative analysis. J Rheumatol 2007;34:2463–5.

77. Leung YY, Tam LS, Kun EW, et al. Comparison of 4 functional indexes in psoriatic arthritis with axial or peripheral disease subgroups using Rasch analyses. J Rheumatol 2008;35(8):1613–21.

78. Lubrano E, Spadaro A, Marchesoni A, et al. The effectiveness of a biologic agent on axial manifestations of psoriatic arthritis. A twelve months observational study in a group of patients treated with etanercept. Clin Exp Rheumatol 2011;29:80–4.

79. Lubrano E, Parsons WJ, Perrotta FM. Assessment of response to treatment, remission, and minimal disease activity in axial psoriatic arthritis treated with tumor necrosis factor inhibitors. J Rheumatol 2016;43:918–23.

80. Haroon M, Ahmad M, Baig MN, et al. Inflammatory back pain in psoriatic arthritis is significantly more responsive to corticosteroids compared to back pain in ankylosing spondylitis: a prospective, open-labelled, controlled pilot study. Arthritis Res Ther 2018;20:73.

81. Baraliakos X, Coates LC, Gossec L, et al. Secukinumab improves axial manifestations in patients with psoriatic arthritis and inadequate response to NSAIDS: primary analysis of the MAXIMISE trial. Ann Rheum Dis 2019;78(Supplement 2): A195.

82. Kavanaugh A, Puig L, Gottlieb AB, et al. Efficacy and safety of ustekinumab in psoriatic arthritis patients with peripheral arthritis and physician-reported spondylitis: post-hoc analyses from two phase III, multicentre, double-blind, placebo-controlled studies (PSUMMIT-1/PSUMMIT-2). Ann Rheum Dis 2016;75: 1984–8.

83. Deodhar A, Gensler LS, Sieper J, et al. Three multicenter, randomized, double-blind, placebo-controlled studies evaluating the efficacy and safety of ustekinumab in axial spondyloarthritis. Arthritis Rheumatol 2019;71(2):258–70.

84. Cuthbert RJ, Bridgewood C, Watad A, et al. Evidence that tissue resident human enthesis gammadeltaT-cells can produce IL-17A independently of IL-23R transcript expression. Ann Rheum Dis 2019;78(11):1559–65.

85. Bohn R, Cooney M, Deodhar A, et al. Incidence and prevalence of axial spondyloarthritis: methodologic challenges and gaps in the literature. Clin Exp Rheumatol 2018;36(2):263–74.

86. Baraliakos X, Braun J. Non-radiographic axial spondyloarthritis and ankylosing spondylitis: what are the similarities and differences? RMD open 2015;1(Suppl 1):e000053.

87. Rudwaleit M, Haibel H, Baraliakos X, et al. The early disease stage in axial spondylarthritis: results from the German Spondyloarthritis Inception Cohort. Arthritis Rheum 2009;60(3):717–27.

88. Akkoc N, Yarkan H, Kenar G, et al. Ankylosing spondylitis: HLA-B*27-positive versus HLA-B*27-negative disease. Curr Rheumatol Rep 2017;19(5):26.

89. Chung HY, Machado P, van der Heijde D, et al. HLA-B27 positive patients differ from HLA-B27 negative patients in clinical presentation and imaging: results from the DESIR cohort of patients with recent onset axial spondyloarthritis. Ann Rheum Dis 2011;70(11):1930–6.

90. Braun J, Bollow M, Sieper J. Radiologic diagnosis and pathology of the spondyloarthropathies. Rheum Dis Clin North Am 1998;24(4):697–735.

91. Ramiro S, Stolwijk C, van Tubergen A, et al. Evolution of radiographic damage in ankylosing spondylitis: a 12 year prospective follow-up of the OASIS study. Ann Rheum Dis 2015;74(1):52–9.

92. Bennett AN, McGonagle D, O'Connor P, et al. Severity of baseline magnetic resonance imaging-evident sacroiliitis and HLA-B27 status in early inflammatory back pain predict radiographically evident ankylosing spondylitis at eight years. Arthritis Rheum 2008;58(11):3413–8.

93. Zeboulon N, Dougados M, Gossec L. Prevalence and characteristics of uveitis in the spondyloarthropathies: a systematic literature review. Ann Rheum Dis 2008; 67(7):955–9.

94. Lim CSE, Sengupta R, Gaffney K. The clinical utility of human leucocyte antigen B27 in axial spondyloarthritis. Rheumatology (Oxford) 2018;57(6):959–68.

Treat to Target in Axial Spondyloarthritis
Pros, Cons, and Future Directions

Jean W. Liew, MD[a], Maureen Dubreuil, MD, MSc[b],*

KEYWORDS

• Treat to target • Disease activity • Axial spondyloarthritis • Ankylosing spondylitis

KEY POINTS

- Treat to target describes a management paradigm that involves choosing a clinically relevant target, assessment with validated measures at a prespecified frequency, and a change in therapy if the target is not met.
- The treat-to-target strategy has been used in other rheumatologic conditions, such as rheumatoid arthritis and psoriatic arthritis, and is advocated in axial spondyloarthritis.
- An ideal outcome measure for a treat-to-target strategy needs to be defined in axial spondyloarthritis, with consideration of existing or potential outcome measures and their attributes.

INTRODUCTION: TREAT TO TARGET

Treat to target describes a disease management paradigm that involves selection of a clinically relevant target, assessment with validated measures at a prespecified frequency, and a change in therapy if the target is not met. Treat-to-target strategies have been incorporated in treatment guidelines and in clinical practice for chronic medical conditions, such as hypertension,[1] type 2 diabetes mellitus,[2] and hyperlipidemia.[3] Treating these diseases to target has been demonstrated to improve important clinical outcomes, such as preventing cardiovascular events and retinopathy.[4–6]

In rheumatology, treat-to-target strategies are recommended for the management of gout, rheumatoid arthritis (RA), and spondyloarthritis (SpA), including psoriatic arthritis (PsA). In gout, the target is a serum uric acid level of less than 6 mg/dL or less than 5 mg/dL in the presence of erosive or tophaceous disease, and levels should be checked in order to titrate urate-lowering therapy.[7] The target and cutoffs were

[a] Division of Rheumatology, Department of Medicine, University of Washington, 1959 Northeast Pacific Street, BB561, Seattle, WA 98195, USA; [b] Section of Rheumatology, Boston University School of Medicine, 650 Albany Street, X201, Boston, MA 02119, USA
* Corresponding author.
E-mail address: mdubreui@bu.edu
Twitter: @rheum_cat (J.W.L.); @Spondy_MD (M.D.)

Rheum Dis Clin N Am 46 (2020) 347–360
https://doi.org/10.1016/j.rdc.2020.01.011
0889-857X/20/Published by Elsevier Inc.

rheumatic.theclinics.com

chosen based on the physiologic level at which monosodium urate precipitates in vivo and the understanding that controlled disease in gout prevents joint damage. In 2014 for RA, the European League Against Rheumatism (EULAR) released treat-to-target guidelines that included 4 overarching principles with the primary goal of optimizing quality of life through decreasing symptoms and joint damage.[8] In order to meet this goal, inflammation should be attenuated via adjusting treatment alongside regular measurements of disease activity. Shared decision making also should be used throughout this process. These guidelines have the backing of multiple randomized controlled trials (RCTs) that compared a treat-to-target or tight control strategy with standard of care in RA.[9] The connection between improved control of inflammation and prevention of joint damage also is established in RA.[10]

The first treat-to-target guidelines for SpA were introduced in 2014[11] and underwent revision in 2017.[12] Both PsA and axial SpA (axSpA) are included but the strength of evidence is greater for the former. Similar to the treat-to-target guidelines for RA, those for SpA include overarching principles and key recommendations. Like the RA guidelines, the overall goal is optimizing quality of life by decreasing symptoms, inflammation, and structural damage by regularly measuring disease activity and adjusting treatment accordingly. In contrast to the RA guidelines, the SpA guidelines include extraarticular manifestations (EAMs) of SpA as possible targets and indicate that imaging also should be considered as an adjunctive form of assessment for disease activity. All imaging modalities (conventional radiograph, computed tomography, magnetic resonance, and ultrasonography) are included, although the guidelines do not specify which sites ought to be assessed. The evidence base for the treat-to-target strategy in PsA rests on 1 RCT, the Tight Control of Psoriatic Arthritis (TICOPA) study[13]; strategy trials in axSpA have been under way but their results have not been published. Furthermore, it is not yet established that the achievement of treatment targets in axSpA would prevent structural damage, EAMs, or co-occurring conditions.

This review focuses on the background for a treat-to-target strategy in axSpA. The potential targets of treatment, which are the available validated measures of disease activity, are discussed. The association of these targets with outcomes of interest, including structural damage, physical function, spinal mobility, and EAMs, as well as the evidence that available treatments can have an impact on these outcomes, are addressed. How treat-to-target strategies have been incorporated into SpA treatment guidelines is reviewed. Finally, treat-to-target RCTs and the research agenda for future studies in axSpA are discussed.

DEFINING THE TARGET: DISEASE ACTIVITY MEASURES

The first necessary step of a treat-to-target strategy is defining the target. The target must be easily measurable in clinical practice, be validated in axSpA patients, and reflect clinical outcomes that are important to both patients and physicians. The 2 most commonly used measures for axSpA in clinical practice are the Bath Ankylosing Spondylitis Disease Activity Index (BASDAI) and the Ankylosing Spondylitis Disease Activity Score (ASDAS). The BASDAI was developed in 1994 and comprises 6 questions addressing 5 major symptoms in AS: fatigue, spinal pain, peripheral joint pain and swelling, localized tenderness, and morning stiffness.[14] Although the BASDAI correlates with other clinical outcomes of interest, such as physical function,[15] and has been used as both an eligibility criterion and outcome in clinical trials, it has major limitations. BASDAI questions pertain only to subjective, patient-reported outcomes and are not specific for symptoms related to inflammation versus other processes; 4 items are given equal weighting; and there is no assessment of extra-articular disease, such as eye, skin, or bowel inflammation.[16] Due to the subjectivity of the items included on the BASDAI, there often is discordance between patient and clinician assessments of the disease activity.[17]

The ASDAS was developed by experts to try to overcome some of the limitations of the BASDAI. ASDAS includes some questions from BASDAI as well as patient and physical global assessments, and laboratory measures (either the C-reactive protein [CRP] or the erythrocyte sedimentation rate [ESR]).[18] The ASDAS has been validated in multiple observational databases and clinical trials as well as in different populations.[19] It has been shown to be responsive to clinical and imaging measures of disease activity, more so than the BASDAI.[20] The ASDAS remains, however, with limitations: it does not incorporate other objective measures of inflammation, such as that found on imaging; and like BASDAI it does not include any assessment of extra-articular disease.[16] ASDAS is challenging to use in US clinical practice because CRP and ESR assessments typically are not available in real time at the point of care. Although ASDAS has validated cutoffs for disease activity categories, there are no validated cutoffs for the BASDAI.

ASAS (then called Assessments in Ankylosing Spondylitis) developed a core set of 5 domains (physical function, pain, spinal mobility, spinal stiffness/inflammation, and patient global assessment) to be assessed in trials and other clinical outcomes studies. Based on this core set, Anderson and colleagues[21] developed standard ASAS response criteria using data from 3 RCTs comparing nonsteroidal anti-inflammatory drugs (NSAIDs) to placebo in AS. The final response criteria included the 4 domains of physical function (measured by the Bath Ankylosing Spondylitis Functional Index [BASFI]), pain (measured by a visual analog scale [VAS]), inflammation (measured with the proxy of morning stiffness), and patient global assessment (measured by VAS). Spinal mobility was excluded due to its poor performance. The ASAS20 and ASAS40 are the commonly used response criteria for primary outcomes in RCTs. An ASAS20 response is defined as greater than or equal to 20% improvement in at least 3 domains with no worsening in the fourth domain. The utility of these response criteria in clinical practice, however, is limited, and they suffer from issues similar to the BASDAI and ASDAS.

In response to the lack of a definition of ankylosing spondylitis (AS) disease severity, ASAS developed an instrument based on the International Classification of Functioning, Disability, and Health model of function and health.[22] The ASAS Health Index (ASAS HI) includes 17 items with dichotomous responses, meant for use in RCTs and in clinical practice. It has been shown to have construct validity, interpretability, reliability, and responsiveness in both axSpA and peripheral SpA populations.[23] A value greater than or equal to 12.0 serves as the cutoff between poor and moderate health, whereas a value less than 5.0 is the cutoff between good and moderate health. The ASAS HI serves as the primary outcome measure in an ongoing treat-to-target trial in axSpA.

For a target to be useful, there should be a clear definition of that target, as has been established for ASDAS inactive disease/remission and low disease activity (LDA). These are defined in **Table 1**. Remission refers to the absence of clinical or laboratory evidence of significant inflammatory disease over a prolonged period of time.[24] It also has been defined as a state in which the disease does not progress.[25,26] In clinical trials, the disease activity states of either inactive disease (ASDAS <1.3) or ASAS partial remission (a value <20 on a scale of 0–100 in all 4 ASAS domains) is used. The main limitation with ASAS partial remission is that it relies partly on the BASFI, and a patient with irreversible structural damage may be unable to fulfill ASAS partial remission criteria.[16]

Table 1
Definitions of remission and low or minimal disease activity

ASDAS inactive disease	ASDAS <1.3
	ASDAS questions
	1. How would you describe the overall level of AS neck, back, or hip pain you have had?
	2. How active was your spondylitis on average?
	3. How would you describe the overall level of pain/swelling in joints other than neck, back, or hips you have had?
	4. How long does your morning stiffness last from the time you wake up?
	5. CRP measured in milligrams per liter
	ASDAS calculation
	$0.1216 * Q1 + 0.1106 * Q2 + 0.0736 * Q3 + 0.0586 * Q4 + 0.5796 \, Ln \, (CRP + 1)$
ASAS partial remission	<20 on a scale of 0–100 in 4 out of 4 domains
	ASAS domains
	1. Physical function (BASFI)
	2. Pain (by VAS)
	3. Inflammation (morning stiffness)
	4. Patient global assessment (by VAS)

Abbreviations: + denotes plus; * denotes times; Ln, natural log.

As conceptually defined at the Outcome Measures in Rheumatology (OMERACT) 6 conference in 2002, MDA comprises both remission and LDA and should be "a useful target of treatment by both patient and physician given current therapy and knowledge."[27,28] After this conference, MDA has been defined and validated in both RA[29] and PsA.[30] MDA for PsA was used as the primary outcome measure in the TICOPA treat-to-target RCT.[31]

WHICH OUTCOMES TO TARGET

Disease activity measures and disease states as defined by these measures are only surrogate targets for the outcomes of interest. In axSpA, a main outcome of interest is irreversible structural damage of the axial skeleton. European cohort studies of axSpA and AS have identified several variables that are independently associated with radiographic progression: baseline syndesmophytes,[32–35] male sex,[33,35] smoking,[34,35] HLA-B27 positivity,[33] and elevated CRP.[34] In long-term extension studies of tumor necrosis factor inhibitor (TNFi) trials, 2-year to 4-year follow-up has shown no benefit of TNFi on the prevention of structural damage in either AS or nonradiographic axSpA.[36–41] The comparator was a historical cohort, the Outcome in AS International Study, whose participants were TNFi-naïve for the first 4 years of follow-up. On the other hand, observational cohort studies with longer term follow-up of 5 years to 8 years have provided evidence that TNFi treatment over this longer duration may slow radiographic progression.[42–44] The data regarding whether NSAIDs have a disease-modifying effect on radiographic progression, either alone or in combination with TNFi, have been mixed.[45–47]

Available therapies for AS and nonradiographic axSpA have shown efficacy on the outcome measures of disease activity, physical function, spinal mobility, and health-related quality of life in RCTs.[48–55] The objective radiographic outcome of structural damage is associated with the outcomes of physical function and spinal mobility.[15,56,57] It is believed that spinal mobility may be determined independently by both reversible inflammation and irreversible structural damage.[57] In long-term extension trials with over 10-year follow-up, measures of physical function and spinal mobility remained stable despite radiographic progression; however, there was no control group in this study.[58]

Magnetic resonance imaging (MRI)-detected inflammation in the sacroiliac (SI) joints and spine may serve as a surrogate for the outcome of structural damage. Whether MRI-detected inflammation should be a target of therapy requires further study. A major hypothesis is that a window of opportunity exists and that radiographic progression can be halted if disease is treated early, particularly with biologic therapy.[59] Studies have shown that the formation of new syndesmophytes at vertebral corners is predicted by the presence of prior inflammatory lesions, in particular lesions of fat infiltration or metaplasia, at the same site.[59–62] Structural lesions (fat metaplasia and ankylosis) seen in the SI joints on MRI also have been found to be associated with future spinal radiographic progression.[63] Finally, MRI-detected inflammation in both the SI joints and the spine are associated with disease activity as measured by the ASDAS and the BASDAI.[64,65] In RA, treat-to-target RCTs specifically looking at whether a target of imaging remission was superior to usual care did not show a benefit.[66,67] Whether the same is true for axSpA remains to be shown.

Beyond the primary outcomes of structural damage, function, mobility, and quality of life, other important outcomes have been rarely addressed in RCTs. These include EAMs and sequelae of long-standing disease, such as cardiovascular disease (CVD) and osteoporosis. The pooled lifetime prevalence of common EAMs in a meta-analysis were uveitis, 26%; psoriasis, 9%; and inflammatory bowel disease, 7%.[68] EAMs have not been studied as secondary outcomes, apart from standard safety assessments, in RCTs. Individuals with axSpA have an increased risk of CVD as well as CVD-related mortality compared with general population comparators of the same age and sex,[69–71] and it is hypothesized that chronic systemic inflammation from axSpA disease activity may be contributing. Whether anti-inflammatory therapy attenuates the CVD risk in axSpA is unclear.[72–75] The pooled prevalence of osteoporosis was 12% to 34% and that of vertebral fractures 11% to 25% in a meta-analysis.[76] In a systematic literature review, Ashany and colleagues[77] found that TNFi in long-term extension trials of 2 years' to 4 years' duration, was associated increased bone mineral density in the hip and lumbar spine but not with a significant change in fracture risk. Outcomes like CVD and osteoporosis require a long duration of follow-up, so they are not easily assessed in RCTs, although may be assessed in prospective cohort studies. Such information would prove valuable for knowing the treatment effects on long-term complications of axSpA.

TREAT-TO-TARGET TRIALS IN RHEUMATOLOGY

In RA and PsA, the treat-to-target approach compared with standard care has been evaluated in key RCTs. In both trials, the intervention arm featured frequent visits with scheduled measurement of disease activity as well as a protocol of treatment titration, addition, or switching. These trials, and their key design characteristics and outcomes, are summarized in **Table 2**.

The Tight Control for Rheumatoid Arthritis (TICORA) study, published in 2004, was conducted in the United Kingdom and included patients with active RA and disease duration of less than 5 years.[9] Subjects were randomized to either intensive therapy, in which a disease activity score (DAS) was performed at each monthly visit, or a routine management arm, in which they were followed every 3 months without measurement of disease activity. The DAS included ESR, joint tenderness, swollen joint

Table 2
Treat-to-target randomized controlled trials in rheumatoid arthritis, psoriatic arthritis, and axial spondyloarthritis

	TICORA	TICOPA	TICOSPA
Study population	Active RA Disease duration <5 y	Active PsA Disease duration <24 mo	axSpA
Study sites	2 UK centers	8 UK centers	18 European sites in France, Belgium, and the Netherlands
Number randomized	111	206	160 anticipated
Duration of study	18 mo	48 wk	12 mo
Intervention group	Tight control, monitored by DAS every 4 wk	Tight control, monitored for MDA every 4 wk	Tight control, monitored for ASAS HI every 4 wk
Comparator group	Standard care, seen every 3 mo	Standard care, seen every 3 mo	Standard care
Treatment protocol for tight control group	Start with sulfasalazine monotherapy Gradually step up to combination DMARD therapy No biologic DMARDs	Start with methotrexate monotherapy Gradually step up with possibility of starting biologic DMARD (adalimumab)	Start with NSAID monotherapy Switch to biologic (TNFi) after 12–16 wk
Primary outcome	Mean decrease in DAS	Proportion with ACR20 response	ASAS HI, comparing follow-up to baseline
Secondary outcomes	EULAR remission ACR20, ACR50, and ACR50 responses Pain score by VAS Physician global assessment Health-related quality of life by HAQ and SF-12 Radiographic progression by van der Heijde-Sharp score Resource utilization analysis	ACR50 and ACR70 responses PASI75 response mNAPSI score BASDAI score Tender joint count, swollen joint count Leeds Dactylitis Index Maastricht Enthesitis Index, Leeds Enthesitis Index Pain score by VAS BASFI score Health-related quality of life by HAQ, PsAQoL, EQ-5D Radiographic progression by van der Heijde-Sharp score Cost-effectiveness analysis	ASDAS major improvement Clinically important improvement in BASDAI50 Change in ASDAS and BASDAI Change in NSAID score Health-related quality of life by WPAI, EQ-5D Resource utilization analysis

Abbreviations: EQ-5D, EuroQoL quality of life instrument; HAQ, health assessment questionnaire; mNAPSI, modified Nail Psoriasis Severity Index; PsAQoL, psoriatic arthritis quality of life; PASI75, psoriasis area severity index with improvement of 75% or greater; SF-12, Short Form 12; WPAI, Work Productivity and Activity Impairment.

count, and patient global assessment of disease activity. The intensive therapy arm followed a protocol in which patients started on sulfasalazine monotherapy and were gradually stepped up on combination disease-modifying antirheumatic drug (DMARD) therapy. Biologics were not used in this trial. The primary outcome of mean decrease in the DAS was significantly higher in the intensive therapy group versus the comparator at 18 months in an intent-to-treat analysis. Secondary outcome measures also were improved with intensive therapy, including health-related quality of life, disability, erosions, and radiographic progression. Adherence was high in this trial. Costs were lower in the intensive therapy group, although this did not reach statistical significance and did not assess subjects' productivity loss or time off work for visits. Although multiple RCTs have demonstrated the strength of a treat-to-target strategy in RA, subsequent studies show that the adoption of this strategy has lagged behind in multiple countries and settings.[78] Barriers include patient and provider adherence, limited access to care, and limited access to biologic medications.

The TICOPA study was also conducted in the United Kingdom, and included PsA patients with disease duration of less than 24 months.[31] Subjects were randomized to a tight control group, which was assessed monthly for MDA criteria, compared with a group receiving standard care assessed every 3 months. The tight control protocol started with methotrexate monotherapy, and, in contrast to TICORA, this did include the possibility of switching to TNFi. The primary finding was that tight control was associated with approximately twice the odds of American College of Rheumatology (ACR) 20 response (odds ratio [OR] 1.91; 95% CI, 1.03–3.55) compared with the standard care. Secondary outcomes, including the more stringent ACR50 and ACR70 response criteria, other measures of disease activity and function, and measures of health-related quality of life, also were significantly different favoring the tight control group. Radiographic progression was similar, however, at follow-up between the 2 groups, likely due to early disease in the study population, with low radiographic damage scores at baseline. Serious adverse events were more common in the tight control group. A cost-effectiveness analysis found that costs of the tight control strategy exceeded the threshold typically allowable by UK guidelines. Ultimately, the use of the treat-to-target strategy from TICOPA received only a conditionally recommendation in ACR treatment guidelines[79] and there are few data on adoption of this strategy in clinical practice.

There have been 2 treat-to-target trials of axSpA. STRIKE (NCT02897115) was a German RCT of axSpA patients meeting the ASAS criteria with symptom duration less than 5 years, who were randomized to treat-to-target versus standard of care. In the treat-to-target arm, they were assessed monthly and the protocol involved starting with an NSAID and escalating to adalimumab. The primary outcome was ASDAS inactive disease at 32 weeks. This trial was unfortunately terminated due to slow recruitment.

TICOSPA (NCT03043846) is a European randomized cluster trial of axSpA patients, comparing tight control with monthly assessments to usual care. The primary outcome is change in the ASAS HI over 1 year. Secondary outcome measures include ASDAS, BASDAI, quality of life, and resource utilization. Enrollment began in 2016 and results are expected in 2020.

TREAT TO TARGET IN SPONDYLOARTHRITIS MANAGEMENT GUIDELINES

In 2017, an international task force published revised recommendations regarding the use of treat to target in SpA .[12] Several recommendations were based on low-level evidence and expert opinion, including the primary recommendation that the target of

SpA management should be clinical remission/inactive disease, including the musculoskeletal disease and EAMs. LDA/MDA was considered allowable as an alternative target of treatment. The recommendations also encouraged consideration of comorbidities, patient factors and drug-related risks, and the results of laboratory or imaging tests in management decisions.

Updated axial SpA treatment guidelines were published by the ACR in collaboration with the Spondylitis Association of America, the Spondyloarthritis Research and Treatment Network in 2019.[80] These updated guidelines did not change the earlier (2015) recommendation to use a validated AS disease activity measure at a regular interval.[81] The 2019 updated guidelines, however, conditionally recommended against use of a treat-to-target strategy in axSpA using a target of ASDAS less than 1.3. The panel noted that a treat-to-target approach in axSpA was supported indirectly by the association of lower disease activity with lesser radiographic progression but lacked direct evidence. The panel cited the costs of a treat-to-target strategy, including the burden on patients and clinicians, as 1 cause for concern.

The most recent PsA treatment guidelines from ACR and the National Psoriasis Foundation (NPF) conditionally recommend use of a treat-to-target strategy for patients with active PsA.[79] The recommendation provided for clinicians to consider not using a treat-to-target strategy among patients for whom a greater burden of adverse events, higher treatment costs, or greater medication burden with tighter control would be a concern. The ACR/NPF guideline development process included a patient panel meeting, during which patients expressed concern for the potential costs of treat to target, including financial (eg, additional copayments) and productivity loss (eg, travel and appointment time).

Although not reviewed by the ACR/NPF panel, patient concerns about the burden of a treat-to-target strategy in PsA were confirmed by a cost-effectiveness analysis by O'Dwyer and colleagues.[82] This study of the PsA treat-to-target strategy from TICOPA from the perspective of the UK National Health System found that the costs of tight control relative to standard care were likely to exceed the threshold allowable by the NHS. The analysis did not incorporate indirect costs to patients, such as productivity loss; incorporating such costs likely would make tight control even less favorable due to its expense. Study investigators suggested that fewer rheumatologist visits would be one strategy to mitigate the costs of tight control.

To date, cost-effectiveness analyses of treat-to-target strategies in axSpA have not been possible, owing to the lack of primary data on the efficacy of such strategies. These remains an unmet need in axSpA.

FUTURE DIRECTIONS AND RESEARCH AGENDA

The goals of a treat-to-target strategy in axSpA require further consideration and evaluation. Existing axial SpA disease activity measures may be used within a treat-to-target framework, but data supporting their use are limited. The inclusion of clinically important disease features, beyond patient-reported outcomes and laboratory measures of inflammation, also should be considered in a treat-to-target approach. This includes discussion of whether imaging evidence of inflammation as well as disease activity in EAMs should be included as targets.

AxSpA researchers should continue to evaluate whether current therapeutic tools are sufficient to reach these targets. As the results of TICOSPA are awaited, which will provide data on whether or not a treat-to-target strategy is superior to standard of care in the management of axSpA, the following questions must be considered:

Is 1 protocol of therapy superior to another? How frequently should disease activity be assessed, and with which measures? If disease is active in 1 domain but not another, how should therapy be adjusted? and Can the costs of tight control and burden to patients be minimized? The most compelling treat-to-target strategies should be assessed in both observational data and with future treat-to-target strategy trials. The challenges to implementing an effective treat-to-target strategy and how to overcome barriers to optimize outcomes in axSpA additionally must be considered.

DISCLOSURE

Dr. J.W. Liew: National Institutes of Health (NIH) T32AR007108. Dr.M. Dubreuil: NIH AR069127 and the Spondylitis Association of America (Bruckel Early Career Investigator Award).

REFERENCES

1. Whelton P, Carey R, Aronow W, et al. 2017 ACC/AHA/AAPA/ABC/ACPM/AGS/APhA/ASH/ASPC/NMA/PCNA guideline for the prevention, detection, evaluation, and management of high blood pressure in adults. J Am Coll Cardiol 2018;71: e127–248.
2. Standards of medical care in diabetes 2019. Diabetes Care 2019;42(Supplement 1):S1–2.
3. Grundy SM, Stone NJ, Bailey AL, et al. 2018 AHA/ACC/AACVPR/AAPA/ABC/ACPM/ADA/AGS/APhA/ASPC/NLA/PCNA Guideline on the Management of Blood Cholesterol: A Report of the American College of Cardiology/American Heart Association Task Force on Clinical Practice Guidelines. J Am Coll Cardiol 2018;73: e285–350.
4. The ALLHAT Officers, Coordinators for the ALLHAT Collaborative Research Group. Major outcomes in high-risk hypertensive patients randomized to angiotensin-converting enzyme inhibitor or calcium channel blocker vs diuretic. JAMA 2002;288:2981–97.
5. Chew EY, Ambrosius WT, Davis MD, et al. Effects of medical therapies on retinopathy progression in type 2 diabetes. N Engl J Med 2010;363:233–44.
6. Ridker P, Danielson E, Fonseca F, et al. Rosuvastatin to prevent vascular events in men and women with elevated C-reactive protein. N Engl J Med 2008;359: 1543–54.
7. Khanna D, Fitzgerald JD, Khanna PP, et al. 2012 American college of rheumatology guidelines for management of gout. part 1: Systematic nonpharmacologic and pharmacologic therapeutic approaches to hyperuricemia. Arthritis Care Res (Hoboken) 2012;64:1431–46.
8. Smolen JS, Breedveld FC, Burmester GR, et al. Treating rheumatoid arthritis to target: 2014 update of the recommendations of an international task force. Ann Rheum Dis 2016;75:3–15.
9. Grigor C, Capell H, Stirling A, et al. Effect of a treatment strategy of tight control for rheumatoid arthritis (the TICORA study): a single-blind randomised controlled trial. Lancet 2004;364:263–9.
10. Breedveld FC, Han C, Bala M, et al. Association between baseline radiographic damage and improvement in physical function after treatment of patients with rheumatoid arthritis. Ann Rheum Dis 2005;64:52–5.
11. Smolen JS, Braun J, Dougados M, et al. Treating spondyloarthritis, including ankylosing spondylitis and psoriatic arthritis, to target: Recommendations of an international task force. Ann Rheum Dis 2014;73:6–16.

12. Smolen J, Schols M, Braun J, et al. Treating axial spondyloarthritis and peripheral spondyloarthritis, especially psoriatic arthritis, to target: 2017 update of recommendations by an international task force. Ann Rheum Dis 2018;77:3–17.

13. Coates LC, Moverley AR, McParland L, et al. Effect of tight control of inflammation in early psoriatic arthritis (TICOPA): A UK multicentre, open-label, randomised controlled trial. Lancet 2015;386:2489–98.

14. Garrett S, Jenkinson T, Kennedy LG, et al. A new approach to defining disease status in ankylosing spondylitis: the Bath Ankylosing Spondylitis Disease Activity Index. J Rheumatol 1994;21:2286–91.

15. Landewé R, Dougados M, Mielants H, et al. Physical function in ankylosing spondylitis is independently determined by both disease activity and radiographic damage of the spine. Ann Rheum Dis 2009;68:863–7.

16. Machado P, van der Heijde D. How to measure disease activity in axial spondyloarthritis? Curr Opin Rheumatol 2011;23:339–45.

17. Spoorenberg A, van Tubergen A, Landewé R, et al. Measuring disease activity in ankylosing spondylitis: Patient and physician have different perspectives. Rheumatology 2005;44:789–95.

18. Lukas C, Landewé R, Sieper J, et al. Development of an ASAS-endorsed disease activity score (ASDAS) in patients with ankylosing spondylitis. Ann Rheum Dis 2009;68:18–24.

19. van der Heijde D, Lie E, Kvien TK, et al. ASDAS, a highly discriminatory ASAS-endorsed disease activity score in patients with ankylosing spondylitis. Ann Rheum Dis 2009;68:1811–8.

20. Pedersen SJ, Sørensen IJ, Hermann KGA, et al. Responsiveness of the Ankylosing Spondylitis Disease Activity Score (ASDAS) and clinical and MRI measures of disease activity in a 1-year follow-up study of patients with axial spondyloarthritis treated with tumour necrosis factor α inhibitors. Ann Rheum Dis 2010;69:1065–71.

21. Anderson JJ, Baron G, van der Heijde D, et al. Ankylosing Spondylitis Assessment Group preliminary definition of short-term improvement in ankylosing spondylitis. Arthritis Rheum 2001;44:1876–86.

22. Kiltz U, van der Heijde D, Boonen A, et al. The ASAS health index (ASAS HI) - A new tool to assess the health status of patients with spondyloarthritis. Clin Exp Rheumatol 2014;32:S105–8.

23. Kiltz U, van der Heijde D, Boonen A, et al. Measurement properties of the ASAS Health Index: Results of a global study in patients with axial and peripheral spondyloarthritis. Ann Rheum Dis 2018;77:1311–7.

24. Baraliakos X, Berenbaum F, Favalli E, et al. Challenges and advances in targeting remission in axial spondyloarthritis. J Rheumatol 2018;45:153–7.

25. Wendling D, Prati C. Remission in axial spondyloarthritis: the ultimate treatment goal? Joint Bone Spine 2016;83:117–9.

26. Sieper J. How to define remission in ankylosing spondylitis? Ann Rheum Dis 2012;71(Suppl 2):i93–5.

27. Kirwan J, Heiberg T, Hewlett S, et al. Outcomes from the Patient Perspective Workshop at OMERACT 6. J Rheumatol 2003;30:868–72.

28. Saag KG. OMERACT 6 brings new perspectives to rheumatology measurement research. J Rheumatol 2003;30:639–41.

29. Wells GA, Boers M, Shea B, et al. Minimal disease activity for rheumatoid arthritis: a preliminary definition. J Rheumatol 2005;32:2016–24.

30. Coates LC, Fransen J, Helliwell PS. Defining minimal disease activity in psoriatic arthritis: a proposed objective target for treatment. Ann Rheum Dis 2010;69: 48–53.

31. Coates LC, Helliwell PS. Treat to target in psoriatic arthritis—evidence, target, research agenda. Curr Rheumatol Rep 2015;17:15–20.

32. Ramiro S, Sepriano A, De Lisboa UN, et al. Spinal radiographic progression in early axial spondyloarthritis: Five-year results from the DESIR cohort. Arthritis Care Res (Hoboken) 2018. https://doi.org/10.1002/acr.23796.

33. Ramiro S, Stolwijk C, Van Tubergen A, et al. Evolution of radiographic damage in ankylosing spondylitis: A 12 year prospective follow-up of the OASIS study. Ann Rheum Dis 2015;74:52–9.

34. Poddubnyy D, Haibel H, Listing J, et al. Baseline radiographic damage, elevated acute-phase reactant levels, and cigarette smoking status predict spinal radiographic progression in early axial spondylarthritis. Arthritis Rheum 2012;64: 1388–98.

35. Maas F, Arends S, Wink FR, et al. Ankylosing spondylitis patients at risk of poor radiographic outcome show diminishing spinal radiographic progression during long-term treatment with TNF-α inhibitors. PLoS One 2017;12:1–12.

36. van der Heijde D, Landewé R, Baraliakos X, et al. Radiographic findings following two years of infliximab therapy in patients with ankylosing spondylitis. Arthritis Rheum 2008;58:3063–70.

37. van der Heijde D, Salonen D, Weissman BN, et al. Assessment of radiographic progression in the spines of patients with ankylosing spondylitis treated with adalimumab for up to 2 years. Arthritis Res Ther 2009;11:1–8.

38. van der Heijde D, Breban M, Halter D, et al. Maintenance of improvement in spinal mobility, physical function and quality of life in patients with ankylosing spondylitis after 5 years in a clinical trial of adalimumab. Rheumatology 2015;54: 1210–9.

39. Braun J, Baraliakos X, Hermann KGA, et al. The effect of two golimumab doses on radiographic progression in ankylosing spondylitis: Results through 4 years of the GO-RAISE trial. Ann Rheum Dis 2014;73:1107–13.

40. van der Heijde D, Baraliakos X, Hermann KGA, et al. Limited radiographic progression and sustained reductions in MRI inflammation in patients with axial spondyloarthritis: 4-year imaging outcomes from the RAPID-axSpA phase III randomised trial. Ann Rheum Dis 2018;77:699–705.

41. Braun J, Baraliakos X, Deodhar A, et al. Secukinumab shows sustained efficacy and low structural progression in ankylosing spondylitis: 4-year results from the MEASURE 1 study. Rheumatology 2018;58(5):859–68.

42. Maas F, Arends S, Brouwer E, et al. Reduction in spinal radiographic progression in ankylosing spondylitis patients receiving prolonged treatment with tumor necrosis factor inhibitors. Arthritis Care Res (Hoboken) 2017;69:1011–9.

43. Molnar C, Scherer A, Baraliakos X, et al. TNF blockers inhibit spinal radiographic progression in ankylosing spondylitis by reducing disease activity: results from the Swiss Clinical Quality Management cohort. Ann Rheum Dis 2018;77:63–9.

44. Mease P, van der Heijde D, Karki C, et al. Tumor necrosis factor inhibition discontinuation in patients with ankylosing spondylitis: an observational study from the US-based Corrona Registry. Rheumatol Ther 2018;5:537–50.

45. Wanders A, van der Heijde D, Landewé R, et al. Nonsteroidal antiinflammatory drugs reduce radiographic progression in patients with ankylosing spondylitis: a randomized clinical trial. Arthritis Rheum 2005;52:1756–65.

46. Sieper J, Listing J, Poddubnyy D, et al. Effect of continuous versus on-demand treatment of ankylosing spondylitis with diclofenac over 2 years on radiographic progression of the spine: Results from a randomised multicentre trial (ENRADAS). Ann Rheum Dis 2016;75:1438–43.

47. Haroon N, Inman RD, Learch TJ, et al. The impact of tumor necrosis factor α inhibitors on radiographic progression in ankylosing spondylitis. Arthritis Rheum 2013;65:2645–54.

48. Davis JC, van der Heijde D, Braun J, et al. Recombinant human tumor necrosis factor receptor (etanercept) for treating ankylosing spondylitis. Arthritis Rheum 2003;48:3230–6.

49. van der Heijde D, Dijkmans B, Geusens P, et al. Efficacy and safety of infliximab in patients with ankylosing spondylitis: Results of a randomized, placebo-controlled trial (ASSERT). Arthritis Rheum 2005;52:582–91.

50. Sieper J, van der Heijde D, Dougados M, et al. Efficacy and safety of adalimumab in patients with non-radiographic axial spondyloarthritis: Results of a randomised placebo-controlled trial (ABILITY-1). Ann Rheum Dis 2013;72:815–22.

51. Landewé R, Braun J, Deodhar A, et al. Efficacy of certolizumab pegol on signs and symptoms of axial spondyloarthritis including ankylosing spondylitis: 24-week results of a double-blind randomised placebo-controlled Phase 3 study. Ann Rheum Dis 2014;73:39–47.

52. Inman RD, Davis JC, Van Der Heijde D, et al. Efficacy and safety of golimumab in patients with ankylosing spondylitis: Results of a randomized, double-blind, placebo-controlled, phase III trial. Arthritis Rheum 2008;58:3402–12.

53. Sieper J, van der Heijde D, Dougados M, et al. A randomized, double-blind, placebo-controlled, sixteen-week study of subcutaneous golimumab in patients with active nonradiographic axial spondyloarthritis. Arthritis Rheumatol 2015;67: 2702–12.

54. Maksymowych WP, Dougados M, van der Heijde D, et al. Clinical and MRI responses to etanercept in early non-radiographic axial spondyloarthritis: 48-week results from the EMBARK study. Ann Rheum Dis 2016;75:1328–35.

55. Baeten D, Sieper J, Braun J, et al. Secukinumab, an interleukin-17A inhibitor, in ankylosing spondylitis. N Engl J Med 2015;373:2534–48.

56. Wanders A, Landewé R, Dougados M, et al. Association between radiographic damage of the spine and spinal mobility for individual patients with ankylosing spondylitis: Can assessment of spinal mobility be a proxy for radiographic evaluation? Ann Rheum Dis 2005;64:988–94.

57. Machado P, Landewé R, Braun J, et al. Both structural damage and inflammation of the spine contribute to impairment of spinal mobility in patients with ankylosing spondylitis. Ann Rheum Dis 2010;69:1465–70.

58. Poddubnyy D, Fedorova A, Listing J, et al. Physical function and spinal mobility remain stable despite radiographic spinal progression in patients with ankylosing spondylitis treated with TNF-α inhibitors for up to 10 years. J Rheumatol 2016;43: 2142–8.

59. Maksymowych WP, Morency N, Conner-Spady B, et al. Suppression of inflammation and effects on new bone formation in ankylosing spondylitis: Evidence for a window of opportunity in disease modification. Ann Rheum Dis 2013;72:23–8.

60. van der Heijde D, Machado P, Braun J, et al. MRI inflammation at the vertebral unit only marginally predicts new syndesmophyte formation: a multilevel analysis in patients with ankylosing spondylitis. Ann Rheum Dis 2012;71:369–73.

61. Baraliakos X, Heldmann F, Callhoff J, et al. Which spinal lesions are associated with new bone formation in patients with ankylosing spondylitis treated with

anti-TNF agents? A long-term observational study using MRI and conventional radiography. Ann Rheum Dis 2014;73:1819–25.

62. Machado PM, Baraliakos X, van der Heijde D, et al. MRI vertebral corner inflammation followed by fat deposition is the strongest contributor to the development of new bone at the same vertebral corner: a multilevel longitudinal analysis in patients with ankylosing spondylitis. Ann Rheum Dis 2016;75:1486–93.

63. Maksymowych WP, Wichuk S, Chiowchanwisawakit P, et al. Fat metaplasia on MRI of the sacroiliac joints increases the propensity for disease progression in the spine of patients with spondyloarthritis. RMD Open 2017;3:23.

64. Machado P, Landewé RBM, Braun J, et al. MRI inflammation and its relation with measures of clinical disease activity and different treatment responses in patients with ankylosing spondylitis treated with a tumour necrosis factor inhibitor. Ann Rheum Dis 2012;71:2002–5.

65. Navarro-Compán V, Ramiro S, Landewé R, et al. Disease activity is longitudinally related to sacroiliac inflammation on MRI in male patients with axial spondyloarthritis:2-years of the DESIR cohort. Ann Rheum Dis 2016;75:874–8.

66. Haavardsholm EA, Aga AB, Olsen IC, et al. Ultrasound in management of rheumatoid arthritis: ARCTIC randomised controlled strategy trial. BMJ 2016; 354:i4205.

67. Dale J, Stirling A, Zhang R, et al. Targeting ultrasound remission in early rheumatoid arthritis: the results of the TaSER study, a randomised clinical trial. Ann Rheum Dis 2016;75:1043–50.

68. Stolwijk C, van Tubergen A, Castillo-Ortiz JD, et al. Prevalence of extra-articular manifestations in patients with ankylosing spondylitis: A systematic review and meta-analysis. Ann Rheum Dis 2015;74:65–73.

69. Bakland G, Gran JT, Nossent JC. Increased mortality in ankylosing spondylitis is related to disease activity. Ann Rheum Dis 2011;70:1921–5.

70. Haroon NN, Paterson JM, Li P, et al. Patients with ankylosing spondylitis have increased cardiovascular and cerebrovascular mortality: a population-based study. Ann Intern Med 2015;163:409–16.

71. Mathieu S, Soubrier M. Cardiovascular events in ankylosing spondylitis: a 2018 meta-analysis. Ann Rheum Dis 2019;78:e57.

72. Dubreuil M, Louie-Gao Q, Peloquin CE, et al. Risk of myocardial infarction with use of selected non-steroidal anti-inflammatory drugs in patients with spondyloarthritis and osteoarthritis. Ann Rheum Dis 2018;77:1137–42.

73. Lee J, Sinnathurai P, Buchbinder R, et al. Biologics and cardiovascular events in inflammatory arthritis: a prospective national cohort study. Arthritis Res Ther 2018;20:171.

74. Tsai WC, Ou TT, Yen JH, et al. Long-term frequent use of non-steroidal anti-inflammatory drugs might protect patients with ankylosing spondylitis from cardiovascular diseases: a nationwide case-control study. PLoS One 2015;10:1–13.

75. Kristensen LE, Jakobsen AK, Askling J, et al. Safety of etoricoxib, celecoxib, and nonselective nonsteroidal antiinflammatory drugs in ankylosing spondylitis and other spondyloarthritis patients: a swedish national population-based cohort study. Arthritis Care Res 2015;67:1137–49.

76. Ramírez J, Nieto-González JC, Curbelo Rodríguez R, et al. Prevalence and risk factors for osteoporosis and fractures in axial spondyloarthritis: a systematic review and meta-analysis. Semin Arthritis Rheum 2018;48:44–52.

77. Ashany D, Stein EM, Goto R, et al. The effect of TNF inhibition on bone density and fracture risk and of IL17 inhibition on radiographic progression and bone

density in patients with axial spondyloarthritis: A systematic literature review. Curr Rheumatol Rep 2019;21. https://doi.org/10.1007/s11926-019-0818-9.

78. van Vollenhoven R. Treat-to-target in rheumatoid arthritis — are we there yet? Nat Rev Rheumatol 2019;15:180–6.

79. Singh JA, Guyatt G, Ogdie A, et al. 2018 American College of Rheumatology/National Psoriasis Foundation guideline for the treatment of psoriatic arthritis. Arthritis Rheumatol 2019;71:5–32.

80. Ward MM, Deodhar A, Gensler LS, et al. 2019 update of the American College of Rheumatology/Spondylitis Association of America/Spondyloarthritis Research and Treatment Network Recommendations for the treatment of ankylosing spondylitis and nonradiographic axial spondyloarthritis. Arthritis Rheumatol 2019; 71(10):1–15.

81. Ward MM, Deodhar A, Akl EA, et al. American College of Rheumatology/Spondylitis Association of America/Spondyloarthritis Research and Treatment Network 2015 recommendations for the treatment of ankylosing spondylitis and nonradiographic axial spondylitis. Arthritis Rheumatol 2016;68:282–98.

82. O'Dwyer JL, Meads DM, Hulme CT, et al. Cost-effectiveness of tight control of inflammation in early psoriatic arthritis: economic analysis of a multicenter randomized controlled trial. Arthritis Care Res 2018;70:462–8.

The Future of Axial Spondyloathritis Treatment

Sinead Maguire, MB, BCh, BAO, LRCSI, MRCPI[a], Raj Sengupta, MD[b],
Finbar O'Shea, MB, BCh, BAO[a],*

KEYWORDS

- Spondyloarthritis • Axial spondyloarthritis • Therapy • Ankylosing spondylitis

KEY POINTS

- Secukinumab, an IL-17 inhibitor, is an effective therapy option for patients with axSpA and has been shown to be associated with decreased radiographic progression of disease.
- Ixekizumab and tofacitinib are approved for treating other forms of inflammatory arthritis and show promise in the treatment of axSpA
- New agents in trials inhibiting IL-17, IL-23, and JAK have shown improved outcomes in axSpA—further trials are needed.

INTRODUCTION

There have been significant developments in the availability of new therapeutic options in axial spondyloarthritis (axSpA) over the last number of years. Different recommendations have been published to reflect this changing landscape. In 2016, the Assessment of SpondyloArthritis International Society/European League Against Rheumatism (ASAS/EULAR) updated their management recommendations for patients with axSpA.[1] More recently, the American College of Rheumatology/Spondylitis Association of America/Spondyloarthritis Research and Treatment Network (ACR/SPARTAN) have updated their recommendations for the treatment of ankylosing spondylitis (AS) and nonradiographic axSpA.[2]

Recommendation 9 of the ASAS/EULAR recommendations confirms the use of an anti-tumor necrosis factor (TNF) agent for patients with persistent high disease activity despite conventional therapy. A similar recommendation is present in the ACR/SPARTAN guidelines.

The biggest change in the treatment landscape in the last few years has been the development of medications that work on an alternative pathway to the anti-TNF agents. Evidence now suggests that interleukin-17 (IL-17) plays a role as an

[a] Department of Rheumatology, St James' Hospital, Ushers Quay, Dublin D08 NHY1, Ireland;
[b] Royal National Hospital for Rheumatic Diseases, Royal United Hospitals, Combe Park, Bath BA1 3NG, UK
* Corresponding author.
E-mail address: FOShea@STJAMES.IE

Rheum Dis Clin N Am 46 (2020) 361–369
https://doi.org/10.1016/j.rdc.2020.01.014
0889-857X/20/© 2020 Elsevier Inc. All rights reserved.

rheumatic.theclinics.com

inflammatory mediator in AS. Since 2016, anti-IL-17 medications have also been included in the ASAS/EULAR recommendations for initial biologic therapy in the management of axSpA. Secukinumab is a recombinant, fully human monoclonal anti-human IL-17A antibody of the IgG1/kappa isotype. Secukinumab has been available for the treatment of axSpA patients for the last 3 years. A significant body of evidence exists for the benefit of secukinumab in axSpA across a series of trials—MEASURE 1 to 5 study program[3–6] (**Table 1**).

This series of studies now has 5-year data demonstrating efficacy of secukinumab in axSpA.[7] In addition, the MEASURE 1 study has shown a low rate of radiographic progression in this cohort. In fact, no radiographic progression (modified Stoke Ankylosing Spondylitis Spine Score change from baseline of <2 units) was seen in 79% of patients receiving secukinumab over 4 years.[8]

Recommendation 10 from the ASAS/EULAR Management guidelines suggest that if an anti-TNF therapy fails, switching to another anti-TNF or an anti-IL-17 agent should be considered. The authors go on to say that in patients with a primary nonresponse to the first anti-TNF agent it may be a more rational approach to switch to another class (specifically an anti-IL-17 agent).

NEW TO MARKET TREATMENTS

TNF blockers have been the cornerstone of treatment of axSpA over the last 2 decades. Aside from biological disease-modifying antirheumatic drugs (bDMARDs), new treatments in the form of small-molecule treatments (targeted synthetic DMARDs) are showing promise in this disease area. One of the first targeted synthetic DMARDs being assessed in axSpA is a Janus kinase (JAK) inhibitor—tofacitinib—which preferentially inhibits signaling via JAK 1 and 3. A preliminary phase II study showed 63% of patients receiving 5 mg bd of tofacitinib achieved an ASAS20 response compared with 40% of patients receiving placebo at 12 weeks[9] (**Table 2**). One hundred and sixty-four patients who had baseline MRI and week 12 follow-up MRI scans during this phase II study showed that 18% patients treated with tofacitinib 5 mg bd achieved MIC (minimal important change) for the Spondyloarthritis Research Consortium of Canada (SPARCC) sacroiliac joint and spine scores compared with 0% of patients receiving placebo. There was a trend for greater clinical improvements in the tofacitinib patients who achieved MIC SPARCC scores.[10] Although no treatment-related serious adverse events were identified in the phase II study, the Food and Drug Administration have recently issued a safety alert regarding an increased risk of pulmonary embolism with tofacitinib 10 mg bd in patients with rheumatoid arthritis.

Table 1
MEASURE 4 study outcomes

	Week	Placebo (%)	Secukinumab 150 mg (%)	P Value	Secukinumab 150 mg + Loading (%)	P Value
ASAS 20	4	39	53.8	.36	49.1	.36
	16	47	61.5	.05	59.5	.06
	52	—	72	—	71.7	—
	104	—	77.5	—	74	—
ASAS40	4	17.9	26.5	.36	29.3	.36
	16	28.2	35.9	.36	38.8	.19
	52	—	54.1	—	51.3	—
	104	—	58.9	—	51.9	—

Table 2
Comparative Assessment of SpondyloArthritis International Society outcomes in trials for tofacitinib and ixekizumab

Treatment		Placebo ASAS20 (%)	Tx Group ASAS20 (%)	Tx ASAS40 (%)	Placebo ASAS40 (%)	P Value
Tofacitinib						
van der Heijde et al,[9] 2017	2 mg bd	41–	52–	42.30–	20–	<.05
	5 mg bd	—	81–	46.20–	—	<.01
	10 mg bd	—	56–	38.50–	—	<.05
Ixekizumab						
COAST-V trial	q2 weeks	40–	69–	52–	18–	<.0001
	q4 weeks	—	64–	48–	—	<.001
COAST-W trial	q2 weeks	30–	50–	31–	13–	.003
	q4 weeks	—	48–	25	—	.017

Note these are not head to head trials. Tx, Treatment

There is a growing body of evidence suggesting that IL-17 is one of the key cytokines in the pathogenesis of axSpA.[11] As previously stated, secukinumab, a monoclonal antibody against IL-17A, has had market authorization for AS treatment since 2016. Phase III studies have shown good efficacy and are described elsewhere in this review. Ixekizumab, another monoclonal antibody against IL-17A, has approval for the treatment of psoriatic arthritis (PsA). Three phase III studies have assessed the efficacy of ixekizumab in axSpA. The COAST-V study assessed the efficacy of ixekizumab 80 mg every 2 or 4 weeks in patients with AS who were DMARD and TNF naive compared with adalimumab or placebo (see **Table 2**).[12] Fifty two percent of patients receiving 80 mg ixekizumab achieved an ASAS40 response compared with placebo. The COAST-W study specifically assessed the efficacy of ixekizumab 80 mg in patients who either failed or were intolerant to TNF blockers as first-line therapy. Thirty one percent of patients treated with ixekizumab 80 mg every 2 weeks exhibited an ASAS40 response at 16 weeks (**Fig. 1**). The COAST-X study is an ongoing phase III study assessing the efficacy of ixekizumab in bDMARD naive nr-axSpA.[13] Preliminary top line data have shown significant improvements in ASAS40 response in patients treated with ixekizumab at weeks 16 and 52 compared with placebo.

TREATMENTS IN TRIALS
Anti-Interleukin-17

Brodalumab
Brodalumab is a human monoclonal antibody against the IL-17 receptor A. It has previously been shown to be effective in the treatment of psoriasis leading to research in psoriatic arthritis. A phase II, randomized, double-blinded, placebo-controlled study was published in 2014 examined the efficacy and safety profile of brodalumab in psoriatic arthritis.[14] One hundred and sixty eight patients were randomized into 2 treatments arms (brodalumab 140 or 280 mg) and 1 placebo group. Patients were followed to week 12, with an open-label extension up to 5 years. Primary outcome was an ACR20 response at week 12 which was seen in 37% of patients in the 140 mg dose group and 39% ($P = .03$) in the 280 mg dose group ($P = .02$). Secondary outcomes were assessed in the extension period of the trial at week 24, showing ACR20 responses continued to increase and were highest in the 280 mg group than the 140 mg group (64% vs 51%). ACR50 and ACR70 response rates continued to improve through to week 52 in the 140 mg group.

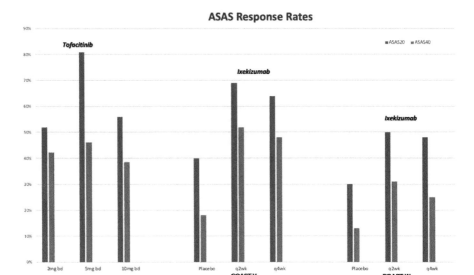

Fig. 1. Comparative ASAS outcomes in trials for tofacitinib and ixekizumab. Note these are not head-to-head trials.

Following this phase III trial, a multicenter, randomized, double-blinded, placebo-controlled study was commenced in axSpA.[15] A total of 159 patients was randomized into a placebo group or a group receiving brodalumab 210 mg and treated at weeks 1, 2, and then every 2 weeks up to week 16. Primary outcome was ASAS40 at week 16, which was found to be higher in the brodalumab group than the placebo group (43.8% vs 24.1%, $P = .018$). Change in the Bath Ankylosing Spondylitis Disease Activity Index (BASDAI) and Bath Ankylosing Spondylitis Functional Index (BASFI) scores were also noted in the treatment group, it is unknown if this was statistically significant. Adverse events rate was comparable between the 2 groups, and no suicidal attempts or ideation was noted during the trial period, which had previously been a concern during the drug's development for psoriasis.

Netakimab
Netakimab is a humanized monoclonal antibody targeting IL-17A. Results of a phase II, randomized, placebo-controlled trial was published out of Russia focusing on safety and pharmacokinetics in patients with active AS. Eighty-nine patients were randomized to receive 40, 80, or 120 mg of subcutaneous netakimab or placebo up to week 12. Rates of ASAS20 response in treatment groups (40/80/120 mg) were 73%, 82%, and 91% versus 43% in placebo group. No dose-dependent toxicity or serious adverse events were recorded.[16]

These results led to the development of the phase III, double-blinded, placebo-controlled, randomized ASTERA trial. This 16-week observational study evaluated the effect of netakimab on patient-reported outcomes in patients with radiographic axSpA up to 16 weeks. ASAS40 response rates at week 16 were superior in the netakimab group compared with the placebo group (40% vs 2.6%; $P<.0001$).[17] Results also demonstrated significant improvement in BASDAI, BASFI, Work Productivity and Activity Impairment response compared with placebo at week 16 ($P<.0001$).[18] Further analysis of the ASTERA patients focused on spinal and sacroiliac inflammation as seen on MRI at baseline and at week 16. Significant improvements with treatment in the Berlin spine score ($P<.0001$) and

SPARCC score (P<.01) were found in the netakimab group compared with the placebo group.[19] Plans for an extension trial to collect data up to 52 weeks are ongoing.

Bimekizumab

Bimekizumab is a monoclonal antibody targeting both IL-17A and IL-17F. Initially trialled in psoriasis, recent trials have been focusing on axSpA. A phase IIb, randomized, double-blind, placebo-controlled, dose-ranging study was done on 303 patients with active AS to assess efficacy and safety.[20] Primary outcome was an ASAS40 dose-response relationship at week 12, which was achieved (P<.01) in this study. Significantly more bimekizumab patients achieved ASAS40 at week 12 than placebo across all doses (P<.05). Patients in the treatment arm also had greater reductions in their BASDAI and AS Disease Activity Score (ASDAS) based on C-reactive protein than those in the placebo arm (P<.001). Similar rates of adverse events were noted in both groups.

Following on from this, a phase IIb, randomized, double-blind, placebo-controlled, dose-ranging study was carried out to assess the impact of bimekizumab on quality of life and patient-reported outcomes[21] in patients with active AS. This 48-week study included 303 patients with active AS randomized into treatment and placebo groups. BASDAI 50 at week 12 was achieved by 23.7% to 47.5% of patients in the treatment group versus 11.9% in the placebo group. All treatment dose groups also reported greater reductions in BASDAI, BASFI, Ankylosing Spondylitis Quality of Life Scale (ASQoL), and Patient's Global Assessment of Disease Activity compared with the placebo group at week 12. Rates of adverse events were similar in both groups.

Anti-Interleukin-23

Guselkumab

Guselkumab is an IgG1 monoclonal antibody that selectively binds to the p19 subunit of IL-23, resulting in inhibition of IL-23 signaling. Several phase III trials have demonstrated guselkumab's efficacy in psoriasis, leading to the development of trials in PsA of which there are currently results available for 2 phase II trials. The randomized phase II trial with guselkumab in PsA patients showed significant improvement in composite indices of disease activity at week 24 compared with placebo.[22] The other trial was a randomized, phase II, placebo-controlled trial, which showed a significant decrease of Routine Assessment of Patient Index Data 3 scores in the guselkumab group at week 24 compared with placebo.[23] Further pharmacodynamic studies have also demonstrated that treatment with guselkumab resulted in rapid reduction in IL-17A and IL-17F. IL-17F changes at weeks 4 and 16 were significantly associated with ACR20 responses at week 24, and IL-17A changes at week 4 and 16 were associated with PASI75 response at week 24 in the guselkumab group.

Tildrakizumab

Tildrakizumab is an IL-23 inhibitor with an anti-p19mAb blocking mechanism. This has been shown to be of therapeutic benefit in psoriasis, which has led to trials in both PsA and axSpA. Both studies are randomized, double-blinded, placebo-controlled phase IIa studies evaluating both efficacy and safety of tildrakizumab. The axSpA trial's primary outcome is to achieve a 40% improvement in a visual analogue scale score from baseline to 24 weeks with a secondary endpoint at 52 weeks.[24] Although the study is now completed, no results are currently available.

Janus Kinase Inhibitors

Filgotinib

Filgotinib is an oral selective JAK 1 inhibitor that has been theorized to have potential therapeutic benefits in many autoimmune conditions. TORTUGA was the first randomized, placebo-controlled, phase II study to examine the efficacy of filgotinib in patients with active radiographic AS.[25] This study recruited 116 adult patients with AS with an inadequate response or intolerance to nonsteroidal anti-inflammatory drugs. Patients were required to have active AS at the time of study commencement for inclusion. The treatment arm received filgotinib 200 mg once daily for a total of 12 weeks. The primary endpoint of change in ASDAS from baseline to week 12 was higher in the filgotinib group (−1.47) than in the placebo arm (−0.57) with a mean difference between groups of −0.87 ($P<.001$). In the filgotinib group (n = 58) versus placebo the following outcomes were achieved at week 12: ASAS20 = 76% versus 40%; ASAS40 = 38% versus 19%; ASAS partial remission 12% versus 3%. Significant improvements in ASQoL, BASDAI, BASFI, Bath Ankylosing Spondylitis Metrology Index (BASMI), SPARCC spine and sacroiliac joint scores were noted in the treatment group compared with the placebo group.

The EQUATOR trial was a randomized, double-blinded, placebo-controlled, phase II trial investigating the efficacy and safety profile of filgotinib in patients with active psoriatic arthritis.[26] Those recruited had previously failed or shown intolerance of at least 1 conventional DMARD before study commencement. The primary endpoint was ACR20 at week 16, which was reached by 80% of the treatment group and 33% of placebo group ($P<.001$). The filgotinib group also demonstrated significantly higher rates of achieving secondary outcomes compared with the placebo group: ACR50 = 48% versus 15%; ACR70 23% versus 6%. No significant difference was detected in rates of adverse events.

Upadacitinib
Upadacitinib is another selective JAK1 inhibitor that has shown efficacy in rheumatoid arthritis. At present there is a phase IIb/III randomized, double-blind, placebo-controlled trial ongoing.[27] This trial is evaluating both efficacy and safety profile in active radiographic axSpA with a primary endpoint of ASAS40 response at week 14. This trial is due to be completed in November 2020.

Unsuccessful Treatments in Axial Spondyloarthritis

Abatacept
Abatacept is a cytotoxic T-lymphocyte–associated antigen 4 immunoglobulin that has been shown to selectively modulate CD80 costimulatory signaling needed for full T-cell activation. A phase II, prospective, open-label study was carried out in patients with active AS.[28] The primary outcome of ASAS40 at week 24 was seen in 13% of anti-TNF-naive patients and no patients in the anti-TNF failure group, with ASAS20 achieved by only 27% and 20% in the respective groups. At week 24 no significant change was detected in BASDAI or ASDAS in either group.

Tocilizumab
Tocilizumab is a humanized monoclonal antibody that binds to IL-6 receptors. BUILDER-1 was a 2-part, phase II/III trial assessing tocilizumab in patients with AS naive to anti-TNF therapy.[29] Patients were randomized into tocilizumab 8 mg/kg or placebo for 12 weeks. ASAS20 response rates at week 12 were similar between treatment and placebo groups ($P = .28$), as was ASAS40 response rates ($P = .27$). The BUILDER-2 trial was planned to be a phase III study on patients with inadequate response to anti-TNF treatment, however this was terminated due to failure of BUILDER-1 to achieve its primary endpoint.

Apremilast
A phase II, double-blind, placebo-controlled, single-center study was carried out in patients with active radiographic axSpA treated with an oral phosphodiesterase

4 inhibitor, apremilast.[30] Patients in the treatment arm achieved higher improvements in BASDAI, BASFI, and BASMI scores at week 12; however, results were not statistically significant. The POSTURE trial was then commenced, which was a phase III, multicenter, randomized, double-blind, placebo-controlled, parallel group study evaluating apremilast in the treatment of active radiographic axSpA.[31] The treatment group failed to achieve a superior ASAS20 response rate at week 16 over placebo and the study was terminated.

Ustekinemab

This humanized monoclonal antibody against the p40 subunit of IL-12 and IL-23 was used in a proof-of-concept study in patients with active AS.[32] Sixty-five percent of patients treated achieved ASAS40 response at week 24, with 75% achieving ASAS20. Three trials of ustekinemab were developed to evaluate efficacy in axSpA.[33] Because of the failure of the first study to achieve its primary endpoint of ASAS40 response at week 24 in the treatment group, studies 2 and 3 were discontinued.

Risankizumab

Risankizumab is a humanized monoclonal antibody against the p19 subunit of IL-23. A phase II, randomized, double-blind, placebo-controlled study was commenced in active patients with AS.[34] Treatment groups did not demonstrate significantly higher proportions of ASAS40 response over placebo leading to trial discontinuation.

SUMMARY

Significant advances have been made in the treatment of axSpA. Improved understanding of the IL-17 pathway has led to the development many medications, including secukinumab, which has been shown to improve patient outcomes in addition to decreasing radiographic progression. Ongoing drug development is focused on the IL-17/IL-23 pathway and JAK inhibitors at present. As the evidence for these medications grow, treatment guidelines will eventually be adjusted to reflect the changing treatment options. This increased range of therapies provides clinicians with greater opportunity to treat axSpA as effectively as possible.

DISCLOSURE

The authors have nothing to disclose.

REFERENCES

1. van der Heijde D, Ramiro S, Landewé R, et al. 2016 update of the ASAS-EULAR management recommendations for axial spondyloarthritis. Ann Rheum Dis 2017; 76:978–91.
2. Ward MM, Deodhar A, Gensler LS, et al. 2019 Update of the American College of Rheumatology/Spondylitis Research and Treatment Network Recommendations for the treatment of Ankylosing Spondylitis and Nonradiographic Axial Spondyloarthritis. Arthritis Rheumatol 2019;71(10):1599–613.
3. Blair HA. Secukinumab: a review in ankylosing spondylitis. Drugs 2019;79(4): 433–43.
4. Marxo-Ortega H, Sieper J, Kivitz A, et al. Secukinumab provides sustained improvements in the signs and symptoms of active ankylosing spondylitis with high retention rate: 3 year results from the phase III trial; MEASURE 2. RMD Open 2017;3(2):e000592.

5. Pavelka K, Kivitz A, Dokoupilova E, et al. Efficacy, safety and tolerability of secu-kinumab in patients with active ankylosing spondylitis: a randomised, double-blind phase 3 study, MEASURE 3. Arthritis Res Ther 2017;19(1):285.

6. Kivitz A, Wagner U, Dokoupilova E, et al. Efficacy and safety of Seckinumab 150 mg with and without loading regimen in ankylosing spondylitis: 104 week results from MEASURE 4 study. Rheumatol Ther 2018;5(2):447–62.

7. Baraliakos X, Braun J, Deodhar A, et al. Long term efficacy and safety of secukinumab 150 mg in ankylosing spondylitis: 5 year results from the phase III MEASURE I extension study. RMD Open 2019;5(2):e001005.

8. Braun J, Baraliakos X, Deodhar A, et al. Secukinumab shows sustained efficacy and low structural progression in ankylosing spondylitis: 4 years results from the MEASURE 1 study. Rheumatology (Oxford) 2019;58(5):859–68.

9. van der Heijde D, Deodhar A, Wei JC, et al. Tofacitinib in patients with ankylosing spondylitis: a phase II, 16-week, randomised, placebo-controlled, dose-ranging study. Ann Rheum Dis 2017;76(8):1340–7.

10. Maksymowych W, van der Heijde D, Baraliakos X, et al. Tofacitinib is associated with attainment of the minimally important reduction in axial magnetic resonance imaging inflammation in ankylosing spondylitis patients. Rheumatology 2018;57:1390–9.

11. McGonagle D, McInnes I, Kirkham B, et al. The role of IL-17A in axial spondyloar-thritis and psoriatic arthritis: recent advances and controversies. Ann Rheum Dis 2019;1–12. https://doi.org/10.1136/annrheumdis-2019-215356.

12. van der Heijde D, Cheng-Chung W, Dougados M, et al. Ixekizumab, an interleukin-17A antagonist in the treatment of ankylosing spondylitis or radio-graphic axial spondyloarthritis in patients previously untreated with biological disease-modifying anti-rheumatic drugs (COAST-V): 16 week results of a phase 3 randomised, double-blind, active-controlled and placebo-controlled trial. Lancet 2018;392(10163):2441–51.

13. A study of Ixekizumab (LY2439821) in Participants with Non-Radiographic Axial Spondyloarthritis (COAST-X) (2019). Available at: www.Clinicaltrials.Gov/Ct2/Show/NCT02757352. Identification number NCT02757352. Accessed 31 Oct 2019.

14. Mease P, Genovese M, Greenwald M, et al. Brodalumab, an anti-IL1RA mono-clonal antibody, in psoriatic arthritis. N Engl J Med 2014;370(24):2295–306.

15. Wei JC, Kim TH, Kishimoto M, et al. Efficacy and safety of Brodalumab, an anti-interleukin-17 receptor A monoclonal antibody in patients with axial spondyloar-thritis: a 16-week results of a phase 3, multicentre, randomised, double blind, placebo-controlled study. Ann Rheum Dis 2019;78:195.

16. Erdes S, Nasonov E, Kunder E, et al. Primary efficacy of Netakimab, a novel interleukin-17 inhibitor, in the treatment of active ankylosing spondylitis in adults. Clin Exp Rheumatol 2020;38:27–34.

17. Gaydukova I, Mazurov V, Erdes S, et al. OP0232 Netakimab reduces the disease activity of radiographic axial spondyloarthritis. Results of the ASTERA study. Ann Rheum Dis 2019;78:193–4.

18. Gaydukova I, Mazurov V, Erdes S, et al. FRI0391 Netakimab improves patient related outcomes in patients with radiological axial spondyloarthritis: results from randomised phase 3 trial (ASTERA). Ann Rheum Dis 2019;78:880–1.

19. Smirnov A, Gaydukova I, Mazurov V, et al. FRI0412 spinal and sacroiliac joints inflammation in patients with radiographic axial spondyloarthritis treated with Ne-takimab—16 weeks results of multicentre, randomised, double blinded, placebo controlled, phase III ASTERA study. Ann Rheum Dis 2019;78:893–4.

20. Van der Heijde D, Gensler LS, Deodhar A, et al. Dual neutralisation of IL-17A and IL-17F with Bimekizumab in patients with active ankylosing spondylitis

(AS): 12-week results from a phase 2b, randomised, double-blind, placebo-controlled, dose-ranging study. Ann Rheum Dis 2018;77:70.

21. Van der Heijde D, Gensler LS, Deodhar A, et al. Dual neutralisation of IL-17A and IL-17F with bimekizumab was associated with improvements in patient reported and quality of life outcomes in patients with active ankylosing spondylitis: results from a phase 2B, randomized, double blind, placebo controlled, dose ranging study. Ann Rheum Dis 2019;78:193.

22. Helliwell P, Deodhar A, Gottlieb A, et al. Comparing composite measures of disease activity in psoriatic arthritis: results from a randomized phase 2 trial with guselkumab. Ann Rheum Dis 2019;78:1843.

23. Deodhar A, Kirkham L, Rahman P, et al. Assessment of disease activity using RAPID3 and evaluation of treatment effect of Guselkumab in patients with PsA: results from a randomized placebo-controlled phase 2 clinical trial. Ann Rheum Dis 2019;78:1838.

24. Efficacy and safety study of SUNPG1622(2019). Available at: https://clinicaltrials.gov/ct2/show/NCT02980705. Identification number NCT02980705. Accessed 31 Oct 2019.

25. van der Heijde D, Baraliakos X, Gensler L, et al. Efficacy and safety of filgotinib, a selective Janus kinase 1 inhibitor, in patients with active ankylosing spondylitis (TORTUGA): results from a randomised, placebo-controlled, phase 2 trial. Lancet 2018;392(10162):2378–87.

26. Mease P, Coates LC, Helliwell PS, et al. Efficacy and safety of filgotinib, a selective Janus kinase 1 inhibitor, in patients with active psoriatic arthritis (EQUATOR): results from a randomised, placebo-controlled, phase 2 trial. Lancet 2018;392:2367e77.

27. A Study Evaluating the Safety and Efficacy of Upadacitinib in Subjects with Active Ankylosing Spondylitis (SELECT Axis 1) (2019). Available at: https://clinicaltrials.gov/ct2/show/NCT03178487. Identification number NCT03178487. Accessed 31 Oct 2019.

28. Song IH, Heldmann F, Rudwaleit M, et al. Treatment of active ankylosing spondylitis with abatacept: an open-label, 24-week pilot study. Ann Rheum Dis 2011;70:1108e10.

29. Sieper J, Porter Brown B, Thompson L, et al. Assessment of short-term symptomatic efficacy of tocilizumab in ankylosing spondylitis: results of randomised, placebo-controlled trial. Ann Rheum Dis 2014;73(1):95.

30. Pathan E, Abraham S, Van Rossen E, et al. Efficacy and safety of apremilast, an oral phosphodiesterase 4 inhibitor, in ankylosing spondylitis. Ann Rheum Dis 2013;72(9):1475–80.

31. Celgene Corporation. Study of apremilast to treat subjects with active ankylosing spondylitis (POSTURE). Bethesda (MD): ClinicalTrials.gov National Library of Medicine; 2000. NLM Identifier: NCT01583374.

32. Poddubnyy D, Hermann KG, Callhoff J, et al. Ustekinumab for the treatment of patients with active ankylosing spondylitis: results of a 28-week, prospective, open-label, proof-of-concept study (TOPAS). Ann Rheum Dis 2014;73(5):817–23.

33. Deodhar A, Gensler LS, Sieper J, et al. Three multicenter, randomized, double-blind, placebo-controlled studies evaluating the efficacy and safety of ustekinumab in axial spondyloarthritis. Arthritis Rheumatol 2019;71(2):258–70.

34. Baeten D, Østergaard M, Wei JC, et al. Risankizumab, an IL-23 inhibitor, for ankylosing spondylitis: results of a randomised, double-blind, placebo-controlled, proof-of-concept, dose-finding phase 2 study. Ann Rheum Dis 2018;77:1295–302.

Axial Spondyloarthritis in the Era of Precision Medicine

Rianne E. van Bentum, MD, Irene E. van der Horst-Bruinsma, MD, PhD*

KEYWORDS

- Spondyloarthritis • Ankylosing spondylitis • Anterior uveitis
- Extra-articular manifestations

KEY POINTS

- In axial spondyloarthritis (axSpA), when a biologic is required, guidelines still recommend to initiate with a tumor necrosis factor-α inhibitor (TNFi), based on long-term experience.
- Extra-articular manifestations (EAMs), such as anterior uveitis, psoriasis, and inflammatory bowel disease (IBD), are common in axSpA
- TNFi generally have a beneficial effect on EAMs, although this might not apply to the effect of etanercept on uveitis or IBD.
- IL-17a are effective in psoriasis treatment, but evidence on uveitis or IBD is contradictory and limited.

AXIAL SPONDYLOARTHRITIS

Axial spondyloarthritis (axSpA) is a chronic inflammatory disease that predominantly manifests in the spine, but can also cause peripheral symptoms, such as enthesitis, peripheral arthritis, or dactylitis. axSpA is classified as radiographic axSpA, with radiographic signs of sacroiliitis, or nonradiographic axSpA, with presence of HLA-B27, clinical SpA characteristics, and/or inflammation of the sacroiliac joints at MRI.[1]

Aside from spinal and articular symptoms, many patients with axSpA suffer from extra-articular manifestations (EAMs), such as anterior uveitis (25%–30%), psoriasis (10%–25%), and inflammatory bowel disease (IBD; 5%–10%).[2–4] These EAMs are considered to be equally prevalent in radiographic and nonradiographic axSpA, although some evidence suggests anterior uveitis to be slightly more common in radiographic axSpA.[2] Treatment with nonsteroidal anti-inflammatory drugs (NSAIDs), disease-modifying antirheumatic drugs (DMARDs), and biologics may have different effects on these EAMs. This should be taken into account when choosing the right option for therapy. This paper first gives an overview of the current treatment recommendations in axSpA and subsequently describes the occurrence and treatment preferences in EAMs.

Department of Rheumatology, Amsterdam University Medical Centre - Location VU University Medical Centre, De Boelelaan 1117, Amsterdam 1081 HV, the Netherlands
* Corresponding author.
E-mail address: ie.vanderhorst@amsterdamumc.nl

Rheum Dis Clin N Am 46 (2020) 371–382
https://doi.org/10.1016/j.rdc.2020.01.013
0889-857X/20/© 2020 Elsevier Inc. All rights reserved.

TREATMENT IN AXIAL SPONDYLOARTHRITIS
Initiation of Treatment

The first step to treat axSpA includes physical therapy and maximum doses of NSAIDs. In addition, this phase includes counseling on the negative effects of smoking and overweight, and the importance of exercise. Patients can respond differently to the different NSAIDs, both regarding efficacy and side effects, although studies do not suggest the preference of one NSAID over another.[5] The use of NSAIDs is contraindicated in patients with IBD. Although the efficacy of DMARDs at the axial manifestations has been disappointing in axSpA, in case of prominent peripheral arthritis, or unavailability of biologics, sulfasalazine or methotrexate could be considered.[6]

If at least two different NSAIDs give an insufficient decrease in disease activity (persistent Ankylosing Spondylitis Disease Activity Score $\geq$2.1 or Bath Ankylosing Spondylitis Functional Index $\geq$4), after at least 3 to 6 months of treatment, the addition of a tumor necrosis factor-α inhibitor (TNFi) is indicated. Several randomized placebo-controlled trials have shown a substantial improvement in disease activity in 60% to 70% of patients for adalimumab, certolizumab, etanercept, golimumab, and infliximab.[7] More recently, interleukin (IL)-17a inhibitors (secukinumab and ixekizumab) have become available for the treatment of axSpA.[6,8] Although head-to-head trials are unavailable, indirect comparison of TNFi and IL-17a shows comparable results.[9] Both the 2016 ASAS-EULAR and 2019 American College of Rheumatology guidelines still recommend to initiate treatment with a TNFi, mostly based on long-term experience with these drugs.[6,10] However, in case of primary nonresponse to TNFi, the guidelines recommend to switch to an IL-17a inhibitor, rather than a second TNFi. Last, IL-23 blockers (eg, ustekinumab) are not effective in axSpA.[11] It is important to note that biologics have been mostly studied in radiographic axSpA, and to a lesser extent in the nonradiographic variant. Some studies suggest that the success rate of TNFi might be slightly lower in the latter, whereas studies on IL-17a inhibitors are still ongoing.

Treatment options for axSpA in general are regarded as safe, if the previously mentioned contraindications for NSAIDs are taken into account. However, concerning biologic agents, TNFi and IL-17a inhibitors induce an increased susceptibility to bacterial infections and could potentially reactivate latent tuberculosis.[12] Therefore, patients treated with biologics might require earlier antibiotic intervention in signs of an infection. In addition, TNFi might be associated with a slightly increased risk of (worsening of) demyelinating diseases or malignancy (mostly of the skin, or potentially lymphoma), although this is rare and evidence is still conflicting (e.g., lymphomas were mostly reported for patients with rheumatoid arthritis, where the disease itself is also associated with an increased risk of lymphoma).[13,14] However, these conditions are considered a relative contraindication to use a TNFi. The evidence on TNFi during pregnancy is limited, but current studies do not suggest an increased risk of adverse pregnancy outcomes. The EULAR recommendations report a safe use of infliximab and adalimumab in the first trimester, and etanercept up to the second trimester, whereas certolizumab can be used throughout the entire pregnancy.[15] The use of IL-17a inhibitors during pregnancy is discouraged because studies in humans are lacking.

Reduction of Treatment

It is still unclear how long TNFi should be continued once remission is achieved. Currently, international treatment guidelines recommend to taper the use of a TNFi in case of sustained low disease activity, to avoid unnecessary overtreatment.[10] A few, mostly small, studies have shown that it is possible to maintain a low disease activity when the use of the TNFi is tapered, wherein reduction of the dose shows better results than discontinuation.[16,17] A recent, noninferiority study has shown that reducing the dose of TNFi by one-third was not inferior to maintaining the standard dose.[18] However, aside from the latter, tapering has been studied limitedly in axSpA, with small patient numbers, mostly retrospective designs and with different tapering protocols.[17] Importantly, there is still a lack of a standardized tapering strategy regarding the best method (dose reduction versus extension of the dosing interval, either at once or gradually) and level of reduction (most studies described a 30%–50% reduction). From a practical point of view, extension of the dose interval would be preferred because it does not require changes of the commercially available injections and is more patient friendly. From both a cost-effective and patient-friendly perspective, in the future, ideally, every patient should receive just as much TNFi as necessary to achieve and maintain treatment effect. Therefore, some studies have evaluated the association between TNFi drug levels and treatment efficacy, attempting to define the optimal cutoff values for TNFi levels. However, although studies in other rheumatic diseases were hopeful, unfortunately in axSpA the evidence for using TNFi levels as a guidance during treatment is still contradictory.[19–21]

EXTRA-ARTICULAR MANIFESTATIONS IN AXIAL SPONDYLOARTHRITIS AND CHOICE OF TREATMENT
Acute Anterior Uveitis

Acute anterior uveitis (AAU) is an acute inflammation of the anterior part of the uvea, involving the iris, ciliary body, and anterior chamber of the eye. Anterior uveitis, just as axSpA, is strongly associated with the HLA-B27 gene, although HLA-B27-negative patients can develop AAU as well. In the general population, the lifetime cumulative incidence is 0.2%, and this is increased to 1.0% in HLA-B27-positive persons.[22] In axSpA, the estimated AAU flare rate is 15 per 100 patient years (TNFi-naive population), with a lifetime risk of approximately 30%, increasing with disease duration.[23,24] Importantly, AAU can be the first presenting symptom of axSpA. In fact, previous studies estimated a prevalence of no less than 40% to 50% of previously undetected axSpA in patients presenting with AAU.[25–28] Because early treatment of axSpA can enhance the prognosis, it is essential that ophthalmologists pay close attention to the presence of back complaints in patients with AAU.

AAU generally occurs in acute unilateral attacks (90%), and is recurrent in 50% of the patients, alternating between eyes. Patients suffer from severe ocular pain, redness of the eye, photophobia, and blurred vision. In up to 20% of the patients, AAU causes complications, such as posterior synechiae (resulting in an irregular pupil), cataract, or glaucoma.[29] AAU generally responds well to local treatment with corticosteroids and mydriatics, and only rarely additional treatment with periocular or oral corticosteroids is indicated. Timely treatment can reduce the risk of complications and if treated adequately, AAU normally resolves within 3 months. Therefore, in patients with axSpA with ocular complains, immediate referral to the ophthalmologist is recommended.

Because AAU has a good long-term prognosis, and flares respond well to local treatment, AAU is in most cases not an indication for preventive (chronic) treatment. However, AAU is invalidating and importantly influences the patient's quality of life. Therefore axSpA treatment should, preferably, also have beneficial effects on the occurrence of AAU.[30] Unfortunately, the first treatment step in axSpA, NSAIDs, are not effective in the treatment or prevention of AAU, although one recent study suggested that the addition of NSAIDs to TNFi treatment might be beneficial.[31] A limited number of retrospective studies suggest a beneficial effect of sulfasalazine and methotrexate in the prevention of HLA-B27-positive AAU.[32-34] However, methotrexate is not effective in the treatment of the axial manifestations of axSpA, and the influence of sulfasalazine is only limited. Therefore, these DMARDs are not part of the standard axSpA treatment.

Fortunately, TNFi, that are effective in the treatment of active axSpA are also effective in the prevention of AAU. Both infliximab and adalimumab have been widely proven to reduce the risk of an AAU flare and recent studies also show beneficial effects for golimumab and certolizumab.[24,35-39] In general, a 40% to 80% reduction in AAU flares per 100 patient-years is reported during TNFi treatment, compared with placebo or the pretreatment period.[24,35-40] Regarding adalimumab, a prospective study in patients with ankylosing spondylitis with a recent history of AAU, and a subanalysis of a multinational clinical study showed an AAU flare reduction of, respectively, 80% and 51% (and 68% in patients with a recent AAU history) during adalimumab.[36,37] Pooled data from several prospective studies in patients treated with infliximab showed a 79% reduction in AAU flares during treatment.[24] Also for certolizumab, a post hoc analysis of a placebo-controlled trial in axSpA suggested 70% fewer AAU flares during certolizumab, compared with placebo.[38] In addition, recently, a prospective study in patients with axSpA with a recent history of AAU has shown an 87% reduction in uveitis flares during 48 weeks of certolizumab treatment.[41] Last, a prospective study on the occurrence of AAU in patients with axSpA during golimumab reported an 80% decrease in AAU flares, compared with the period before TNFi treatment.[39] Studies on the fusion protein etanercept have been contradictory, with some studies suggesting that etanercept might increase the risk of AAU, instead of preventing it.[42,43] However, a comparison of three randomized studies with etanercept in radiographic axSpA still found a lower frequency of AAU flares in comparison with placebo.[44] Unfortunately, adequate comparison of studies remains a challenge because most trials assessed AAU as a secondary outcome and prospective studies mostly focused on one TNFi and had different designs. Nevertheless, a recent study of the Swedish biologic registry has showed a significantly higher AAU rate in etanercept, compared with adalimumab and infliximab (hazard ratio of 3.86 and 1.99, respectively), which suggests etanercept to be slightly less effective in the prevention of AAU, in comparison with other TNFi.[35] In summary, based on current evidence, AAU cannot be regarded a contraindication for the use of etanercept. However, in patients with highly recurrent AAU, a monoclonal antibody is preferred over etanercept.

Lastly, the IL-17a blocker secukinumab was not efficacious in the treatment of other forms of uveitis in three placebo-controlled phase 3 studies.[45] However, its influence on AAU in axSpA still has to be determined, which also applies to ixekizumab and the IL-23 inhibitor ustekinumab.

In conclusion, AAU is the most common EAM in axSpA. Collaboration with an ophthalmologist is important, to improve early recognition of axSpA and to optimize treatment of patients with axSpA with recurrent AAU. In most cases, AAU attacks respond well to local treatment by the ophthalmologist and in most cases there is no indication for preventative treatment of AAU alone. However, TNFi is successful in the reduction of AAU flares in axSpA, with most evidence for the efficacy of adalimumab, infliximab, certolizumab, and golimumab. Therefore, in patients with recurrent AAU and a high axSpA disease activity, requiring a TNFi, a monoclonal antibody is preferred over etanercept (**Table 1**).

Psoriasis

Psoriasis is a rather common skin disease, occurring in up to 11% of adults and resulting in several types of erythematous plaque lesions with silver scale and nail

Table 1
Efficacy of biologics on extra-articular manifestations in axial spondyloarthritis

		Axial SpA	Anterior Uveitis	Psoriasis	Ulcerative Colitis	Crohn Disease
TNF inhibitors	Infliximab	+	+	+	+	+
	Adalimumab	+	+	+	+	+
	Etanercept	+	±	+	-	-
	Golimumab	+	+	+	+	?[a]
	Certolizumab	+	+	+	?[a]	+
Anti-IL-23	Ustekinumab	-	?	+	?	+
Anti-IL-17	Secukinumab	+	-/?	+	-	-
	Ixekizumab	+	?	+	-	-

Abbreviations: +, beneficial effect; ±, uncertain effect; -, no or negative effect; ?, no data available.
[a] Not approved for this indication.

deformities.[46] Multiple Human Leukocyte Antigen types have been connected to the development of psoriasis, and 40% of patients have a first-degree family member with a psoriatic disorder.[47,48]

Approximately 14% to 20% of patients with psoriasis develop arthritis, which occurs more often in European and North and South American patients.[49] Five percent also suffer from axial symptoms, such as sacroiliitis, although the level of radiographic changes is considered to be less severe and more asymmetrical in psoriatic arthritis compared with radiographic axSpA.[50–52] Conversely, of the patients with axSpA (psoriatic arthritis excluded), 5% to 10% develop psoriasis.[2,3]

The skin manifestations of psoriasis generally respond well to topical corticosteroids or psoralen and ultraviolet A light therapy. In case of moderate to severe skin lesions, systemic therapy is indicated, such as methotrexate, apremilast, or biologic agents (TNFi, anti-IL-12/IL-23, anti-IL-17, and anti-IL-23/IL-39).[53,54] Peripheral joint involvement generally responds well to NSAIDs; intra-articular corticosteroid injections (a combination of); DMARDs (methotrexate, leflunomide); and, in case of insufficient response, to biologics.[55]

Contradictory, in patients treated with TNFi, psoriatic lesions of the skin can occur, such as an exacerbation of existing psoriasis, or a new onset of psoriasis, particularly palmoplantar pustulosis. This paradoxic reaction during treatment has been reported for several disease entities (SpA, psoriatic arthritis, rheumatoid arthritis, and juvenile idiopathic arthritis) and for different TNFi. For example, registry data of adalimumab trials in several rheumatic diseases showed an incidence rate of new onset or worsening of psoriasis in less than 0.1/100 patient years,[56] whereas other studies in SpA, Crohn disease (CD), and rheumatoid arthritis reported a prevalence of 1.5% to 6.4% (infliximab, adalimumab, certolizumab, etanercept).[47,57–62] Some studies reported an improvement after switching to another TNFi, whereas others found reoccurrence, suggesting a class effect.[58,61,63] Overall, in general TNFi is effective in the treatment of psoriasis, psoriatic arthritis, and axSpA. However, in patients developing new or worsening psoriasis after the initiation of TNFi, a potential paradoxic reaction should be considered (see **Table 1**).

Inflammatory Bowel Disease

IBDs, including ulcerative colitis (UC) and CD, are primarily treated by the gastroenterologist. Approximately 4% to 10% of patients with axSpA develop IBD, with a recent meta-analysis describing a pooled-prevalence of 4.1% in radiographic and 6.4% in nonradiographic axSpA.[2,3] This highest risk seems to be in the first years after axSpA diagnosis.[64] In addition, approximately 40% to 60% of the patients with SpA have asymptomatic microscopic gut inflammation (of whom two-thirds also have macroscopic lesions), according to ileocolonoscopy studies in patients with SpA without gastrointestinal symptoms.[65,66] One study identified a higher axSpA disease activity, male sex, and less spinal mobility to be associated with these gastrointestinal lesions.[65] Up to 6% to 7% of the patients with chronic gut inflammation develop CD.[67,68] Conversely, of the patients with IBD, up to 20% have asymptomatic sacroiliitis, and 40% suffer from clinical articular symptoms, such as inflammatory back pain, arthritis, and enthesopathy.[69,70] Of the patients with IBD, 10% to 15% and 30% eventually develop, respectively, axSpA and peripheral symptoms within 20 years after diagnosis.[71,72]

In patients with axSpA and IBD, it is recommended to discuss the treatment options with the gastroenterologist, because some axSpA treatments might be less effective for IBD. The use of NSAIDs should be minimized in this group, because NSAIDs can worsen bowel inflammation or increase the risk of IBD complications, although selective cyclooxygenase-2 inhibitors might be safe.[73,74] Although DMARDs are generally not effective in the treatment of axSpA, sulfasalazine has shown some positive effects, in particular on peripheral manifestations, and is also known to reduce inflammatory activity in IBD.[75]

In general, in patients with axSpA and IBD, TNFi are recommended over other biologics. In the treatment of IBD, infliximab, adalimumab, and certolizumab are approved for treatment of CD, whereas infliximab, adalimumab, and golimumab are indicated in UC.[6] Etanercept is not approved for IBD and studies show an increased risk of IBD exacerbations in patients treated with etanercept, compared with infliximab and adalimumab.[76,77] The IL-23 inhibitor ustekinumab has proven to be effective in the treatment of IBD, but is not effective in the treatment of axSpA symptoms.[11] Limited evidence on IL-17a inhibitors (secukinumab, ixekizumab) shows low efficacy on IBD, and suggests that the risk of an exacerbation or new-onset IBD might even be increased (although the pooled prevalence in an analysis of seven trials was still <1%) (see **Table 1**).[78,79] Although a direct comparison between TNFi and IL-17a-inhibitors was not performed, the ASAS-EULAR and American College of Rheumatology guidelines recommend the use of TNF inhibitors in patients with axSpA with IBD.[6,10]

SUMMARY

In axSpA, the first treatment step is an NSAID combined with physical exercises, and if insufficient, a biologic is added within 3 to 6 months. Currently, most experience is obtained with TNFi, all of which have approximately the same efficacy in the treatment of axSpA symptoms. In case of (primary) nonresponse to a TNFi, medication should be switched to preferably an IL-17a inhibitor (secukinumab and ixekizumab), or second TNFi. In patients who have achieved a sustained low disease activity, TNFi tapering is considered, where dose reduction is preferred over drug discontinuation. Unfortunately, standardized tapering schedules are lacking.

Many patients with axSpA suffer from EAMs (anterior uveitis, psoriasis, and IBD), of which uveitis (AAU) is the most common one. In patients with axSpA and EAMs, the effect of axSpA treatment on these EAMs should be taken into account when choosing the appropriate therapy. Overall, most TNFi are efficacious in treating the spinal and extra-articular symptoms, but some differences exist. Importantly, etanercept is contraindicated in case of IBD and seems to be less effective in preventing flares of AAU. In IBD the type of disease (CD or UC) requires different TNFi choices: certolizumab is approved for treatment of CD and golimumab for UC. Until now, IL-17a inhibitors are not recommended in patients with AAU or IBD. Psoriasis generally responds well to all biologics (TNFi, IL-17a inhibitors), but TNFi can induce a paradoxic skin reaction.

Overall, it is recommended that the treatment of axSpA should be individualized, based on the most prominent symptoms and presence of extra-articular and peripheral symptoms.[10]

CONFLICTS OF INTERESTS

The authors declare no conflicts of interest.

REFERENCES

1. Rudwaleit M, van der Heijde D, Landewe R, et al. The development of Assessment of SpondyloArthritis International Society classification criteria for axial spondyloarthritis (part II): validation and final selection. Ann Rheum Dis 2009; 68(6):777–83.
2. de Winter JJ, van Mens LJ, van der Heijde D, et al. Prevalence of peripheral and extra-articular disease in ankylosing spondylitis versus non-radiographic axial spondyloarthritis: a meta-analysis. Arthritis Res Ther 2016;18:196.
3. Stolwijk C, van Tubergen A, Castillo-Ortiz JD, et al. Prevalence of extra-articular manifestations in patients with ankylosing spondylitis: a systematic review and meta-analysis. Ann Rheum Dis 2015;74(1):65–73.
4. van der Horst-Bruinsma IE, Nurmohamed MT. Management and evaluation of extra-articular manifestations in spondyloarthritis. Ther Adv Musculoskelet Dis 2012;4(6):413–22.
5. Kroon FP, van der Burg LR, Ramiro S, et al. Non-steroidal anti-inflammatory drugs (NSAIDs) for axial spondyloarthritis (ankylosing spondylitis and non-radiographic axial spondyloarthritis). Cochrane Database Syst Rev 2015;(7):CD010952.
6. Ward MM, Deodhar A, Gensler LS, et al. 2019 update of the American College of Rheumatology/Spondylitis Association of America/Spondyloarthritis Research and Treatment Network recommendations for the treatment of ankylosing spondylitis and nonradiographic axial spondyloarthritis. Arthritis Care Res (Hoboken) 2019;71(10):1285–99.
7. Callhoff J, Sieper J, Weiss A, et al. Efficacy of TNFalpha blockers in patients with ankylosing spondylitis and non-radiographic axial spondyloarthritis: a meta-analysis. Ann Rheum Dis 2015;74(6):1241–8.
8. Deodhar A, Poddubnyy D, Pacheco-Tena C, et al. Efficacy and safety of ixekizumab in the treatment of radiographic axial spondyloarthritis: sixteen-week results from a phase III randomized, double-blind, placebo-controlled trial in patients with prior inadequate response to or intolerance of tumor necrosis factor inhibitors. Arthritis Rheumatol 2019;71(4):599–611.
9. Poddubnyy D, Sieper J. What is the best treatment target in axial spondyloarthritis: tumour necrosis factor alpha, interleukin 17, or both? Rheumatology (Oxford) 2017;57(7):1145–50.
10. van der Heijde D, Ramiro S, Landewe R, et al. 2016 update of the ASAS-EULAR management recommendations for axial spondyloarthritis. Ann Rheum Dis 2017; 76(6):978–91.

11. Deodhar A, Gensler LS, Sieper J, et al. Three multicenter, randomized, double-blind, placebo-controlled studies evaluating the efficacy and safety of ustekinumab in axial spondyloarthritis. Arthritis Rheumatol 2019;71(2):258–70.

12. Sepriano A, Regel A, van der Heijde D, et al. Efficacy and safety of biological and targeted-synthetic DMARDs: a systematic literature review informing the 2016 update of the ASAS/EULAR recommendations for the management of axial spondyloarthritis. RMD Open 2017;3(1):e000396.

13. Hellgren K, Dreyer L, Arkema EV, et al. Cancer risk in patients with spondyloarthritis treated with TNF inhibitors: a collaborative study from the ARTIS and DANBIO registers. Ann Rheum Dis 2017;76(1):105–11.

14. Cruz Fernandez-Espartero M, Perez-Zafrilla B, Naranjo A, et al. Demyelinating disease in patients treated with TNF antagonists in rheumatology: data from BIO-BADASER, a pharmacovigilance database, and a systematic review. Semin Arthritis Rheum 2011;41(3):524–33.

15. Gotestam Skorpen C, Hoeltzenbein M, Tincani A, et al. The EULAR points to consider for use of antirheumatic drugs before pregnancy, and during pregnancy and lactation. Ann Rheum Dis 2016;75(5):795–810.

16. Almirall M, Salman-Monte TC, Lisbona MP, et al. Dose reduction of biological treatment in patients with axial spondyloarthritis in clinical remission: Are there any differences between patients who relapsed and to those who remained in low disease activity? Rheumatol Int 2015;35(9):1565–8.

17. Navarro-Compan V, Plasencia-Rodriguez C, de Miguel E, et al. Anti-TNF discontinuation and tapering strategies in patients with axial spondyloarthritis: a systematic literature review. Rheumatology (Oxford) 2016;55(7):1188–94.

18. Gratacos J, Pontes C, Juanola X, et al. Non-inferiority of dose reduction versus standard dosing of TNF-inhibitors in axial spondyloarthritis. Arthritis Res Ther 2019;21(1):11.

19. Kneepkens EL, Krieckaert CL, van der Kleij D, et al. Lower etanercept levels are associated with high disease activity in ankylosing spondylitis patients at 24 weeks of follow-up. Ann Rheum Dis 2015;74(10):1825–9.

20. Kneepkens EL, Wei JC, Nurmohamed MT, et al. Immunogenicity, adalimumab levels and clinical response in ankylosing spondylitis patients during 24 weeks of follow-up. Ann Rheum Dis 2015;74(2):396–401.

21. Marsman AF, Kneepkens EL, Ruwaard J, et al. Search for a concentration-effect curve of adalimumab in ankylosing spondylitis patients. Scand J Rheumatol 2016;45(4):331–4.

22. Linssen A, Rothova A, Valkenburg HA, et al. The lifetime cumulative incidence of acute anterior uveitis in a normal population and its relation to ankylosing spondylitis and histocompatibility antigen HLA-B27. Invest Ophthalmol Vis Sci 1991;32(9):2568–78.

23. Frantz C, Portier A, Etcheto A, et al. Acute anterior uveitis in spondyloarthritis: a monocentric study of 301 patients. Clin Exp Rheumatol 2019;37(1):26–31.

24. Braun J, Baraliakos X, Listing J, et al. Decreased incidence of anterior uveitis in patients with ankylosing spondylitis treated with the anti-tumor necrosis factor agents infliximab and etanercept. Arthritis Rheum 2005;52(8):2447–51.

25. Haroon M, O'Rourke M, Ramasamy P, et al. A novel evidence-based detection of undiagnosed spondyloarthritis in patients presenting with acute anterior uveitis: the DUET (Dublin Uveitis Evaluation Tool). Ann Rheum Dis 2015;74(11):1990–5.

26. Juanola X, Loza Santamaria E, Cordero-Coma M, et al. Description and prevalence of spondyloarthritis in patients with anterior uveitis: the SENTINEL interdisciplinary collaborative project. Ophthalmology 2016;123(8):1632–6.

27. Monnet D, Breban M, Hudry C, et al. Ophthalmic findings and frequency of extra-ocular manifestations in patients with HLA-B27 uveitis: a study of 175 cases. Ophthalmology 2004;111(4):802–9.
28. Pato E, Banares A, Jover JA, et al. Undiagnosed spondyloarthropathy in patients presenting with anterior uveitis. J Rheumatol 2000;27(9):2198–202.
29. Gritz DC, Schwaber EJ, Wong IG. Complications of uveitis: the Northern California Epidemiology of Uveitis Study. Ocul Immunol Inflamm 2018;26(4):584–94.
30. O'Rourke M, Haroon M, Alfarasy S, et al. The effect of anterior uveitis and previously undiagnosed spondyloarthritis: results from the DUET cohort. J Rheumatol 2017;44(9):1347–54.
31. Kim MJ, Lee EE, Lee EY, et al. Preventive effect of tumor necrosis factor inhibitors versus nonsteroidal anti-inflammatory drugs on uveitis in patients with ankylosing spondylitis. Clin Rheumatol 2018;37(10):2763–70.
32. Munoz-Fernandez S, Garcia-Aparicio AM, Hidalgo MV, et al. Methotrexate: an option for preventing the recurrence of acute anterior uveitis. Eye (Lond). 2009; 23(5):1130–3.
33. Munoz-Fernandez S, Hidalgo V, Fernandez-Melon J, et al. Sulfasalazine reduces the number of flares of acute anterior uveitis over a one-year period. J Rheumatol 2003;30(6):1277–9.
34. Zu Hoerste MM, Walscheid K, Tappeiner C, et al. The effect of methotrexate and sulfasalazine on the course of HLA-B27-positive anterior uveitis: results from a retrospective cohort study. Graefes Arch Clin Exp Ophthalmol 2018;256(10): 1985–92.
35. Lie E, Lindstrom U, Zverkova-Sandstrom T, et al. Tumour necrosis factor inhibitor treatment and occurrence of anterior uveitis in ankylosing spondylitis: results from the Swedish biologics register. Ann Rheum Dis 2017;76(9):1515–21.
36. Rudwaleit M, Rodevand E, Holck P, et al. Adalimumab effectively reduces the rate of anterior uveitis flares in patients with active ankylosing spondylitis: results of a prospective open-label study. Ann Rheum Dis 2009;68(5):696–701.
37. van Denderen JC, Visman IM, Nurmohamed MT, et al. Adalimumab significantly reduces the recurrence rate of anterior uveitis in patients with ankylosing spondylitis. J Rheumatol 2014;41(9):1843–8.
38. Rudwaleit M, Rosenbaum JT, Landewe R, et al. Observed incidence of uveitis following certolizumab pegol treatment in patients with axial spondyloarthritis. Arthritis Care Res (Hoboken) 2016;68(6):838–44.
39. van Bentum RE, Heslinga SC, Nurmohamed MT, et al. Reduced occurrence rate of acute anterior uveitis in ankylosing spondylitis treated with golimumab: the GO-EASY study. J Rheumatol 2019;46(2):153–9.
40. Deodhar A, Gensler LS, Kay J, et al. A fifty-two-week, randomized, placebo-controlled trial of certolizumab pegol in nonradiographic axial spondyloarthritis. Arthritis Rheumatol 2019;71(7):1101–11.
41. van der Horst-Bruinsma IE, van Bentum R, Verbraak FD, et al. Reduction of anterior uveitis flares in patients with axial spondyloarthritis following 1 year of treatment with certolizumab pegol: 48-week interim results from a 96-week open-label study [abstract]. Arthritis Rheumatol 2019;71(suppl 10). Available at: https://acrabstracts.org/abstract/reduction-of-anterior-uveitis-flares-in-patients-with-axial-spondyloarthritis-following-1-year-of-treatment-with-certolizumab-pegol-48-week-interim-results-from-a-96-week-open-label-study/. Accessed December 9, 2019.
42. Lim LL, Fraunfelder FW, Rosenbaum JT. Do tumor necrosis factor inhibitors cause uveitis? A registry-based study. Arthritis Rheum 2007;56(10):3248–52.

43. Raffeiner B, Ometto F, Bernardi L, et al. Inefficacy or paradoxical effect? Uveitis in ankylosing spondylitis treated with etanercept. Case Rep Med 2014;2014: 471319.

44. Sieper J, Koenig A, Baumgartner S, et al. Analysis of uveitis rates across all etanercept ankylosing spondylitis clinical trials. Ann Rheum Dis 2010;69(1):226–9.

45. Dick AD, Tugal-Tutkun I, Foster S, et al. Secukinumab in the treatment of noninfectious uveitis: results of three randomized, controlled clinical trials. Ophthalmology 2013;120(4):777–87.

46. Michalek IM, Loring B, John SM. A systematic review of worldwide epidemiology of psoriasis. J Eur Acad Dermatol Venereol 2017;31(2):205–12.

47. Alenius GM, Jidell E, Nordmark L, et al. Disease manifestations and HLA antigens in psoriatic arthritis in northern Sweden. Clin Rheumatol 2002;21(5):357–62.

48. Gladman DD, Anhorn KA, Schachter RK, et al. HLA antigens in psoriatic arthritis. J Rheumatol 1986;13(3):586–92.

49. Alinaghi F, Calov M, Kristensen LE, et al. Prevalence of psoriatic arthritis in patients with psoriasis: a systematic review and meta-analysis of observational and clinical studies. J Am Acad Dermatol 2019;80(1):251–65.e19.

50. Jadon DR, Sengupta R, Nightingale A, et al. Axial Disease in Psoriatic Arthritis study: defining the clinical and radiographic phenotype of psoriatic spondyloarthritis. Ann Rheum Dis 2017;76(4):701–7.

51. Helliwell PS, Hickling P, Wright V. Do the radiological changes of classic ankylosing spondylitis differ from the changes found in the spondylitis associated with inflammatory bowel disease, psoriasis, and reactive arthritis? Ann Rheum Dis 1998;57(3):135–40.

52. Alenius GM, Stenberg B, Stenlund H, et al. Inflammatory joint manifestations are prevalent in psoriasis: prevalence study of joint and axial involvement in psoriatic patients, and evaluation of a psoriatic and arthritic questionnaire. J Rheumatol 2002;29(12):2577–82.

53. Nast A, Gisondi P, Ormerod AD, et al. European S3-Guidelines on the systemic treatment of psoriasis vulgaris: update 2015–short version–EDF in cooperation with EADV and IPC. J Eur Acad Dermatol Venereol 2015;29(12):2277–94.

54. Nast A, Spuls PI, van der Kraaij G, et al. European S3-Guideline on the systemic treatment of psoriasis vulgaris: update apremilast and secukinumab–EDF in cooperation with EADV and IPC. J Eur Acad Dermatol Venereol 2017;31(12): 1951–63.

55. Zhang AD, Kavanaugh A. Treat to target in psoriatic arthritis. Rheum Dis Clin North Am 2019;45(4):505–17.

56. Burmester GR, Panaccione R, Gordon KB, et al. Adalimumab: long-term safety in 23 458 patients from global clinical trials in rheumatoid arthritis, juvenile idiopathic arthritis, ankylosing spondylitis, psoriatic arthritis, psoriasis and Crohn's disease. Ann Rheum Dis 2013;72(4):517–24.

57. Baeten D, Kruithof E, Van den Bosch F, et al. Systematic safety follow up in a cohort of 107 patients with spondyloarthropathy treated with infliximab: a new perspective on the role of host defence in the pathogenesis of the disease? Ann Rheum Dis 2003;62(9):829–34.

58. Cullen G, Kroshinsky D, Cheifetz AS, et al. Psoriasis associated with anti-tumour necrosis factor therapy in inflammatory bowel disease: a new series and a review of 120 cases from the literature. Aliment Pharmacol Ther 2011;34(11–12): 1318–27.

59. Kary S, Worm M, Audring H, et al. New onset or exacerbation of psoriatic skin lesions in patients with definite rheumatoid arthritis receiving tumour necrosis factor alpha antagonists. Ann Rheum Dis 2006;65(3):405–7.

60. Rahier JF, Buche S, Peyrin-Biroulet L, et al. Severe skin lesions cause patients with inflammatory bowel disease to discontinue anti-tumor necrosis factor therapy. Clin Gastroenterol Hepatol 2010;8(12):1048–55.

61. Shelling ML, Vitiello M, Lanuti EL, et al. A case of palmoplantar pustulosis induced by certolizumab pegol: new anti-TNF-alpha demonstrates the same class effect. J Clin Aesthet Dermatol 2012;5(8):40–1.

62. Wendling D, Balblanc JC, Briancon D, et al. Onset or exacerbation of cutaneous psoriasis during TNFalpha antagonist therapy. Joint Bone Spine 2008;75(3): 315–8.

63. Afzali A, Wheat CL, Hu JK, et al. The association of psoriasiform rash with anti-tumor necrosis factor (anti-TNF) therapy in inflammatory bowel disease: a single academic center case series. J Crohns Colitis 2014;8(6):480–8.

64. Stolwijk C, Essers I, van Tubergen A, et al. The epidemiology of extra-articular manifestations in ankylosing spondylitis: a population-based matched cohort study. Ann Rheum Dis 2015;74(7):1373–8.

65. Van Praet L, Van den Bosch FE, Jacques P, et al. Microscopic gut inflammation in axial spondyloarthritis: a multiparametric predictive model. Ann Rheum Dis 2013; 72(3):414–7.

66. Leirisalo-Repo M, Turunen U, Stenman S, et al. High frequency of silent inflammatory bowel disease in spondyloarthropathy. Arthritis Rheum 1994;37(1):23–31.

67. Mielants H, Veys EM, Cuvelier C, et al. The evolution of spondyloarthropathies in relation to gut histology. III. Relation between gut and joint. J Rheumatol 1995; 22(12):2279–84.

68. De Vos M, Mielants H, Cuvelier C, et al. Long-term evolution of gut inflammation in patients with spondyloarthropathy. Gastroenterology 1996;110(6):1696–703.

69. de Vlam K, Mielants H, Cuvelier C, et al. Spondyloarthropathy is underestimated in inflammatory bowel disease: prevalence and HLA association. J Rheumatol 2000;27(12):2860–5.

70. Protzer U, Duchmann R, Hohler T, et al. [Enteropathic spondylarthritis in chronic inflammatory bowel diseases: prevalence, manifestation pattern and HLA association]. Med Klin (Munich) 1996;91(6):330–5.

71. Ossum AM, Palm O, Cvancarova M, et al. Peripheral arthritis in patients with long-term inflammatory bowel disease. Results from 20 years of follow-up in the IBSEN study. Scand J Gastroenterol 2018;53(10–11):1250–6.

72. Ossum AM, Palm O, Lunder AK, et al. Ankylosing spondylitis and axial spondyloarthritis in patients with long-term inflammatory bowel disease: results from 20 years of follow-up in the IBSEN Study. J Crohns Colitis 2018;12(1):96–104.

73. Kvasnovsky CL, Aujla U, Bjarnason I. Nonsteroidal anti-inflammatory drugs and exacerbations of inflammatory bowel disease. Scand J Gastroenterol 2015; 50(3):255–63.

74. Takeuchi K, Smale S, Premchand P, et al. Prevalence and mechanism of nonsteroidal anti-inflammatory drug-induced clinical relapse in patients with inflammatory bowel disease. Clin Gastroenterol Hepatol 2006;4(2):196–202.

75. Chen J, Liu C. Sulfasalazine for ankylosing spondylitis. Cochrane Database Syst Rev 2005;(2):CD004800.

76. Braun J, Baraliakos X, Listing J, et al. Differences in the incidence of flares or new onset of inflammatory bowel diseases in patients with ankylosing spondylitis

exposed to therapy with anti-tumor necrosis factor alpha agents. Arthritis Rheum 2007;57(4):639–47.

77. Chitul A, Voiosu AM, Marinescu M, et al. Different effects of anti-TNF-alpha biologic drugs on the small bowel macroscopic inflammation in patients with ankylosing spondylitis. Rom J Intern Med 2017;55(1):44–52.

78. Hueber W, Sands BE, Lewitzky S, et al. Secukinumab, a human anti-IL-17A monoclonal antibody, for moderate to severe Crohn's disease: unexpected results of a randomised, double-blind placebo-controlled trial. Gut 2012;61(12):1693–700.

79. Reich K, Leonardi C, Langley RG, et al. Inflammatory bowel disease among patients with psoriasis treated with ixekizumab: a presentation of adjudicated data from an integrated database of 7 randomized controlled and uncontrolled trials. J Am Acad Dermatol 2017;76(3):441–448 e2.

(Health-Related) Quality of Life as an Outcome in Studies of Axial Spondyloarthritis

Uta Kiltz, MD[a],*, David Kiefer, MD[a], Annelies Boonen, MD, PhD[b]

KEYWORDS

- Axial spondyloarthritis • Health-related quality of life • Functioning and health
- Contextual factors • Life satisfaction

KEY POINTS

- In axSpA, stiffness, pain, mobility limitations, fatigue, and sleep problems are the most prominent health concerns and restrictions that influence the life of patients.
- HRQoL or overall health measurement instruments integrate the broad range of health impairments that affect the daily life of patients in one (composite) measure.
- Health utilities are a specific type of HRQoL instruments that account for preferences of the different aspects of health included in the instruments.
- QoL is a much broader construct compared with overall health or HRQoL and links to happiness or satisfaction with life as a whole.
- Although a large amount of literature studied overall health/HRQoL among persons with axSpA, research on QoL is scarce.

INTRODUCTION

Because axial spondyloarthritis (axSpA) begins in early adulthood, impairments in various aspects of health accompany patients lifelong.[1–5] As a consequence of the different impairments and limitations, patients face restrictions in participation in diverse social roles.[6–8] For the purpose of clinical studies there is an interest to assess the direct consequences of the inflammatory process on specific body functions (eg, pain and stiffness, fatigue, movement functions) and body structures (structural changes in sacroiliac joints or spine), because this information can directly guide drug treatment. However, it is equally important to measure the broader range of impairments that can affect patients, and integrate these into

[a] Rheumazentrum Ruhrgebiet, Herne, Ruhr-University Bochum, Claudiusstr 45, Herne 44649, Germany; [b] Division of Rheumatology, Department of Internal Medicine, Maastricht University Medical Centre (MUMC+), Maastricht and Care and Public Health Research Institute (CAPHRI), Maastricht University, P. Debeyelaan 25, Maastricht 6229 HX, the Netherlands
* Corresponding author.
E-mail address: uta.kiltz@elisabethgruppe.de

Rheum Dis Clin N Am 46 (2020) 383–397
https://doi.org/10.1016/j.rdc.2020.01.017
0889-857X/20/© 2020 Elsevier Inc. All rights reserved.

one measure of overall functioning in daily life. Such tools help to evaluate the overall care provided to patients. Retrieved information can identify unrecognized needs and helps to complete and prioritize the overall management axSpA. To facilitate measurement of the overall impact of a disease on the life of persons, several measurement instruments have been developed. However, complex constructs, such as overall health, cannot be measured currently by objective approaches, and measurement instruments rely invariably on person-reported methods. Information on overall health is retrieved either by relying on a global, implicit assessment of health, or by using composite measures that approach the complex construct more explicitly by integrating its main defining aspects. Initially, measures to assess impact of disease on overall health were called health measurement instruments, but in the 1980s the term "health-related quality life (HRQoL) instruments" was introduced. This term might actually result in misconceptions or wrong expectations about what the available instruments actually measure, because HRQoL measures do not assess quality of life (QoL). Several definitions for QoL have been proposed, and they all point to the individual's perception of life as the core of this concept. Alternative terms related to QoL are "life satisfaction" or "happiness." The World Health Organization defines QoL as "a broad and multidimensional construct that reflects the individuals' perception of their position in life in the context of culture and value systems, and in relation to goals, expectations, standards and concerns." Although this construct is increasingly relevant at the population level, it is a too broad and ill understood construct to be operationalized in health care, where the focus is still on concerns related to medical conditions or health impairments. Because a large amount of evidence revealed that health impairments are the key determinant of a person's QoL, the construct HRQoL evolved in the 1980s.[9] It might be clear that both constructs (QoL and HRQoL/overall health) are distinguishable in two main aspects that are determinant for the development of measurement instruments. First, QoL and HRQoL (or overall health) differ in content. Although HRQoL/overall health focuses on aspects of health, such as seeing, hearing, pain, anxiety, moving around, and work-ability, QoL additionally refers to social well-being, material well-being, self-esteem, and self-determination. Second, the dimension of measurement varies. Although HRQoL is mainly operationalized by assessing the level of impairments and/or limitations (eg, amount of pain, amount of difficulty/ability to get up form a chair), QoL additionally concerns the level of satisfaction with the determining aspects. It is clear QoL is characterized by a higher level of appraisal related to the responder's personal and environmental context (**Table 1**).

In addition the health and HRQoL, alternative names for instruments that integrate the impairments into one health measure, have been proposed. Recently, the International Classification of Functioning, Disability and Health (ICF) proposed the term "functioning" to refer to the health impairments and limitations as a consequence of disease. Functioning was also chosen as the positive alternative for the older construct "disability." According to the ICF health is considered to reflect the experience of disease (functioning) when accounting for the role of contextual factors as facilitator or barriers on functioning and QoL is actually suggested by the ICF research branch to be a personal factor (appraisal). In the current overview, the term "overall health" is used in parallel to HRQoL, because the latter is commonly used. Notwithstanding, we hope to reinstitute the term "overall health" or propose the term "functioning" because these terms better reflects the content and aim of this group of measures. We also want to stimulate the discussion whether more research into true QoL is needed.

Table 1
Similarities and differences in content and dimension of measurement of overall health (or HRQoL) and QoL measurement instruments

	HRQoL (Functioning, Overall Health)	QoL (Life Satisfaction, Happiness)
Content of the construct	Physical health (pain, fatigue, daily activities) Mental health (anxiety, depressive symptoms) Participation (participation in social roles)	
		Material well-being Social-position Self-determination Self-worth
Dimension of measurement	Aimed to be objective (limited influence of personal appraisal and environmental context) Impaired, limited, restricted (difficulty/discomfort) Able to do/perform	Mixed objective and subjective (large influence of personal appraisal and environmental context)
		Satisfied/happy Able to be

FRAMEWORKS RELEVANT TO DEVELOP MEASURES FOR OVERALL HEALTH OR HEALTH-RELATED QUALITY OF LIFE

Health, Well-Being, and Quality of Life According to Patients with Axial Spondyloarthritis

A mixed qualitative-quantitative study investigated whether patients with axSpA (n = 68) consider health, well-being, and QoL to be different constructs and explored whether the view of patients differed from control subjects without SpA (n = 84).[10] Patients scored on all constructs significantly worse on a 0 to 10 numeric rating scale (10 best) compared with control subjects (mean, 6.1–6.3 vs 7.2–7.6; all $P<.01$). Within groups, no significant differences in scores between constructs were found. The quantitative part of the study revealed patients identified more themes related to health, and almost all patients associated health-related themes also with well-being and QoL, whereas this was more rarely the case for control subjects. Emotional functions were relevant to well-being for all participants. Social aspects, work-satisfaction, and financial situation were more frequently related to well-being and QoL by control subjects compared with patients (**Fig. 1**).[10]

Overall, the study indicated that for persons with and without health impairments health, well-being, and QoL are different but related constructs, and that for patient's health constitutes a stronger part of QoL than for individuals without SpA. In this study, well-being and QoL were explored as a separate construct, and findings suggested well-being was considered as an individual experience, whereas QoL related more strongly to social experiences. Of note, patient's fear of side effects contributed to well-being. Remarkably, such aspects as self-determination (being free) or

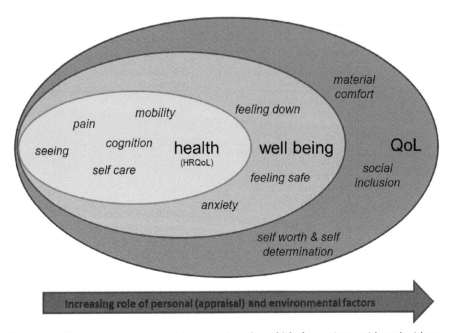

Fig. 1. Health is only a part of well-being and quality of life for patients with and without axSpA. *Data from* van Tubergen A, Gulpen A, Landewe R, et al. Are globals for health, well-being and quality of life interchangeable? A mixed methods study in ankylosing spondylitis patients and controls. Rheumatology (Oxford).2018;57(9):1555-1562.)

self-esteem (discrimination) were not brought forward, likely as a consequence of selection of participants in a country with high respect for human rights.

Which Aspects of Functioning and Health Are Important for Axial Spondyloarthritis

The interest to assess the impact of disease on a person's overall functioning and health emerged only in the second half of the twentieth century. The World Health Organization recognized the need for a model and information system to describe overall functioning and health. In 2001, the ICF was endorsed by the World Health Assembly as the universal framework and classification. The ICF framework adheres to the bio-psycho-social model of disease and recognizes that functioning and health results from a complex interplay of the functioning and disability components, body functions and body structures, and activities and participation, with contextual factors that consist of environmental and personal factors. In addition to the framework, the ICF also offers a universal and hierarchical classification of functioning by means of so-called categories that are seen as the units of health that are necessary to define and classify functioning (**Fig. 2**).[11]

The ICF classification comprises 1545 hierarchical structured categories divided over the previously mentioned ICF components (except for personal factors, for which no classification is as yet available). To make the ICF classification applicable in health care, ICF Core Sets have been developed for specific diseases or specific situations.[12] ICF Core Sets are selections of ICF categories that are necessary to describe the impact of the disease on functioning and health. Disease-specific Core Sets are developed following an elaborate standardized process that includes

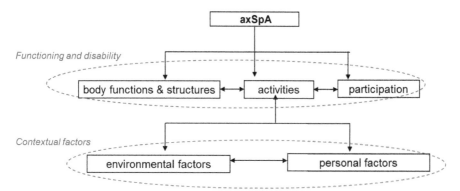

Fig. 2. The bio-psycho-social framework of health of the World Health Organization that is the basis for the International Classification of Functioning, Disability and Health. AS, ankylosing spondylitis. (*Adapted from* (WHO) WHO. The International Classification of Functioning Disability and Health. Vol https://apps.who.int/iris/bitstream/handle/10665/43737/9789241547321_eng.pdf;sequence=1. Geneva2001.)

the perspective of clinicians, health care professionals, researchers, and patients. Two types of Core Sets are distinguished: the Comprehensive ICF Core Sets, which represent the external reference of functioning and is used for research and in rehabilitation settings. The Brief ICF Core Sets are primarily intended for clinical studies. **Table 2** presents the categories (aspects of health) of the brief ICF Core Set for axSpA across the different components.

Because the ICF Core Sets provide information on what to measure, they constitute an evidence-based starting point to develop outcome measurement instruments for functioning and health. The first step toward how to measure is to develop a databank of items measuring each of the ICF health aspects (categories). Using items derived from such effort for axSpA in a best-worse scaling experiment, allowed to rank the aspect of health according to their importance (0%–100%) for patients with axSpA (n = 199).[13] It was shown (**Fig. 3**) that highest relative importance was assigned to pain (b280: 14.2%; 95% confidence interval [CI], 13.8–14.6), sleep (b134: 10.3%; 95% CI, 9.6–11.0), being exhausted (b130: 9.6%; 95% CI, 9.0–10.3), standing (d410: 9.25%; 95% CI, 8.5–10.0), and motivation to do anything that requires physical effort (b455 and d230: 8.7%; 95% CI, 8.1–9.3). Differences between subgroups (man and women; axSpA and peripheral SpA) and between countries were small or in aspects with lower importance. Such information might be worthwhile when deciding whether items should be weighted in a measurement instrument.

Measurement Properties of Person-Reported Measurement Instruments

Although it is essential for any measurement instrument that the content is based on sound theoretic frameworks and represents the perspectives of different stakeholders, the instrument also needs to have appropriate clinimetric measurement properties summarized as validity (truth), reliability and responsiveness (discrimination), and usability (feasibility). Truth captures issues of face, and content validity as described previously, but also construct validity, that is, concordance or discordance with external constructs that are hypothesized to be respectively related or unrelated to overall health of HRQoL. Situations of discrimination can be states at one time (for classification or prognosis) or states at different times (to measure change). Discrimination captures issues of reliability and sensitivity to change. Usability or feasibility refers to constraints of time, money, and interpretability of the instrument. These aspects may be decisive in determining a measure's success.[14] Although content (selection of type and number of items) is essential for validity and psychometric properties, also attribution (disease-specific or generic), answer scale, recall (eg, current or last 4 weeks), and whether or not items are weighted in the final score have a major influence on clinimetrics.

With regard to all measurement characteristics of self-reported instruments, it is important to emphasize they are developed for application in clinical studies. The large intraindividual variations and low ability to detect deterioration make them unsuitable for use with individual patients.

MEASURES OF FUNCTIONING AND HEALTH OR HEALTH-RELATED QUALITY OF LIFE APPLIED IN AXIAL SPONDYLOARTHRITIS

Generic and disease-specific questionnaires have been developed and used to assess possible limitations of overall functioning and health in patients with axSpA. Generic instruments most frequent applied in axSpA are the Short Form-36 (SF-36), the Short Form-12 (SF-12), and the EuroQoL (EQ) thermometer and EuroQoL five dimensions (EQ5D) utility index.[15,16] Disease-specific questionnaires are the Ankylosing Spondylitis Quality of Life (ASQoL) scale, the Assessment of Spondyloarthritis International Society Health Index (ASAS HI), and the ASAS utility index.[15–18] Health utilities are a special type of overall health of HRQoL instruments, because they weigh the value or preference persons have for the different aspects of health that constitute the composite health measure. Overall, generic instruments are less specific for

Table 2		
ICF categories included in the brief ICF core set for axSpA		
ICF Component	**ICF Code**	**ICF Category Title**
Body functions	b280	Sensation of pain
	b710	Mobility of joint functions
	b780	Sensations related to muscles and movement functions (stiffness)
	b130	Energy and drive functions
	b134	Sleep functions
	b152	Emotional functions
	b455	Exercise tolerance functions
Body structures	s760	Structure of trunk
	s740	Structures of the pelvic region
	s770	Additional structures of musculoskeletal system
	s750	Structure of lower extremity
Activities and participation	d230	Carrying out daily routine
	d410	Changing basic body position
	d450	Walking
	d845	Acquiring keeping and terminating a job
	d850	Remunerative employment
	d760	Family relationships
	d930	Recreation and leisure
	d475	Driving
Environmental factors	e110	Products or substances for personal consumption
	e3	Support and relationships

Data from Kiltz U, Essers I, Hiligsmann M, et al. Which aspects of health are most important forpatients with spondyloarthritis? A Best Worst Scaling based on the ASAS Health Index. Rheumatology (Oxford). 2016;55(10):1771-1776.

difficulties experienced by patients with a certain disease but they have the advantage that comparison between disease or with the general population is possible.[19,20]

Generic Instruments Used for Assessing Health-Related Quality of Life in Patients with Axial Spondyloarthritis

EuroQoL Visual Analogue Scale

The EuroQoL Visual Analog Scale (EQ-VAS) thermometer is a single self-reported global question asking respondents to rate current health on a VAS with end points labeled best imaging health (100) and worst imaging health (zero).[16] The EQ-VAS is part of the EuroQoL instrument that also includes the EQ5D health utility (see later). The EQ-VAS is likely underused and underinvestigated in axSpA. The instrument is easy to administer and provides a summary of overall health that is close to the patient's experience. The advantage of being implicit might be considered at the same time a disadvantage, because underlying factors driving the scores remain unclear. Although end-of-scale aversion is a known limitations of the VAS, the instrument is reliable and sensitive to change.

The Short Form-36 and Short Form-12

The SF-36 is a 36-item composite self-report measure designed as a short, generic assessment of health including physical functioning, physical and emotional roles, bodily pain, general health, vitality, social functioning, and mental health.[15] The domain summary scores range from 0 to 100 with higher scores indicating better levels of function and/or better health. The main components of SF-36 are subscores for physical (physical component score [PCS]) and mental health (mental component score [MCS]). The scale scores are calculated by summing responses across scale items and then transforming these raw scores to a 0 to 100 scale.[21] Recall period

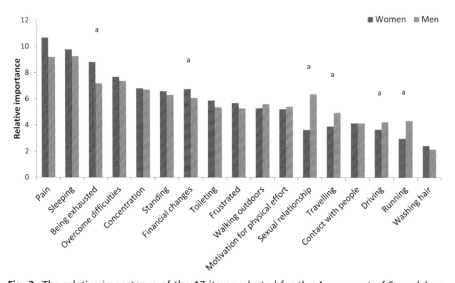

Fig. 3. The relative importance of the 17 items selected for the Assessment of Spondyloarthritis International Society Health Index as revealed in a best-worst scaling experiment separately for men and women. [a] Statistically significantly different. (*Adapted from* Kiltz U, Essers I, Hiligsmann M, et al. Which aspects of health are most important for patients with spondyloarthritis? A Best Worst Scaling based on the ASAS Health Index. *Rheumatology (Oxford)*. 2016;55(10):1771-1776.)

depends which form is being used (standard 4 week, acute form 1 week). The SF-36 has been used to capture health in the general population and a variety of diseases including rheumatologic diseases. The availability of standardized population scores facilitates comparisons between patients and healthy individuals and between diseases. Many studies consistently showed that in patients with axSpA the PCS and MCS are reduced when compared with the general population.[20,22,23] Scores for PCS of patients with axSpA have values between 30 and 50, and for MCS values are between 40 and 50.[20] Overall, the psychometric properties are good for the SF-36. However, its validity has been questioned because presence of severe floor and ceiling effects indicates that it does not capture the full range of health experiences in rheumatologic settings. In general, reliability is better for physical health (intraclass correlation coefficient (ICC) ≥ 0.70) compared with mental health (ICC 0.55).[21] Sensitivity to change for the MCS is low, not only in axSpA but also in other diseases, pointing to an instrument characteristic. According to the SF-36 manual a difference of five points on an SF-36 score is considered "clinically and socially relevant," whereas some trials use a greater than or equal to three-point increase in the SF-36 PCS for an individual patient as a minimal clinically important improvement.[22,24] The SF-12 is a shortened version that contains 12 of the original questions and from which a physical and mental component summary score can be calculated.[25] PCS-12 and MCS-12 were found to be highly correlated with their SF-36-derived counterparts (PCS, $r = 0.94$; MCS, $r = 0.96$), and produce remarkably similar results, in the community sample and across a variety of patient groups. A disadvantage in rheumatology is the absence of questions on vitality (fatigue). For this reason, researchers often add the three vitality questions to their survey.

Disease-Specific Instruments Used for Assessing Health-Related Quality of Life in Patients with Axial Spondyloarthritis

The Assessment of Spondyloarthritis International Society Health Index

The ASAS HI was developed to cover the entire spectrum of possible limitations of global functioning in patients with SpA.[17,26] The content of the ASAS HI was based in the ICF Core Set for axSpA and thus represents perspective of aspects of health typical and important according to patients, health care providers, and researchers. The ASAS HI contains 17 dichotomous items covering represented categories, such as pain, emotional function, sleep, sexual function, locomotion, independence, social life, and working life. The sum score of the ASAS HI is between 0 (good functioning) and 17 points (poor functioning). To differentiate between poor, moderate, and good functional ability, threshold values were determined (good functional ability, <5 points; poor functional ability, ≥ 12 points). An improvement of greater than or equal to three points (smallest detectable change) in an individual patient is considered to be larger than measurement error and thus points to true change.[17] The ASAS HI also includes a nine-item contextual factor set (environmental factors only) and is thus a true health measurement instrument as proposed by the ICF framework and terminology. Although the content validity was guaranteed in its development phase, the clinimetric role in measurement properties should still be evaluated.

The Ankylosing Spondylitis Quality of Life Scale

The ASQoL measures the impact of ankylosing spondylitis (AS) on HRQoL from the patient's perspective.[27] This self-reported questionnaire includes 18 items on domains, such as sleep, mood, motivation, coping, activities of daily living, independence, relationships, and social life.[28] The total score is the sum of the individual, dichotomous responses and ranges between 0 and 18, with higher scores reflecting greater impairment. The questionnaire has been demonstrated to be feasible, reliable, and to have content and convergent validity in patients with axSpA.[29] Content validity is high in this questionnaire because the measure was derived from patient interviews. Patients need between 2 and 16 minutes to complete the questionnaire and it takes less than 1 minute to score the results.[28] High level of reliability was observed for patients with AS (ICC >0.9).[30] The minimal clinically important difference was identified as a change of greater than or equal to three points for both directions, improvement and worsening.[31] However, usability might be interfered by a copyright license.

Health Utilities

Traditional composite health measurement instruments do not account in their scoring for the value persons attach to the different aspects of health included in the instruments. This is surprising, because it has been shown repeatedly that different items in a composite instrument are not equally important for overall health. In choice experiments, respondents are forced to indicate their preference for different health states (ie, combinations of aspects and level of impairments of health). Different preference elicitation methods (ie, choice experiments) are available, such as standard gamble and time trade-off, or more recently best-worse scaling or discrete choice experiments.[32–34] Health utilities are preference-based instruments and valuation approaches that anchor the value (preference) of health states on a 0 to 1 scale, in which zero corresponds to a state equivalent to death and 1 perfect health. Values lower than zero refers to states worse than health. This common scaling between 0 and 1 allows comparison of (changes in) health valuations between conditions. The preference experiments are performed using health states derived from existing health instruments (eg, SF-36 or EuroQoL) and the algorithms derived from the experiments can subsequently convert the scores on the original measures into a health utility index. This health-questionnaire based approach is called an indirect utility valuation. When health utility values are integrated over time (ie, years), quality-adjusted life-years are obtained, which represent the life impact of the disease on valued health. Quality-adjusted life-years are useful when rational choices have to be made by decision makers when allocating resource in health care and to research across different diseases or interventions (eg, in health economic evaluations).

For allocation of societal resources, it is considered appropriate to account for the societal perspective on health preference. Persons that do not suffer from major health problems are invited to value the health profiles of persons with impairments along the choice experiments. Notwithstanding, the patient perspective is increasingly accounted for, because patients know better what it means to live with health impairments.[35] On the same line, disease-specific health utilities are being developed.[36] These disease-specific utility valuation approaches are especially valuable when comparing effects of health preferences of interventions in specific diseases. For example, for patients with axSpA sleep and fatigue are relevant with regard to overall health. Notwithstanding, these aspects of health are not part of most generic health utility valuation approaches.

The generic EuroQoL five dimensions health utility index
The EQ5D provides societal preferences for health states (health utility) across five dimensions of health: (1) mobility, (2) self-care, (3) usual activities, (4) pain/discomfort, and (5) anxiety/depression.[16] Two versions with a difference in response options have been published: a three-level (no problems, some problems, and extreme problems) and five-level version (no problems, slight problems, moderate problems, severe problems, and extreme problems). Individual profiles created using the five

dimensions of the EQ5D are called the EQ5D Health State. Individual scores are converted, based on experiments within the general population, into a summary called the societal EQ5D Index. The EQ5D Index uses a utility-weighted scoring system that has been derived from extensive studies with different countries.[37] In studies, the EQ5D value is given for patents with axSpA with values between 0.6 and 0.8.[8] Overall, the psychometric properties are good for the EQ5D. Among patients with AS, floor effects in the five dimensions ranged from 10.4% (pain/discomfort) to 61.7% (self-care) and ceiling effects ranged from less than 1% (mobility) to 20.2% (pain).[38] Test-retest reliability for the EQ5D Index ranges from ICC of 0.64 to 0.78 for patients with rheumatoid arthritis (no specific values are available for patients with axSpA).[39] The EQ-VAS, by some considered to be a disease-specific and patient preference valuation because the VAS implicitly weighs all aspects of health into one score, is more responsive compared with the EQ5D.[38]

The axial spondyloarthritis–specific Assessment of Spondyloarthritis International Society utility index

Using the 17 health items of the ASAS HI, two consecutive preference experiments were performed among 3099 subjects without SpA to understand the relative importance of each of the 17 items, and rescale them on 0 to 1 utility scale.[40] The societal conversion algorithm indicated a health utility of −0.24 for worst SpA, and 0.88 for best health. The mean utility among 199 patients with SpA was 0.36 (standard deviation [SD], 0.30; range, −0.24 to 0.88) and discriminated well between patients having high or low Bath Ankylosing Spondylitis Disease Activity (BASDAI; ≥4, 0.18 [SD, 0.24] vs BASDAI <4, 0.51[SD, 0.27]; P<.01).

CORE OUTCOMES, CONTEXT, AND REFERENCE SHIFT IN RELATION TO OVERALL HEALTH OR HEALTH-RELATED QUALITY OF LIFE

One of the aims to measure overall health or HRQoL is to understand the relationships between several health outcomes in axSpA, because this helps to identify point of priority in research or care. Based on pretreatment data of 214 patients with AS, hierarchical associations between HRQoL assessed by the SF-36 physical and mental component, physical function (Bath Ankylosing Spondylitis Functional Index), clinical disease activity (BASDAI), spinal mobility (Bath Ankylosing Spondylitis Mobility Index), structural damage (modified Stoke Ankylosing Spondylitis Spinal Score), MRI inflammation, disease duration, age, gender, body mass index, and HLA-B27 were explored. The resulting model is visualized in **Fig. 4**. Physical function and disease activity were independently associated with the physical component of SF-36 and

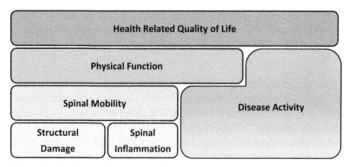

Fig. 4. The hierarchal relationship among key outcome measures in axSpA.

physical function also, but to a lesser extent, with the mental component of SF-36. Physical function was also independently associated with measures of spinal mobility and disease activity. Spinal mobility was an intermediate variable between structural damage and physical function.

Increasingly, contextual factors receive attention in outcome research. Contextual factors are factors that are not the outcome, but should be considered, because they are essential when interpreting the outcome or the effect of the intervention on the outcome. Contextual factors can distort, confound, or modify work outcomes. The ICF additionally states contextual factors do not belong to the functioning and disability component, and distinguishes personal and environmental factors. Limited research is available on the role of contextual factors in axSpA. One study examined the effect of gender among 216 patients with axSpA in the OASIS longitudinal study.[41] In multivariable analysis, male gender was significantly associated over time with a better ASQoL (B = -1.18; 95% CI, -2.17 to -0.20; P = .02), and in a separate model with a higher mSASSS over time (B = 8.24; 95% CI, 4.38 to 12.09; P<.01). Another study among 522 patients with axSpA from Canada and Australia explored the cross-sectional association between nationality, ethnicity, marital status, education, employment, and helplessness, adjusted for disease activity and physical function (BASDAI and Bath Ankylosing Spondylitis Functional Index) in relation to ASQoL and EQ5D. Contextual factors explained 37% and 47% of the variance in EQ5D and ASQoL.[8] Helplessness and employment were the most important contextual factors. When ASQoL was the outcome, employment had a positive effect on ASQoL among higher educated persons and helplessness had a negative impact on EQ5D among lower educated persons. It is surprising that no studies evaluated the role of side effect on QoL of patients. Specifically, it is not clear whether side effects are sufficiently represented in current measures to reflect the impact on patient's functioning and health. Another outstanding (research) question is which contextual factors are modifiable and could receive attention in clinical care. A special form of systematic bias (distortion/confounding) in outcome assessment is response shift. Response shift helps to explain the disconnect that can be observed when the disease worsens objectively over time, but patients report stable or even better outcome. Biologic response modification in response to stress has been advocated as a potential pathway, but also psychological reinterpretation of the impairments and limitations, called response shift, has been proven. In this psychological pathway, response shift can occur when patients reconceptualize the target construct, reprioritize the aspects within the construct, or redefine the standard of measurement (the maximum for optimal health is recalibrated). In axSpA adaptation or response shift has not been evaluated for overall health or HRQoL, but was studied for well-being (the Bath Ankylosing Spondylitis Global Assessment among 86 patients with axSpA that had been treated for on average 3.3 years with infliximab).[42] Patients re-evaluated (after 3.3. years) their well-being on a 0 to 10 numeric rating scale (10 very severe effect on well-being) when starting treatment with infliximab 3.3 years earlier using a retrospective assessment (the so-called "then-test"). Using the then-test, patients rated their overall well-being at the start of infliximab 7.2 (SD = 2.3), and the actual score at that time was 7.0 (SD = 1.6; P = .45). Time elapsed did not influence the then-test (P = .13) and there was also not influence of age, gender, or disease duration on the gap between initial and retrospective assessment. As patients remembered correctly the impact of axSpA on well-being, the then-test in this specific study setting could not prove evidence of adaptation or response shift in axSpA. It cannot be excluded that patients remembered how they well adapted and accounted for this in their retrospective score.

QUALITY OF LIFE IN AXIAL SPONDYLOARTHRITIS

The Bath Ankylosing Spondylitis Global Assessment was introduced by Jones in 1996 to measure the effect of axSpA on the respondents' well-being.[43] It consists of two items scored on a 0 to 10 VAS (10 very severe effects, the first estimating well-being over the last week, and the second over the last 6 months). Construct validity with other patient-reported outcomes was moderate to good (r = 0.40–0.74), test–retest reliability was good (r = 0.84 for 1 week; r = 0.93 for 6 months), and satisfactory sensitivity to change was reported (pre-post difference, -1.54 point; standardized error of mean, 0.31; P = .001).[43] The minimal clinically important difference from the patient's perspective has been reported as 15 mm or 27.5%, with a sensitivity of 0.61 and specificity of 0.74, determined using receiver operating characteristic curve analyses.

One study compared QoL between 246 patients with axSpA and 510 control subjects without axSpA using Satisfaction Work Life Scale (SWLS).[44] The SWLS was created in 1985 and addresses the individual's cognitive judgment of their satisfaction with their life as a whole across five dimensions (eg, the condition for my life are excellent, I'm satisfied with my life; If I could live my life over, I would change almost nothing).[45] Each statement is assigned scores from one to seven. The study aimed to test the hypotheses that participation in social roles participation contributes to life satisfaction. Patients with axSpA were more frequently (extremely) dissatisfied with life (17.9% vs 8.6%). Less physical difficulty or higher satisfaction with interpersonal relations and with leisure activities were associated with higher SWLS, and this was somewhat stronger in patients than in control subjects. In employed control subjects, but not in employed patients, satisfaction with work participation was independently associated with SWLS. Income was associated with SWLS only in control subjects. The study speculated that personal relationships and leisure activities, which are typically ignored when treating AS, might help to improve the reduced life satisfaction.

SUMMARY

QoL is essentially different from HRQoL. Although HRQoL refers to the various impairments and limitations that patients experience in daily life as a consequence of their health condition, QoL aims to evaluate the satisfaction with life as a whole. The term "overall health" measurement instruments would be a more evident and transparent term than HRQoL measurement instruments. Several self-reported instruments to assess overall health have been developed and validated for application in axSpA. The health utility measures mainly differ from other available multi-item measures for overall heath, by accounting for the importance individuals have for the various aspects of health (preference valuation). Head to head comparison of instruments is lacking, but given their individual validity, the choice for clinical studies should be based on content and feasibility in the specific study. Evidence confirms overall health in axSpA is hierarchically the resultant of disease activity, spinal mobility, and physical function, which are driven themselves by inflammation and radiographic damage characterizing etiopathology of axSpA. Limited evidence on the role of contextual factors points to the relevance of education and helplessness, a personality trait. A currently ongoing research project will answer the question whether and how a contextual factor item set needs to be taken into account when interpreting HRQoL outcomes.

Only few studies address QoL in axSpA and limited evidence indicates satisfaction with life is reduced when compared with the general population. This study pointed to the importance of relationships with family and friends for QoL of patients. More research into well-being and QoL is needed, followed by a discussion of what the role of health care is in relationship to improving the nonhealth component of QoL.

Current measures for overall health have been developed to assess outcome at the group level and the large intraindividual variations and low ability to detect deterioration preclude use in individual patients. In an era where self-reported health measurement instruments are increasingly used in clinical practice, validity of measurement at the individual level should receive more attention. Experience-based sampling,[46] computer-assisted testing, and individualized questionnaires[47] are promising instruments to serve this goal.

DISCLOSURE

Authors have nothing to disclose.

REFERENCES

1. Singh JA, Strand V. Spondyloarthritis is associated with poor function and physical health-related quality of life. J Rheumatol 2009;36(5):1012–20.
2. Packham J. Optimizing outcomes for ankylosing spondylitis and axial spondyloarthritis patients: a holistic approach to care. Rheumatology (Oxford) 2018; 57(suppl_6):vi29–34.
3. Kiltz U, van der Heijde D. Health-related quality of life in patients with rheumatoid arthritis and in patients with ankylosing spondylitis. Clin Exp Rheumatol 2009; 27(4 Suppl 55):S108–11.
4. Kiltz U, Baraliakos X, Karakostas P, et al. Do patients with non-radiographic axial spondylarthritis differ from patients with ankylosing spondylitis? Arthritis Care Res (Hoboken) 2012;64(9):1415–22.
5. Braun J, Sieper J. Ankylosing spondylitis. Lancet 2007;369(9570):1379–90.
6. Dagfinrud H, Mengshoel AM, Hagen KB, et al. Health status of patients with ankylosing spondylitis: a comparison with the general population. Ann Rheum Dis 2004;63(12):1605–10.
7. Ward MM. Health-related quality of life in ankylosing spondylitis: a survey of 175 patients. Arthritis Care Res 1999;12(4):247–55.
8. Gordeev VS, Maksymowych WP, Evers SM, et al. Role of contextual factors in health-related quality of life in ankylosing spondylitis. Ann Rheum Dis 2010; 69(1):108–12.
9. Guyatt GH, Feeny DH, Patrick DL. Measuring health-related quality of life. Ann Intern Med 1993;118(8):622–9.
10. van Tubergen A, Gulpen A, Landewe R, et al. Are globals for health, well-being and quality of life interchangeable? A mixed methods study in ankylosing spondylitis patients and controls. Rheumatology (Oxford) 2018;57(9):1555–62.
11. WHO. The International Classification of Functioning Disability and Health. Available at: https://www.who.int/classifications/icf/en/. Geneva2001. Accessed February 26, 2020.
12. Selb M, Escorpizo R, Kostanjsek N, et al. A guide on how to develop an International Classification of Functioning, Disability and Health Core Set. Eur J Phys Rehabil Med 2015;51(1):105–17.
13. Kiltz U, Essers I, Hiligsmann M, et al. Which aspects of health are most important for patients with spondyloarthritis? A best worst scaling based on the ASAS Health Index. Rheumatology (Oxford) 2016;55(10):1771–6.
14. Beaton DE, Maxwell LJ, Shea BJ, et al. Instrument selection using the OMERACT Filter 2.1: the OMERACT methodology. J Rheumatol 2019;46(8):1028–35.
15. Ware JE Jr, Sherbourne CD. The MOS 36-item short-form health survey (SF-36). I. Conceptual framework and item selection. Med Care 1992;30(6):473–83.

16. EuroQol Group. EuroQol–a new facility for the measurement of health-related quality of life. Health Policy 1990;16(3):199–208.

17. Kiltz U, van der Heijde D, Boonen A, et al. Measurement properties of the ASAS Health Index: results of a global study in patients with axial and peripheral spondyloarthritis. Ann Rheum Dis 2018;77(9):1311–7.

18. Kiltz U, van der Heijde D, Boonen A, et al. The ASAS Health Index (ASAS HI): a new tool to assess the health status of patients with spondyloarthritis. Clin Exp Rheumatol 2014;32(5 Suppl 85):S-105–108.

19. Weinstein MC, Torrance G, McGuire A. QALYs: the basics. Value Health 2009; 12(Suppl 1):S5–9.

20. Boonen A, Patel V, Traina S, et al. Rapid and sustained improvement in health-related quality of life and utility for 72 weeks in patients with ankylosing spondylitis receiving etanercept. J Rheumatol 2008;35(4):662–7.

21. Busija L, Pausenberger E, Haines TP, et al. Adult measures of general health and health-related quality of life: Medical Outcomes Study Short Form 36-Item (SF-36) and Short Form 12-Item (SF-12) Health Surveys, Nottingham Health Profile (NHP), Sickness Impact Profile (SIP), Medical Outcomes Study Short Form 6D (SF-6D), Health Utilities Index Mark 3 (HUI3), Quality of Well-Being Scale (QWB), and Assessment of Quality of Life (AQoL). Arthritis Care Res (Hoboken) 2011; 63(Suppl 11):S383–412.

22. Davis JC Jr, Revicki D, van der Heijde DM, et al. Health-related quality of life outcomes in patients with active ankylosing spondylitis treated with adalimumab: results from a randomized controlled study. Arthritis Rheum 2007;57(6):1050–7.

23. Braun J, McHugh N, Singh A, et al. Improvement in patient-reported outcomes for patients with ankylosing spondylitis treated with etanercept 50 mg once-weekly and 25 mg twice-weekly. Rheumatology (Oxford) 2007;46(6):999–1004.

24. Ware JE Jr, Kosinski M, Gandek B. SF-36 health survey. Manual and interpretation guide. Lincoln (RI): Quality Metric Inc; 2000.

25. Jenkinson C, Layte R. Development and testing of the UK SF-12 (short form health survey). J Health Serv Res Policy 1997;2(1):14–8.

26. Kiltz U, van der Heijde D, Boonen A, et al. Development of a health index in patients with ankylosing spondylitis (ASAS HI): final result of a global initiative based on the ICF guided by ASAS. Ann Rheum Dis 2015;74(5):830–5.

27. Doward LC, Spoorenberg A, Cook SA, et al. Development of the ASQoL: a quality of life instrument specific to ankylosing spondylitis. Ann Rheum Dis 2003; 62(1):20–6.

28. Zochling J. Measures of symptoms and disease status in ankylosing spondylitis: Ankylosing Spondylitis Disease Activity Score (ASDAS), Ankylosing Spondylitis Quality of Life Scale (ASQoL), Bath Ankylosing Spondylitis Disease Activity Index (BASDAI), Bath Ankylosing Spondylitis Functional Index (BASFI), Bath Ankylosing Spondylitis Global Score (BAS-G), Bath Ankylosing Spondylitis Metrology Index (BASMI), Dougados Functional Index (DFI), and Health Assessment Questionnaire for the Spondylarthropathies (HAQ-S). Arthritis Care Res (Hoboken) 2011;63(Suppl 11):S47–58.

29. Jenks K, Treharne GJ, Garcia J, et al. The ankylosing spondylitis quality of life questionnaire: validation in a New Zealand cohort. Int J Rheum Dis 2010;13(4): 361–6.

30. Haywood KL, M Garratt A, Jordan K, et al. Disease-specific, patient-assessed measures of health outcome in ankylosing spondylitis: reliability, validity and responsiveness. Rheumatology (Oxford) 2002;41(11):1295–302.

31. Richard N, Haroon N, Tomlinson GA, et al. Ankylosing spondylitis quality of life: defining minimal clinically important change. Ann Rheum Dis 2018;77(Suppl 2):645.

32. Bansback N, Harrison M, Brazier J, et al. Health state utility values: a description of their development and application for rheumatic diseases. Arthritis Rheum 2008;59(7):1018–26.

33. Bansback N, Brazier J, Tsuchiya A, et al. Using a discrete choice experiment to estimate health state utility values. J Health Econ 2012;31(1):306–18.

34. Porter ME. A strategy for health care reform: toward a value-based system. N Engl J Med 2009;361(2):109–12.

35. De Wit GA, Busschbach JJ, De Charro FT. Sensitivity and perspective in the valuation of health status: whose values count? Health Econ 2000;9(2):109–26.

36. Petrillo J, Cairns J. Converting condition-specific measures into preference-based outcomes for use in economic evaluation. Expert Rev Pharmacoecon Outcomes Res 2008;8(5):453–61.

37. Gignac MA, Cao X, McAlpine J, et al. Measures of disability: Arthritis Impact Measurement Scales 2 (AIMS2), Arthritis Impact Measurement Scales 2-Short Form (AIMS2-SF), The Organization for Economic Cooperation and Development (OECD) Long-Term Disability (LTD) Questionnaire, EQ-5D, World Health Organization Disability Assessment Schedule II (WHODASII), Late-Life Function and Disability Instrument (LLFDI), and Late-Life Function and Disability Instrument-Abbreviated Version (LLFDI-Abbreviated). Arthritis Care Res (Hoboken) 2011; 63(Suppl 11):S308–24.

38. Haywood KL, Garratt AM, Dziedzic K, et al. Generic measures of health-related quality of life in ankylosing spondylitis: reliability, validity and responsiveness. Rheumatology (Oxford) 2002;41(12):1380–7.

39. Hurst NP, Kind P, Ruta D, et al. Measuring health-related quality of life in rheumatoid arthritis: validity, responsiveness and reliability of EuroQol (EQ-5D). Br J Rheumatol 1997;36(5):551–9.

40. Essers I, Hiligsmann M, Kiltz U, et al. Development of one general and six country-specific algorithms to assess societal health utilities based on ASAS HI. RMD Open 2019;5(1):e000872.

41. Webers C, Essers I, Ramiro S, et al. Gender-attributable differences in outcome of ankylosing spondylitis: long-term results from the Outcome in Ankylosing Spondylitis International Study. Rheumatology (Oxford) 2016;55(3):419–28.

42. Essers I, van Tubergen A, Heldmann F, et al. Do patients with ankylosing spondylitis adapt to their disease? Evidence from a 'then-test' in patients treated with TNF inhibitors. RMD Open 2015;1(1):e000164.

43. Jones SD, Steiner A, Garrett SL, et al. The Bath Ankylosing Spondylitis Patient Global Score (BAS-G). Br J Rheumatol 1996;35(1):66–71.

44. van Genderen S, Plasqui G, van der Heijde D, et al. Social role participation and satisfaction with life: a study among patients with ankylosing spondylitis and population controls. Arthritis Care Res (Hoboken) 2018;70(4):600–7.

45. Diener E, Emmons RA, Larsen RJ, et al. The satisfaction with life scale. J Pers Assess 1985;49(1):71–5.

46. Vachon H, Rintala A, Viechtbauer W, et al. Data quality and feasibility of the Experience Sampling Method across the spectrum of severe psychiatric disorders: a protocol for a systematic review and meta-analysis. Syst Rev 2018;7(1):7.

47. Bacalao EJ, Greene GJ, Beaumont JL, et al. Standardizing and personalizing the treat to target (T2T) approach for rheumatoid arthritis using the Patient-Reported Outcomes Measurement Information System (PROMIS): baseline findings on patient-centered treatment priorities. Clin Rheumatol 2017;36(8):1729–36.

Patient's perspective

The Patient's Perspective on the Burden of Disease in Ankylosing Spondylitis

Lisa See, BA

KEYWORDS

- Ankylosing spondylitis • axSpA • Patient perspective • Nontraditional therapies
- Exercise

KEY POINTS

- A patient's 50-year perspective of living with ankylosing spondylitis.
- Traditional and nontraditional treatments of ankylosing spondylitis.
- Challenges to receiving a diagnosis of ankylosing spondylitis.
- Physical and emotional outcomes after receiving a diagnosis of ankylosing spondylitis.
- Importance of exercise for ankylosing spondylitis patients.

When Dr Michael Weisman asked me to contribute an essay for this collection, I was flattered, but I also reminded him that I am not a doctor and I have not done any medical research. He laughed, and said, "I know that!" He requested I write something personal about my experiences as an ankylosing spondylitis (AS) patient, and that is what I have tried to do. Going back over my 51 years with AS, I see that I have had a lot of adventures—some good, some bad, some funny, and a few creepy, depressing, scary, uplifting, and even inspiring. Nothing I write here is meant to be critical of the doctors or treatments I have had. Some doctors and treatments were better than others, though. I have hardly been perfect, either. As an AS patient, I have at times been dubious, gullible, optimistic, sad, scared, and stubborn.

I was 13 when I first started having back problems. My family lived in Topanga Canyon, California. My mom was a bit of a hippie. Taking me to what she called a regular doctor was not her cup of tea, so she took me to visit what would be the first of many chiropractors. The adjustments gave me some relief but not enough. I still woke up nearly every night with my lower back in spasms. I was stiff. I may have been moderately athletic in elementary school—I was a fast runner and I was not bad at playing first base—but these things hurt my body too much now that I was in junior high. Complaining did not get me anywhere. My mother was a magical thinker.

15332 Antioch St. #67 Pacific Palisades, CA 90272
E-mail address: LSee@LisaSee.com
Twitter: @Lisa_See (L.S.)

Rheum Dis Clin N Am 46 (2020) 399–405
https://doi.org/10.1016/j.rdc.2020.01.012
rheumatic.theclinics.com
0889-857X/20/© 2020 Elsevier Inc. All rights reserved.

If I had a sore throat, it was because I was swallowing my emotions and therefore my words. If my back hurt, it was because I did not want to bear the weight of my responsibilities, like taking out the trash or doing my homework.

There came a day when my mom realized that my visits to the chiropractor were not helping me all that much, whereas at the same time I was not getting any closer to what she saw as the deeper emotional source of my physical issues. She broke down and took me to a regular doctor. The pediatrician bent me this way and that. Although I was only 13, I could no longer touch my toes. Once the examination was done, the doctor announced with something like awe, "You have the back of a 90-year-old man" ("man," not even a woman), This was followed by, "You will never be able to bear children." The doctor gave me a list of don'ts: Don't go horseback riding. Don't jog or run. Don't do any sports that would have a jarring impact on my spine. I was not prescribed painkillers, which was a good thing, but I also was not prescribed any other type of medication or physical therapy. This was 1968. Was he unable to make a diagnosis because he was not accustomed to seeing arthritic diseases in his pediatric practice, because I was a girl (when the common wisdom at the time was that AS was a man's disease), or because my mom seemed so flakey, and, by extension, I must have been flakey too? I do not know. What I do know is that the source of my problems remained a mystery, and my prognosis seemed, even at that age, rather grim.

Spring ahead to 1974. I was 19, going to college but living at home. I had gotten stiffer, and I continued to wake up in the middle of the night with my lower back muscles in spasms. We lived in an old, funky, 2-story cabin. To get from my bedroom to the main part of the house, I had to walk outside. One morning I awoke in terrible pain. I hobbled outside, wound my way upstairs, entered the house, and fainted on the kitchen floor. The pediatrician, whom I was still seeing, announced that I had lumbago and sciatica. He said I should stay in bed, which I did for the next 6 weeks. I lay on my back with my legs propped up on pillows. Not moving, I now know, was the worst thing I could have done.

My mother was desperate. She became convinced I would spend the rest of my life as an invalid. (There was a part of me—still a teenager, remember—that was rather enchanted by the idea, thinking of all the invalids in literature: Camille, Clara in *Heidi*, Pollyanna, Beth in *Little Women*, and Colin in *The Secret Garden*.) My mother may have been flighty in some ways, but she also has a PhD, was a single mother supporting my sister and me through her writing and teaching as an English professor, and was a woman who never gave up through all the hardships in her life, of which there were many. She wrangled every person she could think of to see what, if any, treatments might help me. I was caravanned down to Orange County to have electromagnetic field therapy. I was driven out to the desert to soak in hot springs and mud baths to draw out toxins. I was taken to a new set of chiropractors. Some crystals may have passed over me once or twice. I returned to my pediatrician, who only repeated what he had said years before—that I would never be able to bear children. This time he added that I would never be able to walk without a limp. Bottom line: nothing helped. I was flat on my back in bed, hopeless.

One night while out to dinner, my mother overheard a couple at the next table talking about an acupuncturist—recently arrived in the United States—who was introducing the ancient technique at a local university medical school and secretly giving treatments at his home. (This was still 1974. In 1976, California became the eighth state to license acupuncture.) My mom leaned over and asked how to reach this Chinese doctor, whom I will call Dr Yee. The diner outlined an elaborate system of calling a number, letting it ring so many times, hanging up, calling back, letting it ring another specific number of times, and then calling back again. My mother followed the instructions and got an appointment.

I could barely walk. I mean, barely. I had already been in bed, except for visits to various traditional and nontraditional doctors, for 6 weeks. My mother drove me to a tract house in the San Fernando Valley. She stayed in the living room, while Dr Yee's pretty, young wife led me to their baby's bedroom, outfitted with a crib, changing table, and twin bed. I was told to take off all my clothes and lay on the bed. (Because acupuncture was not practiced in the state, no one—apart from that man in the restaurant—had any experience with it. Neither my mother nor I questioned the fully naked request.) Dr Yee came in, spoke to me for a few minutes, and then brought out the longest needles I had ever seen. The deepest one went several inches into my hip. Dr Yee left me alone. Laying there, not moving and hoping there would not be an earthquake, I felt something I had not felt in weeks, no, years. It was a total absence of pain. The doctor returned, pulled out the needles, and left me to get dressed. I walked out of that house without a limp.

The relief did not last, however, and I returned twice a week for treatments. I improved so quickly that I was able to attend classes again. I started driving again too. One day when I arrived at the house, Mrs Yee and the baby were out. This time Dr Yee led me to the master bedroom, where I was told to take of all my clothes, as usual. And, as usual, once I was settled, Dr Yee came in and inserted the needles. Later, after he pulled them out, he sat on the edge of the bed. I remember this so clearly: the big mirror on the ceiling, his matching white patent leather belt and shoes, and the earnest look on his face. "Now that I have cured you," he said, "I must have sex with you."

I was stark naked, on the man's marital bed, but somehow I had the wherewithal to say, "We don't do things like that in this country!"

As a 19 year old, I talked my way back into my clothes and out the door. He began calling me at home. Would I like to take a ride in his Citroën? (No.) Would I like to have lunch? (No.) Did I want him to heal me? (Yes.) My mother came up with a solution: she asked one of her students, a Vietnam veteran who had served in the Marines, to accompany me to all future acupuncture appointments.

Now I know that this episode was my first major flare-up, but I had no such knowledge then, because I still did not have a diagnosis. Life went on. I continued my college work. I went to parties and discos. My dad—an anthropology professor—got a new job, which came with good insurance benefits. Although I had not lived with him since I was 3 years old, he put me on his policy and got me in to see an orthopedist at Kaiser Permanente. The doctor confirmed things I already knew: I had the back of an old man, and I would never be able to bear children, because he could see on my radiographs that my sacroiliac bones were fused. He came up with a treatment plan, which included a stretching routine and regular sit-ups. I was religious about my physical therapy, which seemed to help, especially if I did my exercises at night just before bed. I was still to follow that initial list of don'ts, however: no horseback riding, running, jogging, etc.

After 2 years in college, I left to travel around Europe for a few years. I came home, graduated, started writing, drifted away from doing my exercises and stretches, and began to get tighter and stiffer. When I met my future husband, I was 25 years old and I could just barely touch my knees. I was in unrelenting, low-grade pain, but I had lived with it so long that I did not think much about it. The constant inflammation took a toll on my body, though. When I got married, I weighed 44.4kg. (It was not until years later that my husband would confide that when we married he expected that I would 1 day end up an invalid—in a wheelchair if I was lucky, bedridden if I was not.) I am happy to say that I gave birth to 2 children. I am not going to say it was a walk in the park, but, thankfully, all the dire predictions failed to occur. After my second son was born, I was exhausted, achy, and unable to sleep because my back hurt so much. I went to my general practitioner. I listed my complaints. He looked at me and not unkindly said, "What do you expect? You're a mother with young children." I felt slightly vindicated when the bloodwork he had ordered came back and revealed that my thyroid levels were low. He suspected Hashimoto disease. I have been on thyroid medications ever since, which improved some symptoms but did not ease my aching back.

That is how things remained for another 5 years or so. Then there came a night when my husband and I were at a dinner party. Just as when my mother had overheard someone talking about the acupuncturist, on this night I eavesdropped on a conversation about a doctor who seemed to perform miracles on people with back and neck pain. I made an appointment. A new round of radiographs were taken, and, finally, I got my diagnosis. The way the doctor explained it, there had recently been 2 young men who had died in motorcycle accidents. Radiographs showed that their sacroiliac joints were fused. Their deaths, and this discovery, led to a way to diagnose AS.

Just now, having looked up the history of AS, I must doubt the veracity of this story, but at the time it made sense to me. It also made sense when the doctor said that on average it took much longer for women than for men to be diagnosed. In the 1970s, as I understand it, it took men 3 years to 4 years to receive a diagnosis, whereas for women the average was 10 years. I was in my mid-30s. In my case, it had taken approximately 20 years. I was prescribed Indocin, as well as physical and occupational therapy, and given a pamphlet suggesting I might struggle with the diagnosis and that I could benefit from joining a support group. On the one hand, I was relieved. I could finally put a name to the pain I had suffered. AS was not something in my head or some mysterious way my body was trying to communicate, as my mother had always told me. The Indocin worked amazingly well. (In the coming years, I would also try Celebrex, Mobic, and Vioxx, all of which produced side effects while not working as well for me as Indocin did.) On the flip side, after all the years of uncertainty, I did indeed struggle with the diagnosis. The word, *disease*, did not sit well with me. Instead of trying to deal with my feelings, I told my husband I was not the type of person who joined support groups. I went ahead with the physical therapy and occupational therapy—some techniques of which I use to this day.

When this doctor retired, I was at long last referred to a rheumatologist. He was horrified that I had been on a nonsteroidal anti-inflammatory drug (NSAID) for 20 years. I did not react well when he gave me a stern lecture, informing me that I had been taking Indocin for far too long and that, although I had never had a reaction to the drug, if I ever did, I probably would have a stomach hemorrhage and die. "You'll never get to the hospital in time," he warned. This should have scared me. This should have inspired me to consider other medications. Instead, I was so mad that I immediately looked for another rheumatologist. Let me note for the record that I have not always been the best patient. But you could also look at this another way: in all the years I had been taking Indocin, not a single doctor, including my personal physician, had ever mentioned anything about side effects that might include stomach hemorrhage, let alone death. And, unless he had a better idea, I needed that Indocin.

My second rheumatologist prescribed lansoprazole to protect my stomach from potential NSAID damage. She spoke to me about the new biologics, which sounded promising. But when I heard that I would have to give myself a shot...forget that! She also mentioned that Cedars-Sinai Medical Center here in Los Angeles was looking for AS patients willing to participate in a national clinical study. In Los Angeles, the study was being overseen by Dr Weisman. Would I be interested in finding out more about it? Absolutely! By this time, I knew of Dr Weisman's reputation but had been told he was not accepting new patients. If I joined the study, he would see me, if only for a few minutes, every time I came in to have my blood drawn, have radiographs, or have measurements taken.

My participation was not entirely self-motivated. After my own adventures and misadventures, and after all the information and misinformation I had received over the years, I wanted to be a part of something that might create new ways to diagnose the disease, possibly change perceptions of who might get it, and look at the differences between how the disease presents in men and women (or if these differences are more a function of gender biases). Most important, I hoped that by participating in the study, I could be part of a cure, at best, and better understanding of the disease, at least, in case my children, grandchildren, or great-grandchildren should find themselves with back pain and stiffness as they entered puberty. I am proud to say that when additional studies came up, I prevailed on my parents and my sons to participate along with me. They all did.

I am a writer by profession. I go on the road for 6 weeks to 12 weeks a year on extensive—and grueling—book tours. On a typical day, I fly to a new city, speak at a lunch event, speak at an evening event, maybe do an interview or 2, shake lots of hands, sign piles of book, and get plenty of impromptu hugs from fans. In other words, I am in an environment of high stress, not enough rest, with a heightened exposure to germs. In 2011, when my novel *Dreams of Joy* was published, it debuted at number 1 on *The New York Times* bestseller list. When something like that happens, the publisher doubles down. My tour was extended. I did even more events. I was in Raleigh, North Carolina, when I developed a cough. By the time I got to Atlanta, I was very sick. But everyone was relying on me, so I kept traveling. Whenever I flew back to Los Angeles, I would see my personal physician. I was prescribed antibiotics and different medications to help with the cough. I continued to travel hard and put out a lot of energy doing events. I lost weight. I started to have pain in what felt like every joint. My knees, wrists, and fingers were swollen, hot, and pink. My hips, neck, and back felt like they were on fire. It hurt to sit. It hurt to lay down. It hurt to move. I was exhausted.

When the tour ended, I saw my rheumatologist. My bloodwork showed a high level of inflammation. Actually, all my bloodwork looked bad. She did more tests. We tried all the usual treatments, plus cortisone injections. I did not improve. If anything, I got worse. I developed the symptoms and markers for Reynaud disease. My rheumatologist was sure that 1 or more new autoimmune diseases were emerging—Sjögren syndrome, rheumatoid arthritis, lupus, or rhupus. I was told it might take as long as 5 years to get a conclusive diagnosis.

If I have learned anything over all these years, it is that I need to be proactive about my care. It is important to try different treatments. It is important to get second opinions and sometimes third opinions. It also is important for a patient to keep his or her own medical records. (Now these can be accessed more easily online, but in the past I had to request copies of test results.) The next time I had an appointment for the AS study, I brought the file I had kept for the previous 20 years with me. When Dr Weisman came in for his usual quick visit, I asked him to look at my file and inquired if he would consider taking me on as a patient. He said yes to both. He told me not to worry. Those other diseases were not on my horizon. I was, however, having a serious flare-up of my AS.

It was through Dr Weisman's encouragement that I finally agreed to take Enbrel. He said it might take months before I felt a difference. For me, relief from my symptoms was immediate, and I kick myself to this day for being so resistant to giving myself a shot, which turned out to not be a big deal after all. For someone like me, who travels a lot, there are challenges to having to take a medication that requires refrigeration. I realize that now some of these requirements have been relaxed; nevertheless, patients must be careful with how they handle delivery and storage of this drug. (It cannot, for example, be delivered to your front door and wait all day in the sun for you to come home. Believe me, no patient wants to pay the out-of-pocket replacement cost for a single injection, let alone a box of 4 injections.) This refrigeration requirement has led to some interesting experiences. I have been invited to store my medicine in hotel kitchens and bar refrigerators across the country as well as in South America and Asia. I have had conversations with chefs, bartenders, maîtres d's, general managers, and hostesses. I have been given sneak peeks of what is coming up on dinner menus and been treated more than once to the house cocktail.

It has been a long and circuitous route. I still do not sleep very well, and many nights I can be found sleeping seated on the couch with my back and neck supported by pillows. The fatigue I feel—from lack of sleep, too much stress, and a daunting workload—may or may not be worse than what other AS patients experience. I feel fortunate compared with people like my father's cousin, who did not receive a diagnosis of AS until a few years ago, when she was 85 years old. She had lived in pain for the vast majority of her life, not knowing why.

I try to cover all bases in my care. I watch what I eat to avoid—or at least cut down on—foods known to cause inflammation, and I try to rest for an hour in the late afternoon before resuming work. I do not dwell on the ways the disease can manifest in the eyes, bowel, or heart, but that does not mean I do not watch out for symptoms. I now have an ophthalmologist and a cardiologist. I am my mother's daughter, so I also have a naturopath, chiropractor, acupuncturist, and Chinese traditional medicine doctor. (I would not go—or pay the money—if I was not helped by their treatments to some extent.) A few years ago, I started working privately with a Pilates instructor, who said the goal should be for me to touch my toes within 2 years. Although I thought the idea was far-fetched, I agreed to try. I not only met the goal of touching my toes but also, on a good day, I can get my palms flat on the floor. Now, in addition to hiking, tennis, and Pilates, I have added yoga. My current goal is to keep being able to touch my toes until the day I die. (So much for a back like a 90-year-old man!)

Now, when I learn of someone who has been diagnosed with AS, I always offer to talk to them. Usually, they are upset to have a disease. They are scared, having looked up various outcomes on the Internet. They ask me a variety of questions: Will I end up bent over like a pretzel, or will my case be mild? Will I be able to work? Will I be able to travel? Will I be able to take care of my family? Will I be able to rock climb, skydive, garden, knit, or golf? I cannot give them definitive answers. I can only share what I have learned from my own experiences. Try different treatments, because you never know what will work for you or help you, even if it is for a short time, even if it is only from the placebo effect. Trust your doctors but be willing to move on—and up—to new ones if, and when, you can. Remember doctors can be wrong. They are only human, after all. Understand that every new physician you see—whether a gynecologist or neurologist—will doubt your diagnosis, as still happens to me to 30 years after finally receiving mine. (These days it is easier to prove to a new physician with the results from an antinuclear antibody or HLA-B27 test.) Keep your freezer stocked with icepacks and bags of frozen peas to reduce inflammation but know that sometimes only a heating pad will give you relief. Most important, remember that although the disease is now a part of you, it does not define you. Try to look at AS as an adventure, with plenty of twists, turns, and discoveries along the way. And always remember to thank the people who help you—whether physical therapists, yoga instructors, nutritionists, or rheumatologists—for their insights, patience, persistence, and encouragement. Then thank your body, flaws and all, for getting you through another day.

DISCLOSURE

The author has nothing to disclose.

AS Patient
How to Cope with the Lifelong and Changing Disease Challenges

Dieter Wiek

KEYWORDS

- Late diagnosis • Medication • Disclosure • Eye problems • Physiotherapy
- Self-help group

KEY POINTS

- Early diagnosis can prevent disabilities and lead to a better health outcome.
- Exercises are essential to maintaining mobility and functionality.
- Developing a medication plan with a doctor in a cooperative and confidential manner supports a good health outcome.
- Patient organizations offer self-management and enable the exchange of thoughts.

THAT'S ME
October 2019

Age: 72 (**Fig. 1**)
Weight: 86 kg
Profession: retired grammar school teacher/school director
Marital status: married, no children
Illness: ankylosing spondylitis (AS) for more than 50 years
HLA-B27 positive

Illness Status: October 2019

My spine is almost totally fused.

My current disease status has been influenced by 2 key events apart from my AS illness:

- In 2011, I fell on my back and broke several vertebrae. This meant 2 operations.
- I had osteoarthritis problems with my left hip for several years. A hip operation has reduced the pain, but numbness in the thigh and lack of mobility are key problems

HOW MY ILLNESS DEVELOPED

- Looking back, I was very athletic. I played handball in winter, in summer I enjoyed athletics, and in my free time I played soccer.

E-mail address: dieter_wiek@web.de

Rheum Dis Clin N Am 46 (2020) 407–415
https://doi.org/10.1016/j.rdc.2020.01.015
0889-857X/20/© 2020 Elsevier Inc. All rights reserved.

rheumatic.theclinics.com

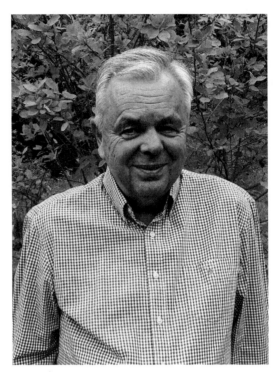

Fig. 1. Author portrait: "That's me."

- When I was 16, I felt I had injured my right ankle after a long jump competition. I contacted different doctors and they all made different diagnoses. One orthopedic gave me corticoid injections several times that did not help in the long run. Within 3 months, then, after the first symptoms, my right knee and my left elbow were swollen, and I could not move them properly. From the first symptoms to the point I ended in hospital took 6 months.
- I stayed in hospital for 25 weeks; my body had totally changed due to intense corticoid therapy. Due to hospitalization and rehabilitation, I could not go to school for 1 year. My first diagnosis was rheumatoid arthritis (RA) (**Fig. 2**).
- The RA symptoms slowly disappeared, with ups and downs. At the beginning of my 20s, I suffered more from low back pain, my cervical spine hurt, and my mobility was again and again more limited.
- I was diagnosed with AS when I went to a rheumatology clinic in my mid-20s. I went to physiotherapy regularly; in summer, I went to a spa in Italy; my medication was indomethacin (Amuno) (**Fig. 3**).
- At the beginning of my 30s, I felt I had to change my therapy concept. So, I joined a self-help group that offered hydrotherapy and group physiotherapy courses, although it was quite far away from my home. I spent my summer holidays in a rehabilitation clinic (**Fig. 4**).

VOLUNTARY WORK

I have worked as a volunteer locally, on the national level, and for a couple of years for European League Against Rheumatism. Let me sum up the top questions that patients have asked me in consultation hours:

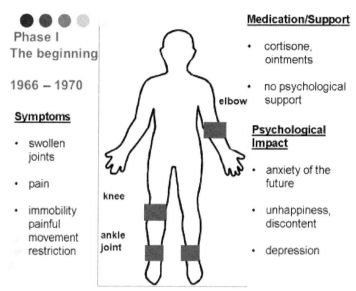

Fig. 2. Phase I, the beginning.

Q: Where do I find a good rheumatologist? Can you recommend one?

I always explained what options she/he has. When asking the patient after having consulted the rheumatologist, it is obvious what a good rheumatologist is as patients see it. This is someone who is competent, listens to the patient, communicates with the patient, and understands the illness impact on the patient's social life. The key points are competence and empathy.

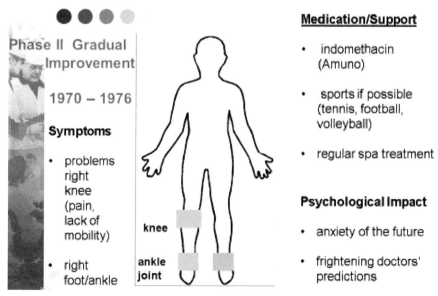

Fig. 3. Phase II, gradual improvement.

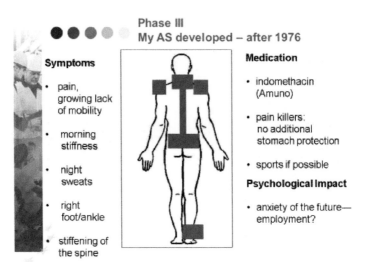

Fig. 4. Phase III, my AS developed.

Q: The medication my rheumatologist recommended has got lots of side effects; that scares me. What alternative medication is there causing less harm?

Lots of patients do not trust the medicine when reading the package insert and then consult nonmedical practitioners. I have always pointed out that due to inflammation there is the danger of irreversible physical damage.

Q: How can I influence my illness through nutrition? Is there a special diet for me? Can fasting cure me, because the inflammatory substances may then be washed away?

We have always offered different lectures about nutrition, diets, and fasting courses, where patients were supervised by a doctor. So, the message could only be: This is evidence-based and what we know, and just find out what is good for you.

Q: Should I notify my employer of my illness?

Disclosure is a very serious problem, especially for manual workers. Without any disability status and/or legal protection, there is the danger of being fired. The individual situation of the employed patient has to be explored. Job retraining and/or workplace adaptations have to be taken into account.

POINTS TO CONSIDER

In the following, a few key issues are outlined from a nonmedical patient perspective.

Late Diagnosis

In my case, it took several years until I received the right diagnosis. I do not want to complain, because this was in the 1960s. Data prove that even today a diagnosis often is made with enormous delay. There are many different reasons for this. But this long disease duration due to diagnostic delay has to be prevented, because only then will it be possible to avoid disabilities, optimize the health outcome for patients, and reduce costs for a country's health care system and economy.

All stakeholders in the health care system are challenged here.

Medical Therapy/Drug Treatment

Initially, in the 1960s, when doctors thought I had RA, I received high doses of corticoids that changed my appearance totally.

After being diagnosed with AS, I tried different nonsteroidal anti-inflammatory drugs and then took indomethacin for many years. From time to time, depending on the doses, I had serious stomach side effects. My voluntary work showed me that even in the 1970s and 1980s some doctors did not see the dangers of side effects on the stomach and did not prescribe proton pump inhibitors if needed, which is common today.

I only took a disease-modify antirheumatic drug for about 9 months (sulfasalazine), when I suffered from serious peripheral involvement (left ankle) and could hardly walk.

When cyclooxygenase-2 inhibitors got onto the market, I first took Viox; then, when it was taken from the market, I switched to Arcoxia, as needed.

I have never tried biologics because the inflammation is rather low and my pain is not due to any inflammation process. I know that for most patients biologics mean a new quality of life.

I think patients nowadays should be informed about medication opportunities; about the potential side effects, in particular the cardiovascular and gastrointestinal risks; and what measures can be taken to avoid or minimize side effects.

Another key issue nowadays is the switching of patients from biologic originators to biosimilars. According to my experiences, the switching is being done totally differently. Some doctors just maintain that the name of the product has changed; some give a sheet of paper that explains what a biosimilar is and why it is as good as the originator; and some doctors inform and even involve rheumatology nurses. I think it should be the aim that after information and education doctor and patient achieve a shared decision.

Eye Problems: Uveitis/Iritis

In the first 30 years after being diagnosed I suffered from a uveitis attack quite regularly, even often in my holidays when I was somewhere abroad. Pain and sensitivity to light forced me to consult a doctor. Only once, both eyes were affected.

Based on my experience and being aware of the symptoms, I now have the medication with me (steroid eye drops and dilating drops), especially when traveling in countries outside of Europe. I can only recommend that, in particular, when visiting less advanced countries. You have to consult an eye doctor for an eye examination, but the advantage is you can start with the medication and sometimes the eye doctor becomes superfluous, if the inflammation is not too serious.

Foot Problems

Foot problems have been common to me since diagnosed and have always been changing but have become less compared with the first 25 years of illness duration. Either pain under the heel and/or the arch and/or at the back of the heel caused serious problems in daily life.

So, for many years I only have only bought and worn shoes where I can use my orthopedic insoles and those shoes that possessed good shock absorbency.

I feel that we pay lots of money for all kinds of body lotions, perfumes, and so forth, but we neglect our feet that carry our weight all our life.

I would like to recommend caring for your feet, buying quality shoes, and using bespoke insoles, which I assume may be more difficult for fashion-conscious ladies.

Psychological Impact

When I was diagnosed with AS in a rheumatology clinic and was surrounded by patients with serious structural damage, irreversible spinal fusion, and different kinds of deformities, I felt depressed for months, although my illness was not obvious.

I remember a situation as a young teacher when I visited another school with colleagues to learn about team teaching. There I realized at once an elderly AS colleague in the teachers' room, his spine stiffened and bent forward. I swore to myself that I would not teach with this kind of health status and posture, because I remembered when I was a pupil how a handicapped teacher was ridiculed and teased by pupils, although, to my mind, his teaching was good.

Despite pharmacologic and nonpharmacologic therapies, I could not prevent the spinal fusion. It took me several years to cope with this changing of my body. Having accepted my illness at a certain stage, I felt much better; there was no use concealing my illness. For my pupils, my health status was never a talking point; the quality of my teaching and the way I supported them were essential. But there were great challenges. When entering the classroom for the first time and getting into contact with pupils for the first time, I had to radiate self-confidence and self-assurance and show that I was the boss.

I think if structural damages and deformities occur, a patient goes through different stages of coping strategies. These phases often are associated with pain, which increases the impact on the person's psyche. Lots of patients need psychological support to cope with their illness and manage these crises.

Hazards

Driving

For those with a (completely) fused neck, the ability to drive safely (**Fig. 5**) is seriously affected. I have always experienced that doctors do not touch this very relevant aspect of safety—safety for self but also for fellow citizens. A patient should check what support is useful, so that mobility can be preserved (**Fig. 6**).

Fractures

A couple of years ago, I slipped and fell onto my back. I broke several vertebrae; 2 operations caused a longer stay in hospital and rehabilitation (**Fig. 7**).

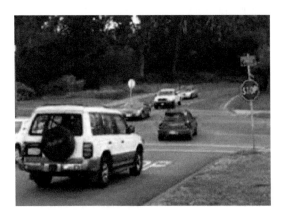

Fig. 5. Driving.

A   B   C

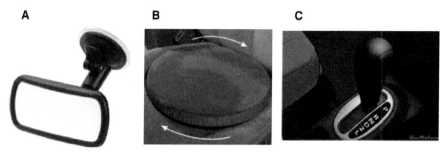

Fig. 6. Some helpers: (A) extra mirrors, (B) swivel car cushion, and (C) automatic transmission.

Aspects

It is a necessity to create awareness of the dangers implied when falling or in cases of a car crash.

Surgery

If the hips are affected, which happened to me as well, a hip replacement may be needed (**Fig. 8**). To my mind, good physical exercises before the hip replacement are essential for a good outcome.

Physical Therapy/Hydrotherapy

It is essential to do certain exercises every day like stretching, postural exercises, deep breathing, and different motion exercises for the spine. Ideally, it is good to learn a program of 15 minutes to 20 minutes and practice these exercises every morning.

 As we all know how difficult it is to achieve sustainability and overcome laziness, it is of great help to join a patient group once or twice a week. Doing these exercises in a group with a qualified physiotherapist means fun, and this improves mobility, reduces stiffness and pain, and often even helps to sleep much better.

 There are times, however, when it is needed to consult an individual physiotherapist, especially at times of flares.

Fatigue

Again and again, fatigue has been a serious problem for me and I know it is relevant for lots of patients. I was quite lucky because I often could set up my daily routine

A   B   C

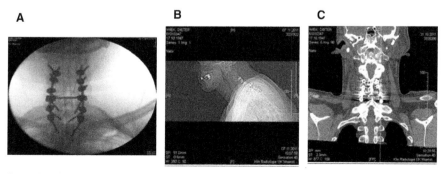

Fig. 7. (A–C) Vertebrae fractures radiographs.

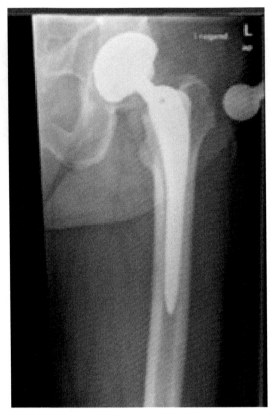

Fig. 8. Hip radiograph.

accordingly. A lot of different factors like sleep disturbances, pain, physical limitations, and feeling depressed contribute to fatigue.

Rest periods and relaxation techniques but also exercises and fresh air help overcome this tiredness. Employers should be aware of this problem, allow short breaks, and see that the AS patient's overall performance will not be less.

Working with Ankylosing Spondylitis

When I got ill at the age of 17 and had very difficult health issues in my 20s, it was my top priority to have a qualified job that enabled me to organize at least a part of the day according to my needs. And that is what I always communicated in consultation hours: for young people seriously affected, a professional qualification is the best way of getting into a job and staying in work. This is crucial for a successful life. It means income, recognition, acceptance, and being an integrated member of society.

When the disease progresses, workplace adaptations may be needed, more working time flexibility and so forth, but with reasonable adjustments, there is a good chance of staying well in work.

Self-Management

Nowadays we live in an information age; smartphones enable access to endless information and make it possible to communicate with others affected.

Nevertheless, I personally believe that it is quite useful to join a self-management course. It is essential to learn about

- Medication options
- Nonpharmacologic interventions
- Comorbidities
- How AS can affect joints, eyes, or other parts of the body
- Why breathing exercises are so important and smoking is not good for you
- How working with AS can be managed

These are just some relevant examples that contribute to better self-management.

Patient Organization—Should I Join?

I have been engaged in a patient organization for more than 30 years. There are good reasons for joining:

- Most organizations offer regular gym exercise groups and/or hydrotherapy, self-management courses, and so forth.
- When attending these activities, you talk to people who understand you and you exchange your views and experiences with them.
- You are updated about research and the most effective treatment.
- With your membership you support the organization's campaigning and lobbying activities for better health care for AS patients.

DISCLOSURE

Nothing to disclose.

Moving?

Make sure your subscription moves with you!

To notify us of your new address, find your **Clinics Account Number** (located on your mailing label above your name), and contact customer service at:

Email: **journalscustomerservice-usa@elsevier.com**

800-654-2452 (subscribers in the U.S. & Canada)
314-447-8871 (subscribers outside of the U.S. & Canada)

Fax number: **314-447-8029**

Elsevier Health Sciences Division
Subscription Customer Service
3251 Riverport Lane
Maryland Heights, MO 63043

*To ensure uninterrupted delivery of your subscription, please notify us at least 4 weeks in advance of move.

Printed and bound by CPI Group (UK) Ltd, Croydon, CR0 4YY

08/05/2025

01864691-0006